Humidification in the Intensive Care Unit

Antonio M. Esquinas

Editor

Humidification in the Intensive Care Unit

The Essentials

Second Edition

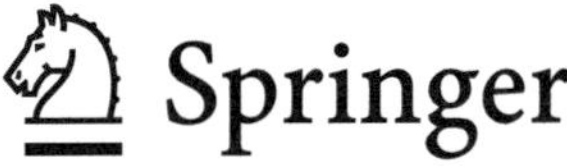

Editor
Antonio M. Esquinas
Intensive Care Unit
Hospital General Universitario Morales Meseguer
Murcia, Spain

ISBN 978-3-031-23955-7   ISBN 978-3-031-23953-3   (eBook)
https://doi.org/10.1007/978-3-031-23953-3

Preface

The significant number of patients with acute respiratory failure requiring various forms of treatment with oxygen therapy, nasal high flow, non-invasive ventilation and invasive mechanical ventilation due to various epidemiological causes and high hospital demand, especially in intensive care units in the last decade, and the significant development of new equipment and technologies are a constant in daily medical practice, and widely contrasted by various medical specialties that care for these patients with severe respiratory failure.

However, despite this important clinical and technological advance, the practice and knowledge of humidification in critically ill patients continues to be the subject of research and technological innovation. This continuous interest in the knowledge of humidification is based on some essential clinical questions, which we still do not know, such as (a) the evaluation of a correct indication, monitoring and definition of standard evaluation of results and complications regarding adequate humidification, (b) how our humidification practice can impact on our daily clinical objectives and, finally, what are the terms and role of adequate or inadequate humidification? This situation is a more complex one, if these questions are translated to the complexity of the critically ill patient admitted to intensive care units for respiratory failure with a complex humidification pathophysiology.

Despite these and other questions about excellence in humification in critically ill patients, we believe that this second edition in its sections and chapters continues to provide the healthcare professional with an updated vision, basic concepts and new lines of research in the future.

It is necessary to propose new models of clinical and technological analysis on the practice and technique of humification, especially in critical ill patients, that incorporate an adequate number of variables or factors, and that can be included in a single universal model of "excellence" of perfect humidification in critical patients.

To this end, we hope that this second edition will serve as a bridge to the goal of adequate training and clinical practice of humidification in critically ill patients.

As Editor of this second edition of *Humidification in the Intensive Care Unit: The Essentials*, I would like to thank all the authors for their collaboration.

Murcia, Spain   Antonio M. Esquinas

Contents

Part I

Humidification and Devices

Heated Humidification Devices

Antonietta Coppola, Anna Annunziata,
and Giuseppe Fiorentino

1.1 Introduction

During normal breathing, the upper airways condition inspired gases in order to prevent dryness and damage to the mucosae. During mechanical ventilation (MV) , the inspired gases are dry, and there are numerous studies that have demonstrated the negative effect of dry gases on the respiratory tract. The lack of adequate conditioning may thicken airway secretions, which increases the airway resistance, reduces the gas exchange effectiveness and increases the risk of respiratory infections [1]. For these reasons, gas delivered during MV must be warmed and humidified to avoid serious complications related to dry gases [2]. Humidification is recommended for every patient receiving invasive MV, and it is considered the standard of care according to the American Association for Respiratory Care [1]. There is no clear consensus on humidification during non-invasive ventilation, but humidification is highly suggested to improve comfort [1]. Several types of humidifiers have been produced for clinical use, each with advantages and disadvantages. Humidification devices can be divided into active heated humidifiers (HHs), which are devices heated by warm water; passive humidifiers (PHs) such as heat and moisture exchangers (HMEs), which capture the heat of exhaled air and release it at the next inspiration; and hot water humidifiers.

1.2 Active Heated Humidifiers

Active heated humidifiers (HHs) allow air passage inside a heated water reservoir and are usually placed in a ventilator circuit in the inspiratory limb. Air and water vapour travel along the inspiratory limb and reach the patient's airway. This system

A. Coppola (✉) · A. Annunziata · G. Fiorentino
UOC fisiopatologia e riabilitazione respiratoria, A.O.dei Colli- Ospedale Monaldi, Naples, Italy

A. M. Esquinas (ed.), *Humidification in the Intensive Care Unit*,
https://doi.org/10.1007/978-3-031-23953-3_1

needs the addition of water traps due to the accumulation of water vapour condensate, which is formed when the temperature of the inspiratory limb decreases. These humidifiers have sensors at the outlet of the humidifier and at the Y-piece, near the patient. This sensor provides continuous feedback to a central regulator to guarantee a determined temperature at the distal level. When the temperature is too high or too low, the alarm system is triggered. In an ideal system, the alarm should be triggered by humidity levels, but it is actually triggered only based on temperature. The temperature setting is usually 37 °C. HHs have different techniques for humidification and different designs. They are divided into bubble, passover, counter-flow and inline vapouriser.

In bubble humidifiers, a gas is pushed through a tube in the bottom of water container. The gas forms bubbles because it escapes from the distal end and gains humidity as it rises from the water surface. These devices could have a diffuser that breaks gas into smaller bubbles. The vapour content is influenced by the size of bubbles, the gas–water interface, the amount of water in the container and the flow rate. In this case, slower flows guarantee more time for gas humidification. Bubble humidifiers may be unheated or heated. Heated bubble humidifiers are designed to work with high flow rates (100 L/min) and provide high humidity. They are usually used in oxygen delivery systems. These humidifiers give a high resistance to flow generating an increase in work of breathing. A problem with these humidifiers is that they may generate microaerosols, but it is not clinically significant regarding the risk of healthcare-associated pneumonia [3]. Bubble humidifiers are less used now than they had been in the past.

Passover humidifiers are the most used in both non-invasive and invasive MV because of their lower flow resistance and absence of microaerosols. In these devices, gas passes over a heated water reservoir carrying vapour to the patient. There are other types of passover humidifiers: hydrophobic and wick humidifiers. In hydrophobic passover humidifiers, dry gas passes through a hydrophobic membrane that allows the passage of water vapour but not liquid water. Aerosols and bubbles are not generated. In wick humidifiers, the gas enters a water reservoir and passes through a wick that has a distal end immersed in water. The wick pores provide the gas–water interface that allows for greater humidification with respect to simple passover humidification. The water in the reservoir is supplied manually or through a feed system that guarantees a constant water level. The gas enters and travels through the wick, but it is not submerged underneath the water surface, so bubbles are not generated. In this device, a temperature is guaranteed by a temperature probe placed near the Y-piece of the ventilator. This could generate a condensate in the tube, increasing resistance. Incremented resistance increases peak pressure in volume-controlled modes and decreases volume delivered in pressure-controlled modes. Nevertheless, to reduce the risk of condensation, the AARC clinical guidelines recommend the use of gas delivered at 37 °C and 100% humidity [1].

In an inline vapouriser, water vapour is injected into the gas of the inspiratory circuit, using a small plastic capsule. Gas is supplemented by a disc heater in the capsule. A peristaltic pump delivers water to the capsule. The amount of water is set by a clinician based on minute ventilation and can be adjusted constantly.

In a counter-flow humidifier, the water is heated outside the vapouriser and pumped to the top of the humidifier and through small-diameter pores to reach a large surface area, from where the gas flows in the counter direction. Air is moisturised and warmed during the passage through the chamber. In a study on an artificial lung, Schumann et al. [4] demonstrated that the counter-flow device requires less to breathe with respect to heated passover humidifiers and HMEs. These humidifiers are promising but more studies are needed to evaluate their benefits.

1.3   Passive Humidifiers

The working principle for PHs is based on their capacity to retain heat and humidity during expiration and to deliver at least 70% of the inhaled gas during subsequent inspiration. It is a passive system because all heat and moisture are derived entirely from the patient and no energy is added to the system. This 'passive' function can be achieved by different mechanisms, and the classification of these devices is based on their mechanism.

There has been growing acceptance of PHs in recent years because of their low cost, simple operation and elimination of condensate from the breathing circuit [1]. Concern over adverse ventilator effects of PHs has mainly been aimed at the increased resistance imposed by the foam or paper insert. The working principle of PHs implies that a higher volume of condenser material will yield better device performance. For this reason, the 'ideal' dead space for a humidifier is approximately 50 mL [5].

Their performance ultimately depends on a number of factors such as ambient temperature, inspiratory and expiratory flow rates, surface area and water vapour content of the medium. These humidifiers are inexpensive, easy to use and silent and do not require water or an external energy source, temperature monitor or alarms. Moreover, there is no danger of over-hydration, hyperthermia or burns. As disadvantages, they can deliver only limited humidity, contribute insignificantly to temperature preservation and are less effective than AHs, especially when intubation lasts for several days. When the dead space increases, it may be necessary to augment the tidal volume, which would increase the work of breathing [6].

The simplest passive humidifiers are the heat and moisture exchangers. Heat and moisture exchangers (HMEs) are also called artificial noses because they act as nasal cavity in gas humidification. HMEs operate passively by storing heat and moisture from the patient's exhaled gas and releasing it to the inhaled gas. They are simple condensers constructed with elements made of disposable foam, synthetic fibre or paper, with a significant surface area that can generate an effective temperature gradient through the device delivering heat on each inspiration. A condenser element retains moisture from every exhaled breath and returns it back to the next inspired breath. These humidifiers are placed between the patient and Y-piece of ventilator, increasing resistance in the airflow during expiratory and inspiratory phase, which makes the humidifier part of the instrumental dead space [1].

Initially, simple HMEs were made from condenser made of metallic elements with a high thermal conductivity, and they recaptured 50% of a patient's exhaled moisture, providing a humidification of 10–14 mgH$_2$O/L at tidal volume [7]. They created high resistance during ventilation and are no longer used. Newer types of HMEs are hydrophobic, hygroscopic, filtered or pure hygroscopic HME.

Hydrophobic HMEs use a water-repellent element with a large surface area and low thermal conductivity that maintains higher temperature gradients than in the case of simple HMEs. Hydrophobic membranes have small pores and are pleated to increase the surface area. At usual ventilatory pressure, they allow the passage of water vapour but not liquid vapour. They have efficient bacterial and viral filters. High ambient temperature may impair their performance. Combined hygroscopic and hydrophobic HMEs are made with synthetic fibre. A hygroscopic chemical product (calcium chloride or lithium chloride) is added inside the hydrophobic HME, which absorbs expired water vapour and delivers it to the inspired gas, optimising the delivery of humidity. The synthetic fibre also helps to decrease the accumulation of condensation in a device-dependent position. Pure hygroscopic HMEs have only the hygroscopic compartment. During expiration, vapour is condensed in the element as well as in the hygroscopic salts, and during inspiration, vapour is obtained from the salt. They provide humidity between 22 and 34 mgH$_2$O/L. Despite the theoretical advantages of hygroscopic HMEs compared with hydrophobic devices, researchers found no differences in the quantity of tracheal aspirates, mucus viscosity, atelectasis, tracheal tube occlusion, bacterial colonisation and ventilator-associated pneumonia (VAP) [8].

In purely hydrophobic HMEs, the condenser is made of a water-repellent element as a hydrophobic membrane with low thermal conductivity that maintains higher temperature gradients than in the case of simple HMEs. They allow passage of water vapour but not liquid water. Adding a filter to a hydrophobic or hygroscopic HME produces a heat and moisture exchange filter (HMEF).

The applied filter can operate based on mechanical or electrostatic filtration, so the filters can be incorporated into pleated or electrostatic filters. Pleated filters have low electrostatic charges but denser fibres, so they represent a barrier for viruses and bacteria. The nature of the membrane causes turbulent airflow, increasing the deposition of viral and bacterial particles on the internal side of the filter. Moreover, they increase airflow resistance. Electrostatic filters have less dense fibres but high electrostatic charges, and they depend on an electric field. Bacteria and viruses have an electric charge, so they get trapped inside the electric field of the filters. They are characterised by large pores and work based on electric fields, contributing very little to the humidification process and increasing resistance [9]. For this reason, they are used to protect patients from bacteria and viruses [2].

HMEs vary considerably in terms of performance and durability [10, 11]. Some devices perform suboptimally leading to increased airway resistance and tracheal tube occlusion from retained secretions. Lellouche et al. [11] independently tested the performance of 48 p-HMEs and showed only 37.5% performed well (AH ≥ 30 mgH$_2$O/L) with 25% performing poorly, providing AH of 4 mgH$_2$O/L. This finding has been replicated elsewhere [12]. While some manufacturers use the gravimetric method to test performance (as employed by the international standard ISO 9360 11), which involves weighing the humidifier before and after the period of operation under strictly controlled conditions, others use the psychrometric method. Although there is little discrepancy between both methods in vitro [10, 11], only a psychrometric test can be used in patients, and future devices should be benchmarked against this technique in vivo. Current evidence suggests that HMEs that can deliver gases with an AH of >30 mgH$_2$O/L have a low risk of tracheal tube occlusions, while those providing AH of 30 mgH$_2$O/L have a longer lifespan, extending to 48 h [13] or even as long as 1 week in certain patients without any increase in the risk of tracheal tube occlusion or bacterial colonisation [14]. However, further testing of devices that consistently achieve AH > 30 mgH$_2$O/L in vivo and determining the durability of each device are needed.

An important characteristic of HME filters is that there is no problem with tube condensation, preventing the development of ventilator-associated pneumonia, but in well-maintained circuits, this factor is controversial. The presence of secretions and blood in the device increases the airway resistance and work of breathing. Aerosol medication cannot be administered, and HMEs should be removed from the device.

1.4   Active Heat and Moisture Exchangers

Active heat and moisture exchangers (aHMEs) include a regular HME but place a small heater between the HME and the patient that vapourises added water, converting them from passive to active and increasing the humidification capacity. There are various existing models. The Humid-Heat® device (Gilbeck AB, Sweden) is a hygroscopic HME that allows water to drip onto a heated paper element that acts as a wick. They have pre-set values for humidity and temperature, but the minute volume of the ventilator must be set. The HME Booster® (Medisize, Belgium) features a heater covered with a Gore-Tex® membrane. Water is added to the surface of the heater and vapourised, allowing passage through the membrane, a phenomenon that regulates the amount of water vapourised. The heating unit is incorporated between the patient and the HME. The Performer device has a metal plate placed between two hydrophobic and hygroscopic membranes; it is heated by an external source that has three temperature levels: 40, 50 and 60 °C. Water is provided at one end of the humidifier, reaching the two membranes and the metal plate that heats it. The water vapour produced increases the vapour content in the inspired gas. The Hygrovent Gold is an active hydrophobic HME. There is a heating element and a water line that provides water in the HME. These devices have the advantage such as they run dry and the HME functions normally. There is an increased flow resistance with this active device.

1.5 Hot Water Humidifiers

Hot water humidifiers (HWH) are considered the gold standard in humidification. They deliver gas at 37 °C with an AH of 44 mgH_2O/L, but in clinical use, they may only deliver AH between 35 and 40 mgH_2O/L [15]. They comprise a heating element that heats the water within a chamber. Dry gas is then passed through this chamber over the hot liquid surface or bubbled through the water to become humidified. The temperature within the chamber is thermostatically controlled, which allows fully saturated gas to be produced at a variety of temperatures. They are more efficient in providing humidification compared with passive HMEs, but the risks are greater, and they are more expensive. The main risks are overheating, causing inhalational burns, and the possibility of water condensing within the inspiratory limb of the ventilator tubing as gas cools, leading to bacterial colonisation. This may be reduced by incorporating heated wires within the walls of the tubing. The risk of colonisation may also be reduced by increasing the temperature of the water bath up to 45–60 °C (continuous pasteurisation) [16], adding antibacterial agents to the water or breathing circuit tubing [17] or maintaining a closed sterile system. Increasing temperature poses an increased risk of inhalational thermal injury. Antibacterial agents are rarely used due to the risk of ingestion, and maintaining a closed sterile system is difficult to achieve. Unless visibly soiled, breathing circuits need not be replaced routinely [18], and unnecessary manipulations and breaks in circuit tubing should be avoided.

References

1. American Association for Respiratory Care, Restrepo RD, Walsh BK. Humidification during invasive and noninvasive mechanical ventilation: 2012. Respir Care. 2012;57(5):782–8.
2. Branson RD, Chatburn RL. Humidification of inspired gases during mechanical ventilation. Respir Care. 1993;38:461–8.
3. www.cdc.gov/hicpac/pdf/guidelines/HApneu2003guidelines.pdf
4. Schumann S, Stahl CA, Möller K, Priebe H-J, Guttmann J. Moisturizing and mechanical characteristics of a new counter-flow type heated humidifier, BJA. Br J Anaesth. 2007;98(4):531–8. https://doi.org/10.1093/bja/aem006.
5. Plotnikow GA, Accoce M, Navarro E, Tiribelli N. Humidification and heating of inhaled gas in patients with artificial airway. A narrative review. Acondicionamiento del gas inhalado en pacientes con vía aérea artificial. Revisión narrativa. Rev Bras Ter Intensiva. 2018;30(1):86–97. https://doi.org/10.5935/0103-507x.20180015.
6. Al Ashry HS, Modrykamien AM. Humidification during mechanical ventilation in the adult patient. Biomed Res Int. 2014;2014:715434. https://doi.org/10.1155/2014/715434.
7. Vargas M, Chiumello D, Sutherasan Y, et al. Heat and moisture exchangers (HMEs) and heated humidifiers (HHs) in adult critically ill patients: a systematic review, meta-analysis and meta-regression of randomized controlled trials. Crit Care. 2017;21(1):123. https://doi.org/10.1186/s13054-017-1710-5.
8. Thomachot L, Viviand X, Arnaud S, Boisson C, Martin CD. Comparing two heat and moisture exchangers, one hydrophobic and one hygroscopic, on humidifying efficacy and the rate of nosocomial pneumonia. Chest. 1998;114:1412–8.

9. Vandenbroucke-Grauls CM, Teeuw KB, Ballemans K, Lavooij C, Cornelisse PB, Verhoef J. Bacterial and viral removal efficiency, heat and moisture exchange properties of four filtration devices. J Hosp Infect. 1995;29(1):45–56.
10. Lellouche F, Taille S, Lefrancois F, Deye N, Maggiore SM, Jouvet P, et al. Humidification performance of 48 passive airway humidifiers. Comparison with manufacture data. Chest. 2009;135:276–86.
11. Branson RD, Davis K. Evaluation of 21 passive humidifiers according to the ISO 9360 standard: moisture output, dead space and flow resistance. Respir Care. 1996;41:736–43.
12. Guillaume T, Boyer A, Etienne P, Salah A, de Lassence A, Dreyfuss D, et al. Heat and moisture exchangers in mechanically ventilated intensive care unit patients: a plea for an independent assessment of their performance. Crit Care Med. 2003;31:699–704.
13. Thomachot L, Vialet R, Viguier JM, Benjamin S, Roulier P, Claude M. Efficacy of heat and moisture exchangers after changing every 48 hours rather than 24 h. Crit Care Med. 1998;26:477–81.
14. Ricard JD, Le Miere E, Morkowicz P, Lasry S, Saumon G, Djedaini K, et al. Efficiency and safety of mechanical ventilation with heat and moisture exchanger changed only once a week. Am J Respir Crit Care Med. 2000;161:104–9.
15. Lellouche F, Taille S, Maggiore SM, Qader S, L'Her E, Dey N, et al. Influence of ambient and ventilator output temperatures on performance of heated wire humidifiers. Am J Respir Crit Care Med. 2004;170:1073–9.
16. Redding PJ, McWalter PW. Pseudomonas fluorescence cross infection due to contaminated humidifier water. Br Med J. 1980;281:275.
17. Yousefshahi F, Khajavi MR, Anbarafshan M, Khashayar P, Najafi A. Sanosil, a more effective agent for preventing the hospital-acquired ventilator associated pneumonia. Int J Health Care Qual Assur. 2010;23:583–90.
18. Long MN, Wickstrom G, Grimes A, Benton CF, Belcher B, Stamm AM. Prospective, randomized study of ventilator- associated pneumonia in patients with one versus three ventilator circuit changes per week. Infect Control Hosp Epidemiol. 1996;17:14–9.

Heat and Moisture Exchangers (HMEs)

2

Jean-Damien Ricard, Alexandre Boyer, and Didier Dreyfuss

HMEs were first described in the mid-1950s and the early 1960s and have undergone considerable development since the beginning of the 1970s [1]. The basic principle of all HMEs lies in their capacity to retain heat and moisture during expiration and deliver these to the incoming dry medical gas during the subsequent inspiration. This passive function can be achieved by different mechanisms.

The first HMEs were simple condensers, made with metal elements with a large surface area such as rolled wire gauze or stainless steel tubes. Because of the high density and thermal conductivity of metal, no effective temperature gradient was achieved across the device. Metal elements of the condenser were then replaced by disposable foam, plastic, or paper. Increased moisture output was further achieved by coating the condenser element with a hygroscopic chemical (calcium or lithium chloride), which chemically adsorbs expired water vapor that is then returned to the inspired gas. These HMEs were called hygroscopic condensers. Deriving from the field of filtration, hydrophobic HMEs were also used to heat and humidify inspired gas. The very large surface area of pleated, water-repellent ceramic of the first hydrophobic HMEs along with its low thermal conductivity enabled an important temperature gradient to develop within the HME that favored heat and moisture retention. Finally, hygroscopic and hydrophobic elements were used in a single

J.-D. Ricard (✉)
INSERM U1137, UFR de Médecine, Université Paris Cité, Paris, France

AP-HP, Hôpital Louis Mourier, DMU ESPRIT, Service de Médecine Intensive Réanimation, Colombes, France
e-mail: jean-damien.ricard@aphp.fr

A. Boyer
Service de Réanimation Médicale, CHU Bordeaux, Bordeaux cedex, France

D. Dreyfuss
INSERM U1137, UFR de Médecine, Université Paris Cité, Paris, France

A. M. Esquinas (ed.), *Humidification in the Intensive Care Unit*,
https://doi.org/10.1007/978-3-031-23953-3_2

"

HME to create a "combined" HME. The hygrometric performance of these various HMEs differs considerably, with hydrophobic HMEs exhibiting the poorest humidity outputs (risk of endotracheal tube occlusion) and combined HMEs the highest, although recent measurements indicate that some purely hygroscopic HMEs provide comparable values of absolute humidity to that of combined HMEs [2, 3].

2.1 Active Heat and Moisture Exchangers

New devices have been designed to boost humidifying performances of HMEs [4]. Briefly, these devices, which are added to the circuit between the HME and the endotracheal tube, consist of a ceramic heating element fed by an electrical energy source that vaporizes water (fed into the system by a side port) into the airway. They enable a 3–4 mgH$_2$O/L increase in absolute humidity delivered by the HME [4], although the actual clinical benefit of this increase has, to date, not been demonstrated.

2.2 Clinical Use

Apart from certain specific situations, HMEs or heated humidifiers can equally be used to heat and humidify inspired gases [1]. Despite this, practices differ considerably among countries [5, 6]. A survey found that HMEs were used for all patients in 63% of French ICUs, whereas this was the case in only 13% of Canadian ICUs [6].

Conversely, heated humidifiers were primarily used in 60% of Canadian ICUs and in only 20% of French ICUs. These results may account for some of the difference in cost of mechanical ventilation between the two countries [5]. Rationalizing the choice of a given humidifying device should help decrease costs in mechanical ventilation without impeding quality of care.

2.3 Efficacy

Several important aspects must be taken into account when analyzing the effectiveness and outcome of inspired gas conditioning. These include:

The avoidance of endotracheal tube occlusion (which is the worst and most feared complication of inadequate gas conditioning), and this aspect is directly linked to the performance of the humidifying device in terms of heat and humidity delivery.

The avoidance of spreading microorganisms (and in particular multidrug-resistant organisms), and this is directly linked to the humidifying device's capacity to prevent respiratory tubing contamination.

The addition of minimal resistance and dead space. The practicability of using the device.

The minimal maintenance necessary to ensure optimal use of the device. The minimal cost associated with the purchase and the long-term use of the device.

According to this list, the ideal humidifier can be defined as a device providing adequate levels of humidification whatever the ventilator and patient conditions, in an automatic manner, which is safe (i.e., electric shock-free, with no or limited connections that could be faulty), protects the environment from the patient's pathogens, and is easy to use, maintenance-free, and inexpensive.

2.4   Ensuring Adequate Humidification

The adequate level of humidification can be defined as a level where there is no excessive heat or water loss by the respiratory tract. The difficulty arises when one tries to set the minimum value of absolute humidity a device should deliver. This may be useful when selecting and comparing different devices. Although ranges as wide as 25–35 mgH_2O have been suggested in the past, the figure of 30 mgH_2O/L is recommended [7], that is, a clinician wishing to select an appropriate humidifying device should make sure that this device delivers at least 30 mgH_2O/L absolute humidity. Another definition of adequate humidification includes avoiding endotracheal tube occlusion. Some may argue that restricting adequate humidification to the risk of endotracheal occlusion is overly simplistic. One must bear in mind, however, that it is the worst and most feared side effect of insufficient humidity and can be sometimes fatal [8]. There is no doubt that 20 years ago, HMEs and heated humidifiers were not equivalent in terms of humidity output. In 1988, Cohen et al. alerted clinicians of the risk of endotracheal tube occlusions associated with the use of HME [9]. Two years later, Martin et al. reported a fatal case of endotracheal tube occlusion with an HME [8]. Several other publications confirmed the increase in endotracheal tube occlusion risk with HMEs in comparison with heated humidifiers. These studies, however, all used purely hydrophobic HMEs whose performances, when measured, display low values for absolute humidity [2, 10]. It has been shown that endotracheal tube occlusion occurs after a gradual reduction in the tube's inner diameter by clots of secretions along the inner surface of the tube [11]. This reduction was found to be significantly greater with a purely hydrophobic HME than with a heated humidifier or a combined (hydrophobic and hygroscopic) HME [11]. Although hygrometric measurements were not performed simultaneously in this study [11], it seems evident that inner diameter reduction (and thus ultimately endotracheal tube occlusion) is dependent on the amount of humidity delivered by the humidifying device. Indeed, humidity measurements of the devices used by Villafane et al. [11] have been made by others, and the results are consistent with their findings (i.e., the hydrophobic HMEs that suffered the greater inner diameter reduction displayed the poorest humidity output [10]). This leads to the question of hygrometric and clinical performance.

Although heated humidifiers undisputedly deliver greater values for absolute humidity than HMEs [10], there is to date no evidence for any benefit of these greater values in terms of clinical outcome, including endotracheal tube occlusion.

Table 2.1 displays the incidence of endotracheal tube occlusion reported in recently published studies. It is important to note that (1) endotracheal tube

Table 2.1 Endotracheal tube occlusion rates in studies comparing heated humidifiers and heat and moisture exchangers

First author, year	No. of patients	No. of ETT obstructions	
		HH	HME
Branson, 1993	120	0	0
Dreyfuss, 1995	131	0	1
Branson, 1996	200	0	0
Villafane, 1996	23	1	0
Boots, 1997	116	0	0
Hurni, 1997	115	1	0
Kollef, 1998	310	0	0
Thomachot, 1998	29	0	0
Kirton, 1998	280	1	0
Lacherade, 2002	370	5	1
Jaber, 2004	60	2	1

HH heated humidifier, *HME* heat and moisture exchanger

occlusion rates have drastically dropped in comparison with earlier studies [9, 12, 13], (2) endotracheal tube occlusion is also reported with the use of heated humidifiers, and (3) the incidence of endotracheal tube occlusion no longer appears to be greater with HMEs than with heated humidifiers. In one study, the incidence was greater with heated humidifiers than with HMEs [14]. To conclude, HMEs have considerably evolved since their first appearance on the market. They are no longer associated with more frequent endotracheal tube occlusion than heated humidifiers and ensure safe and efficient inspired gas conditioning [15]. Their practicability and cost-effectiveness are by far superior to heated humidifiers, explaining why they should be used in first intention in most patients requiring mechanical ventilation.

References

1. Ricard J-D. Humidification. In: Tobin M, editor. Principles and practice of mechanical ventilation. New York: McGraw-Hill; 2006. p. 1109–20.
2. Davis K Jr, Evans SL, Campbell RS, Johannigman JA, Luchette FA, Porembka DT, Branson RD. Prolonged use of heat and moisture exchangers does not affect device efficiency or frequency rate of nosocomial pneumonia. Crit Care Med. 2000;28:1412–8.
3. Boyer A, Thiery G, Lasry S, Pigné E, Salah A, de Lassence A, Dreyfuss D, Ricard J-D. Long-term mechanical ventilation with hygroscopic heat and moisture exchangers used for 48 hours: a prospective, clinical, hygrometric and bacteriologic study. Crit Care Med. 2003;31:823–9.
4. Thomachot L, Viviand X, Boyadjiev I, Vialet R, Martin C. The combination of a heat and moisture exchanger and a booster (TM): a clinical and bacteriological evaluation over 96 h. Intensive Care Med. 2002;28:147–53.
5. Cook D, Ricard JD, Reeve B, Randall J, Wigg M, Brochard L, Dreyfuss D. Ventilator circuit and secretion management strategies: a Franco-Canadian survey. Crit Care Med. 2000;28:3547–54.
6. Ricard JD, Cook D, Griffith L, Brochard L, Dreyfuss D. Physicians' attitude to use heat and moisture exchangers or heated humidifiers: a Franco-Canadian survey. Intensive Care Med. 2002;28:719–25.

7. American Association for Respiratory Care. AARC clinical practice guideline: humidification during mechanical ventilation. Respir Care. 1992;37:887–90.
8. Martin C, Perrin G, Gevaudan MJ, Saux P, Gouin F. Heat and moisture exchangers and vaporizing humidifiers in the intensive care unit. Chest. 1990;97:144–9.
9. Cohen IL, Weinberg PF, Fein IA, Rowinski GS. Endotracheal tube occlusion associated with the use of heat and moisture exchangers in the intensive care unit. Crit Care Med. 1988;16:277–9.
10. Ricard J-D, Markowicz P, Djedaïni K, Mier L, Coste F, Dreyfuss D. Bedside evaluation of efficient airway humidification during mechanical ventilation of the critically ill. Chest. 1999;115:1646–52.
11. Villafane MC, Cinnella G, Lofaso F, Isabey D, Harf A, Lemaire F, Brochard L. Gradual reduction of endotracheal tube diameter during mechanical ventilation via different humidification devices. Anesthesiology. 1996;85:1341–9.
12. Misset B, Escudier B, Rivara D, Leclercq B, Nitenberg G. Heat and moisture exchanger vs heated humidifier during long-term mechanical ventilation. A prospective randomized study. Chest. 1991;100:160–3.
13. Roustan JP, Kienlen J, Aubas P, Aubas S, du Cailar J. Comparison of hydrophobic heat and moisture exchangers with heated humidifier during prolonged mechanical ventilation. Intensive Care Med. 1992;18:97–100.
14. Lacherade J, Auburtin M, Souffir L, van de Low A, Cerf C, Rebuffat Y, Reizzega S, Ricard J-D, Lellouche F, Lemaire F, Brun-Buisson C, Brochard L. Ventilator-associated pneumonia: effects of heat and moisture exchangers and heated water humidificators. Intensive Care Med. 2002;28:S132.
15. Ricard JD. Gold standard for humidification: heat and moisture exchangers, heated humidifiers, or both? Crit Care Med. 2007;35:2875–6.

Main Techniques for Evaluating the Performances of Humidification Devices Used for Mechanical Ventilation

François Lellouche

Evaluation of the humidity of the gases delivered to patients has allowed an improvement and a progressive diversification of the humidification devices used during mechanical ventilation. The main techniques to evaluate the performances of the heat and moisture exchangers (HMEs) and of the heated humidifiers (HH) in terms of humidification are mainly used in research. The technique of the visual evaluation of condensation on the flex tube or on the humidification chamber's wall is feasible at the patient bedside but has several limitations. Many techniques to measure the moisture of gases exist. The most frequently used in the clinical setting are the psychrometric method and the capacitance hygrometers usable on patients (during invasive or non-invasive ventilation) or on benches. The gravimetry (used by the standard ISO 9360) has technical limitations and can be used only on bench. Psychrometry and capacitance hygrometers are generally used for clinical research, whereas the manufacturers of the humidification systems often use the gravimetry. This may explain the differences in performance evaluation found for humidification device assessment [1, 2]. However, the large differences found between the manufacturer's claim and the measured humidity call into question the validity of the ISO standard for detecting underperforming devices [1, 3].

F. Lellouche (✉)
Centre de recherche de l'Institut Universitaire de Cardiologie et de Pneumologie de Québec-Université Laval, Québec, QC, Canada
e-mail: francois.lellouche@criucpq.ulaval.ca

A. M. Esquinas (ed.), *Humidification in the Intensive Care Unit*,
https://doi.org/10.1007/978-3-031-23953-3_3

3.1 Visual Evaluation of Condensation

3.1.1 Condensation in the Flex Tube

A simple way to evaluate if the gases administered to the patients are correctly humidified is to visually seek if condensation exists in the flex tube of the endotracheal tube. Indeed, if there is a difference between gas temperature in the circuit and the room temperature, the gas cools along the circuit, involving an increase in the relative humidity and possibly a condensation on the wall if the dew point temperature is reached. This technique was validated by two teams; they showed a good correlation between condensation and the absolute humidity of gases delivered by the tested HME [4, 5]. This simple technique can be used with both HME and HH, but it remains vague and can only give an idea of the level of relative humidity of gases. Under no circumstances, however, it allows to accurately evaluate the gas water contents.

3.1.2 Condensation on the Humidification Chamber's Inner Wall

With the heated humidifiers, it is possible to determine indirectly if the gas reaches a high relative humidity by examining condensation on the walls of the humidification chamber. This technique was validated for relatively low room temperatures (between 22 and 24 °C) [6]. Indeed, low room temperatures are required to get a sufficient difference of temperature with the gas circulating in the humidification chamber. While cooling by contact with the wall, the relative humidity of the gas can raise, and condensation on the wall will occur at the dew point. On the contrary, with high room temperature, the delta between ambient and chamber temperature is not enough to lead to condensation. In this case, there is no correlation between condensation on the wall and the level of gas humidification [6] (Fig. 3.1). Consequently, this technique is useless when ambient temperatures are high, conditions that lead to heated wire humidifier dysfunction [6].

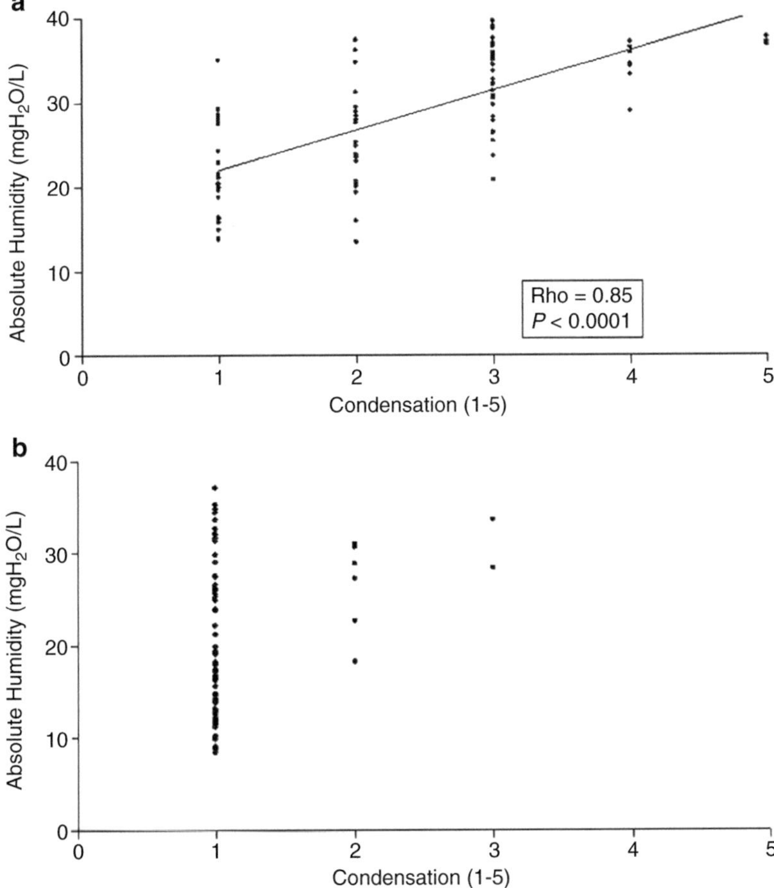

Fig. 3.1 (**a** and **b**) Visual evaluation of condensation on the heated humidifier humidification chamber [6]. A close correlation exists between visual evaluation of the condensation (based on a condensation scale; see below) and heated wire humidifier performance (absolute humidity (mg H_2O/L) of inspiratory gases) when ambient air is low enough (22 to 24 °C) (**a**). However, there is no correlation when ambient air is high (28 to 30 °C) (**b**). *Scale for visual evaluation of condensation*: the level of condensation on the humidification chamber wall can be assessed by visual inspection as follows: 1, dry; 2, vapor; 3, vapor with a few small droplets; 4, numerous droplets not covering the entire wall; 5, numerous droplets covering the wall almost completely. This scale has been used in several studies [5, 6]

3.2 Techniques to Measure the Hygrometry of Gases During Mechanical Ventilation

3.2.1 What Is Hygrometry?

Hygrometry characterizes the quantity of moisture of air, namely, the quantity of water vapor present in the air (or in another gas). It does not take into account the water present in liquid or solid form.

Definition of humidity: humidity or moisture expresses the presence of a mixture of dry air and water vapor in ambient air. In general, moisture refers to the "rate of moisture" expressed in % which refers to the relative humidity. The determination of this measurement is related to conditions, such as the temperature and the pressure. The rate of moisture in a volume of air is generally expressed by one of the following parameters (Fig. 3.2):

- *Absolute humidity* (AH) or water content of a gas which defines the quantity of water vapor (i.e., gaseous state or steam) contained within a certain volume of this gas. It is generally expressed in mgH_2O/L. The maximum water content of a gas increases with its temperature (Fig. 3.3).

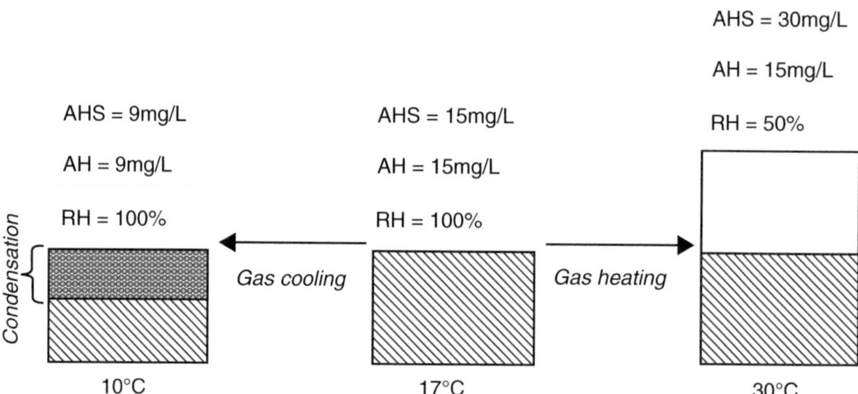

Fig. 3.2 Schematic representation of relative humidity (RH), absolute humidity (AH), and absolute humidity at saturation (AHS) with different temperatures. At 17 °C, a gas is completely saturated with water vapor; the water content (AH) is equal to AHS. This temperature corresponds to the dew point. By cooling down gas at 10 °C, condensation occurs. By warming up the gas, the water content (AH) remains the same, but since gas can contain more water with a higher temperature, the relative humidity diminishes. The hatched lines represent the quantity of water vapor in comparison with the complete volume of gas. This volume is artificially separated from the rest of the gas (in white) which is a volume of dry gas without water vapor

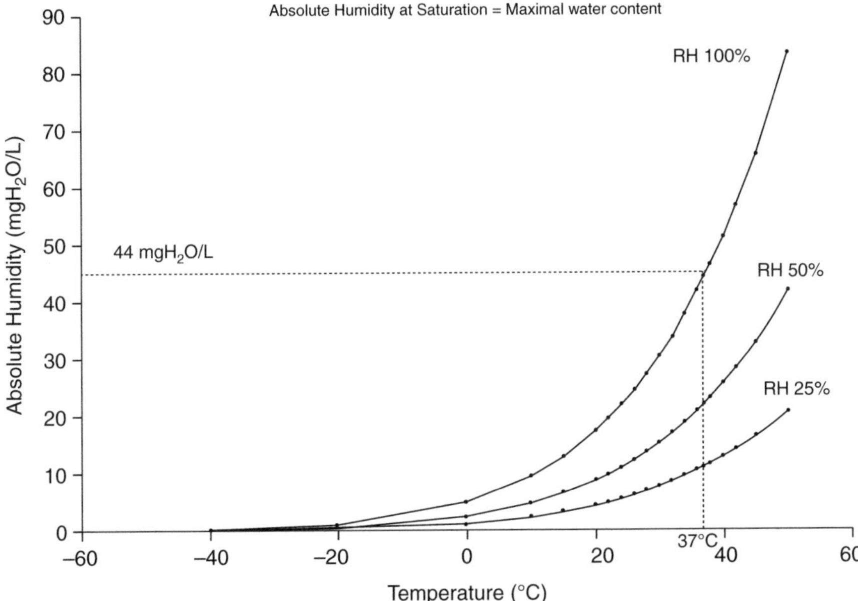

Fig. 3.3 Presentation of the air water contents (i.e., absolute humidity (in mgH$_2$O/L)) according to its temperature and according to the relative humidity of the air (RH). The curves of 25, 50, and 100% of saturation or relative humidity (RH) are represented. At 100% of relative humidity, the water content corresponds to the maximum water contents (i.e., absolute humidity at saturation (AHS)). At 37 °C, water content of the gas is 44 mgH$_2$O/L with 100% of relative humidity (gas completely saturated with vapor water), and it is 22 mgH$_2$O/L with 50% of RH and 11 mgH$_2$O/L with 25% of RH

- *Dew point temperature*: it is the temperature for which at constant pressure, it is necessary to cool down a mass of humid air to reach the saturation of this steam gas. When the gas is further cooled, condensation appears. Knowing this temperature makes it possible to determine the humidity of air, thanks to the tables and diagrams like the Mollier diagram (Fig. 3.3). A parameter associated with this concept is the *absolute humidity at saturation* (AHS) (or maximal water content) which corresponds to the absolute humidity or water content, when the gas is saturated. The absolute humidity at saturation depends on the gas temperature (Fig. 3.3) [7].
- *Relative humidity* (RH) is defined as the ratio of absolute humidity with the absolute humidity at saturation of this gas: RH = (AH/AHS) × 100.

A gas containing steam contains a quantity of energy (enthalpy) or latent heat, which will be released at the time of the passage of the gas state to the liquid state (condensation). On the contrary, during the evaporation of gas, energy is required and the temperature of the gas decreases.

3.2.2 Psychrometry

3.2.2.1 Working Principles of Psychrometry

The psychrometric method comes from the exploitation of the Mollier diagram. The work of Mollier completed at the nineteenth century highlighted the relation between temperature and humidity relative to a given pressure. The Mollier diagram directly resulting from its research shows this relation. In spite of the limited means of its author at the time of this research, the Mollier diagram remains a reference. In particular, the psychometric method that is used for the majority of hygrometric measurements presented here is based on this work. The diagrams are valid for a given pressure. The influence of the pressure for a clinical application is negligible, because of the low amplitude of the barometric variations. Thus, measurements to be carried out only take into account the temperature as a variable (Fig. 3.4).

There are a great number of moisture sensors, relying on very complex principles (reserved with applications in laboratory) like hygrometer with radioactive isotopes and on very simple principles like the hair hygrometer, based on the principle of lengthening of a hair with moisture [8].

Psychrometer is one of the oldest hygrometers, invented by Regnault, around 1845. Its principle is based on the Mollier diagram and the measure of a difference in temperature between a "dry" temperature sensor and a "wet" temperature sensor.

A psychrometer consists of two temperature probes, wet and dry, placed in the gas for which humidity is assessed. One of the thermometers, called "wet" thermometer, is maintained wet with the help of a cloth soaked with water. The other, called "dry" thermometer, measures the temperature of the gas. Through contact with air, the water of the fabric evaporates if the gas is not already saturated with water, which causes a cooling of the wet thermometer until a balanced temperature. Knowing these two temperatures makes it possible to determine the rate of humidity relative to the abacuses means, derived from the Mollier diagram.

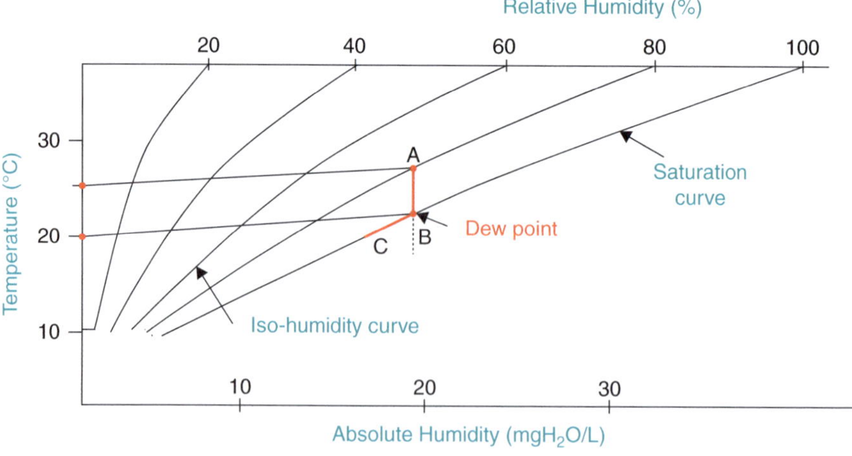

Fig. 3.4 The Mollier diagram

In the medical field which interests us, psychrometry was used in many studies [2, 5, 9–26], and the use of this technique was well described [13, 22].

Two temperature sensors – dry and wet – are placed on the inspiratory way (generally in the event of measurement of the inspiratory gas hygrometry) or on the expiratory way (in the event of measurement of the expiratory gas hygrometry). The temperatures must be measured after the steady state is reached, after 15 min to 3 h (in particular when measurements relate to heated humidifiers with compensation system). The psychrometric method is based on the comparison of the dry and wet temperatures. The dry probe is put first (ventilator side), and the humid probe, encircled with a sterile piece of cloth soaked in water, is put about 1 cm ahead of the dry probe (patient side) (Fig. 3.5). The vaporizing of the water on the humid probe depends on the relative humidity of the gas (the more the gas is "dry" or has a low relative humidity, the more vaporization occurs, leading to the cooling of the probe). The gradient of temperature between both probes varies in a converse manner proportional to the relative humidity of gas. There is no gradient of temperature between the dry and humid probe when the gas is saturated with a relative humidity of 100%.

Relative humidity (RH) is calculated in reference to a psychrometric diagram taking into account differences between the temperatures of the two probes [27].

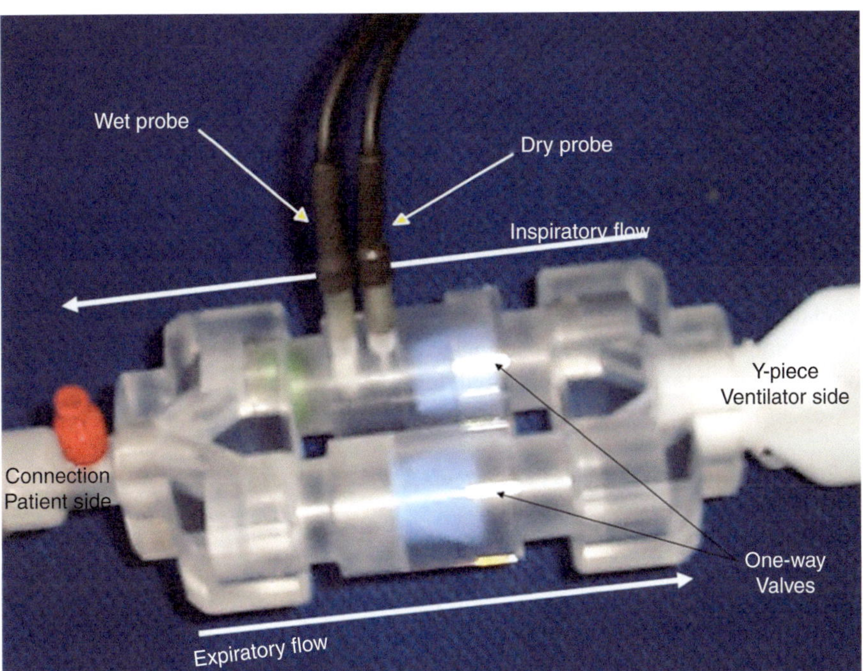

Fig. 3.5 Flow separator used for psychrometric studies. This separator is required due to the low response time of this hygrometer. It allows analyzing only inspiratory (most often) or expiratory gas without mixing of the flows. The additional dead space is minimal as the gases are separated; however, resistive proprieties must be taken into account during the measurements

The absolute humidity at saturation (AHS) is acquired by the following expressions:

$$AHS = 16.451563 - 0.731\,T + 0.03987\,T_2\,(mgH_2O\,/\,L),$$
$$\text{for a dry temperature from } 24.1 \text{ to } 38°C$$

$$AHS = 6.0741 + 0.1039\,T + 0.02266\,T_2\,(mgH_2O\,/\,L),$$
$$\text{for a dry temperature from } 10 \text{ to } 24.1°C$$

where T is the temperature of the dry probe.

Absolute humidity (AH) is acquired by the following formula and by knowing the relative humidity (RH) and absolute humidity at saturation (AHS):

$$AH = (AHS \times RH)\,/\,100\,(mg\,H_2O\,/\,L)$$

The response time of this psychrometer for a gas at a speed of 1 m/s was measured in 1.25 s for 50% of equilibration and 4.1 s for 90% of equilibration of the temperature. The response time (63% of the equilibrium time) is in the order of 2 s [13]. Considering that the relatively long response time does not allow the separation of inspiration and expiration in normal breathing conditions, a flux separator should be used, allowing separating inspiratory gases from expiratory gases (Fig. 3.5). It allows the non-"pollution" of inspiratory gases with expiratory gases during measurement.

The temperature probes are placed on the inspiratory or expiratory ways, according to the type of measurement. The calibration of this machine is based on the calibration of the temperature probes. Furthermore, before every series of measurements, the measured temperatures by the two temperature probes of the psychrometer (prior to the soaking in water of the humid probe) should be compared with a standard temperature acquired with a high-precision thermometer, placed at the same level as both assessed temperature probes. The value of the highest temperature in the inspiratory canal should be considered in the course of several cycles after equilibrium. Certain teams use the medium inspiratory temperature [13, 22].

3.2.3 Comparison of Psychrometry with Other Techniques

3.2.3.1 Studies Using the Psychrometry

The psychrometric technique was used by numerous teams [2, 5, 9–26]. The first measurements which we acquired with the psychrometric method showed a very good reproducibility of measurements compared with data beforehand published for identical systems of humidification. For instance, the hygrometric performance evaluation of the Hygrobac DAR HME made by different teams found data very close [5, 22, 28]. Also, within our laboratory, the reproducibility of measurements accomplished for the same system was very good with weak standard deviations (usually lower in 1 mgH₂O/L) [1, 6, 29–31].

By comparing the psychrometric measurements provided in the literature with other techniques to measure hygrometry, it appears a good correlation between measurements accomplished with psychrometry and those performed with other techniques. The most frequent alternative techniques to measure the performances of the humidification systems are the gravimetry (bench studies only) and the capacitance hygrometer which also allows making measurements in mechanically ventilated patients.

3.2.3.2 Studies Using the Gravimetry

Gravimetry is one of the techniques used for the evaluation of the humidification systems. A method was developed and recommended by the norm ISO 9360 [32]. It is based on weight difference of a semi-closed system over a given period (normally of 2 h) and assesses the loss of water in the system which consists of a lung, the humidification system to be tested [26, 33–38], and a model simulating a patient with a saturated expiratory gas (Fig. 3.6). Results are normally expressed in mgH$_2$O/L of water loss/hour. Knowing the value of exhaled humidity and minute ventilation, it is possible to determine the absolute humidity of the delivered gas.

This method is used mainly by the manufacturers to test the humidification systems on bench. The major limitation of this technology is that it cannot be directly used with patients. The other limitation is that it requires high-precision equipment for the weighing of the system and for the measurements of inspired and expired volumes at different levels of temperature and humidity. The study of Branson and Davis is the most exhaustive among those having used this technology [33]. These authors assessed the performances of 21 HMEs with the gravimetric method according to norm ISO 9360. It is possible to make the comparison with our bench study [1] for four HMEs tested in the same conditions of ventilation (tidal volume of 500 mL, respiratory rate of 20 breaths/min) (Table 3.1). Most of the other HMEs were different or with a reference that did not allow making identification with certainty.

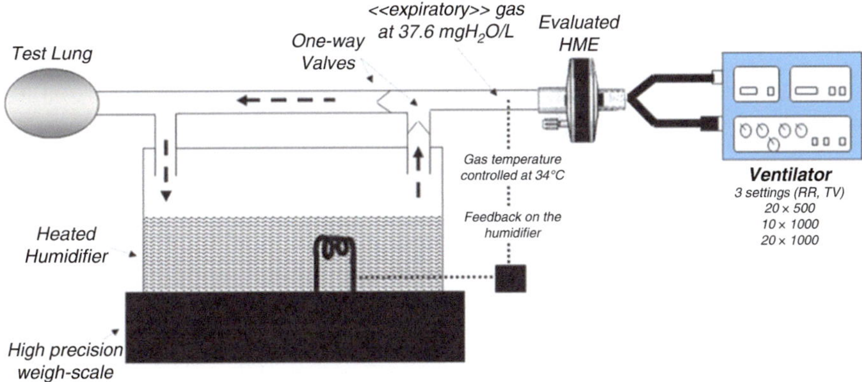

Fig. 3.6 Gravimetric method to measure hygrometry according to the norm ISO 9360 [33]

The most important difference in measurements was with Hygroster (-7.5%) but remains weak. For other HMEs, the difference is minimal: Hygrobac (-2.5%), Hygrobac S ($+4.2\%$), and Portex 1200 ($+0.2\%$). When used by the companies, the differences between psychrometry and gravimetry are very high as shown in several studies [1, 3].

The main advantage of the psychrometry is that it can be used on patients as well as on bench, allowing a clinical validation of the model.

3.2.3.3 Studies Using Capacitance Hygrometer

This hygrometer was described for this usage for humidification system evaluation in 1983 by Tilling [39]. The sensor is a fine polymeric film with electrodes positioned on each side. According to relative humidity, the water steam is absorbed on the polymeric film, which changes its capacitance. These hygrometers are usually not expensive. Their main flaw is to have a significant drift, which often requires frequent calibrations. Moreover, considering that the response time is very quick, the given values (maximum, minimum, and medium value) make the analysis of results very difficult.

This hygrometer was used by several teams [19, 40–43], but results are difficult to compare with other hygrometers considering the quick response time of this hygrometer, the values of absolute humidity being given in maximum, minimum, or average (Table 3.2). It seems that the medium value is the one which gets closer to most psychrometric data, except in the case of Pall Ultipor used in the study of Martin et al. [19].

Table 3.1 Comparison of the results for absolute humidity measurements (in mgH_2O/L) acquired for several HMEs evaluated with gravimetry [33] and psychrometry [1]

	Hygrobac	Hygrobac S	Hygroster	Sims Portex 1200
Branson (1996) [33]	32.5	29.6	33.2	27.2
Lellouche (2009) [1]	31.7	31.2	30.7	27.8

Table 3.2 Comparison of results obtained from identical HME with a capacitance hygrometer [19, 40, 42, 43] and with the psychrometric method [1]. For data coming from the capacitance hygrometer, the maximum, mean, or minimum available values of absolute humidity (in mgH_2O/L) are displayed. The Pall filter tested was BB2215, whose performances are very close to the BB50 [5]

	Humid-Vent Light	Pall Ultipor BB50	MaxiPleat
Martin [19]	Mean: 32.9 ± 3.1 Minimum: 29.0 ± 5.0	Mean: 31.0 ± 3.8 Minimum: 22.0 ± 6.6	
Thomachot [43]	Mean: 29.3 ± 3.4		
Thomachot [42]	Mean: 32.6 ± 2.5		
Boisson [40]			Maximum: 34.0 ± 2.4 Mean: 22.9 ± 2.8
Lellouche (2009) [1] (psychrometric method)	30.8 ± 0.3	21.8 ± 1.5 (BB2215)	20.1 ± 0.6

3.2.4 Limitations of the Psychrometric Method

The psychrometric method has nevertheless some limitations which are necessary to know. It is possible that the ambient temperature has an influence on measurement. Indeed, at the level of the separator of flux, there can be thermal exchanges between the gas passing in this piece and surrounding air, particularly when the difference in temperature between these gases is important. To restrict this phenomenon, it is possible to use an isothermic foam around the separator of flux. The use of the medium rather than maximum temperature could also restrict this phenomenon. Another problem linked to the piece which separates inspiratory gases from expiratory gases is the high resistance, especially in the inspiratory way. Inspiratory resistance was measured at 19.6 cmH$_2$O for 1 L/s and expiratory ones at 4.8 cmH$_2$O for 1 L/s. Due to the inspiratory resistance, in patients ventilated with assist-control ventilation in volume, the peak pressures increase and in patients ventilated with a pressure mode, the volumes delivered by the ventilator are reduced with the presence of the flow separator. In the first case, it is necessary to increase the high pressure alarms, and in the second event, it is necessary to increase the level of assistance to about 5–10 cmH$_2$O to obtain an equivalent tidal volume. Due to the expiratory resistances, there can be a risk of expiratory flow limitation. Usually, the duration of the measurements does not exceed 15 min to attain the steady state, which limits this potential issue. In practice, we did not have problem of poor tolerance in the course of numerous measurements, probably due to the selection of the patients. The patients included had to have a relative respiratory stability (FiO$_2$ ≤ 80%) as well as hemodynamic stability (epi- or norepinephrine ≤2 mg/h).

Another limitation shared by most of the hygrometric measurements is the inability to assess systems producing nebulizations. Indeed, psychrometry measures the vapor of water contained in a gas, while nebulization draws away micro-droplets under liquid form. These droplets make the dry probe wet, which distorts measurements. This limitation also exists with other methods using sensors (hygrometer with capacitance, dew point hygrometers).

3.2.5 Limitations of the Gravimetric Method (and ISO 9360)

Manufacturers usually state the humidity output of their devices based on ISO 9360 method. Thiery et al. suggested that independent hygrometric measurements are required to evaluate humidification devices [2]. The authors found markedly lower performances with psychrometric measurements in patients with Hygroster than those specified by the manufacturer: 27.3 ± 2.2 mgH$_2$O/L vs. 33.4 mgH$_2$O/L, respectively. Lellouche et al. evaluated on bench 48 HMEs and filters and compared the humidity performances claimed by the manufacturers using the ISO 9360 method and humidity measured by the psychrometric method [1]. The authors found large differences between humidity performances specified by manufacturers using the ISO 9360 method and the humidity measured on bench by the psychrometric method. The mean difference in absolute humidity between the two methods was 3.0 ± 2.7 mgH$_2$O/L, with 36% of the device having a difference greater than 4 mgH$_2$O/L, and the maximum difference was 8.9 mgH$_2$O/L. Recently, we compared manufacturer's claim (based on ISO 9360 method) and psychrometric measurements of HME responsible for endotracheal tube occlusions in patients mechanically ventilated for COVID-19 [3]. We measured unacceptably low humidity output (mean 25.8 ± 0.9 mgH$_2$O/L) despite the fact that manufacturers reported a reassuring humidity of 32.8 ± 1.6 mgH$_2$O/L. The mean difference between claimed and measured humidity in this small series was 6.4 ± 1.4 mgH$_2$O/L. None of the HME involved in endotracheal tube occlusion had a humidity delivered above 30 mgH$_2$O/L with psychrometric measurements, while they all passed the test with the ISO 9360. In other words, the ISO standard fails to protect patients from an underperforming HME.

3.3 Benches for Measurements of Hygrometry (for HME, "Active" HME, and Heated Humidifiers)

The bench evaluation of HME and "active" HME requires simulating a physiological model that provides saturated exhaled gas as for a patient with a normal core temperature. According to the literature data, exhaled gases are saturated with vapor water at 32 °C in the endotracheal tube at the teeth level [44, 45], which corresponds to a water content of 34 mgH$_2$O/L (Fig. 3.7). These values of absolute expiratory humidity are concordant with those found in the study assessing expiratory humidity in patients with hypothermia and normal core temperatures [30]. The simulation of saturated expiration can be performed with a heated humidifier (Fig. 3.8).

Several studies are published using a model with simulation of expiratory saturated gases going from 32 to 37 °C, which corresponds to gas absolute humidity between 34 and 44 mgH$_2$O/L [26, 33–38, 46–49]. We performed a bench study to compare different filters and HME in stable and controlled situations [1] (Fig. 3.8).

The bench evaluation of the *heated humidifier* performances is easier. The heated humidifier to test is installed on a ventilator with different settings (Fig. 3.9). The circuit of the ventilator is connected to a test lung (at Y-piece), the latter being changed regularly to avoid the accumulation of water. Different temperatures are measured (ambient temperature, ventilator output temperature, inlet chamber temperature) by a high-precision thermometer, and temperatures measured by the humidifier are also recorded (heater plate temperature, outlet chamber temperature, temperature at the Y-piece) [6].

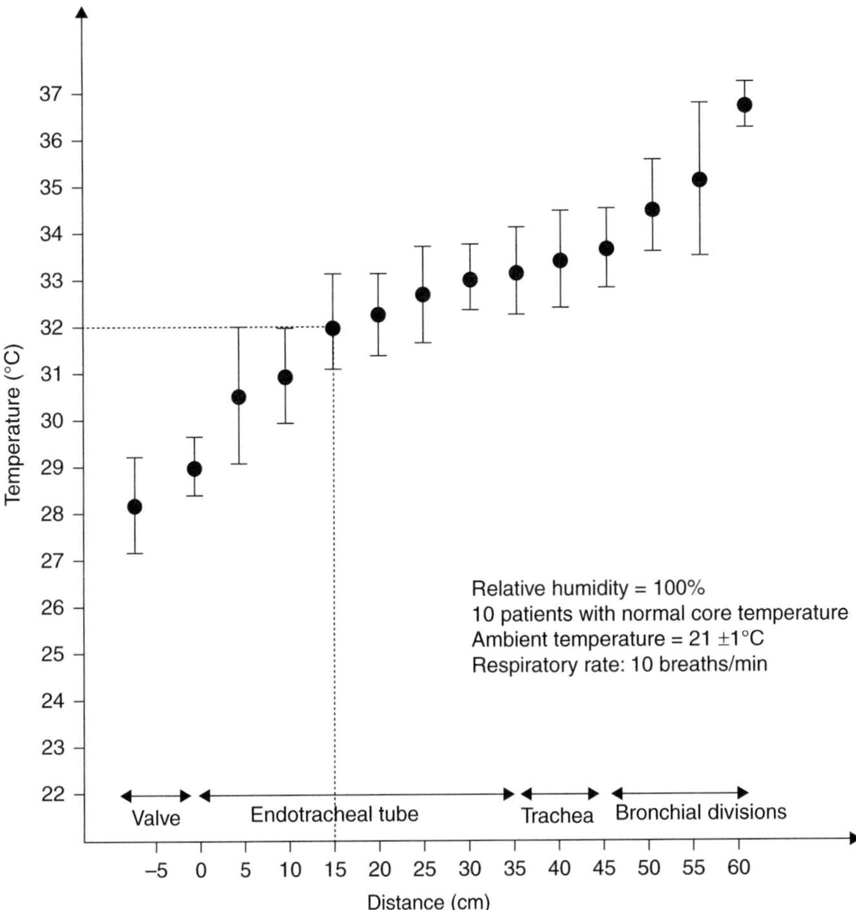

Fig. 3.7 Expiratory gas temperature in ten patients during anesthesia. In dotted lines is the gas temperature in the endotracheal tube at the level of the teeth. (Adapted from Dery et al. [45])

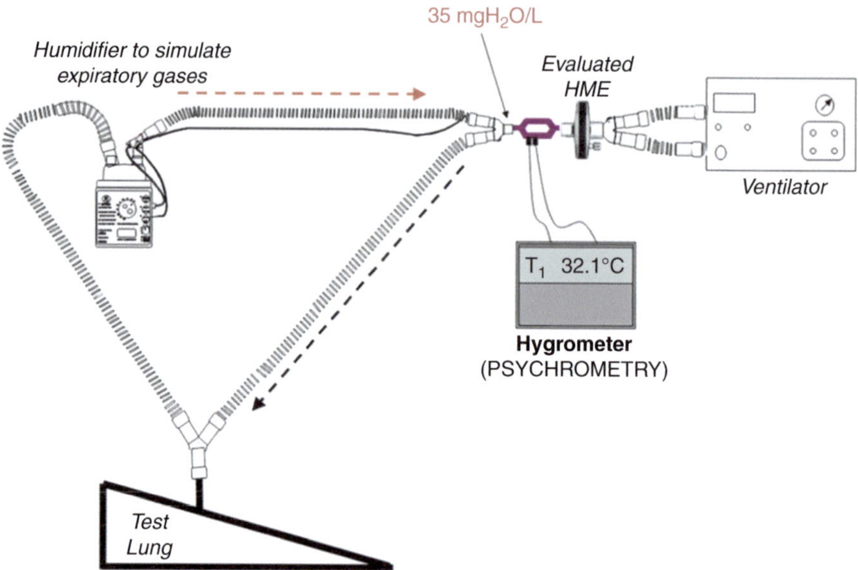

Fig. 3.8 Hygrometric bench test apparatus used to measure the humidification performances of HMEs and antibacterial filters. A driving ventilator delivered controlled cycles (respiratory rate set at 20 breaths/min with a tidal volume of 500 mL and a positive end-expiratory pressure of 5 cmH$_2$O). A heated humidifier (MR730) was connected to the expiratory limb of the model and was set to deliver gases with a water content of 35 mgH$_2$O/L at the Y-piece. A circuit with heated wire was used after the humidification chamber. The (ambient) temperature should be maintained constant between 24.5 °C and 25.5 °C. The system can be installed in a space isolated (like an incubator) to keep this constant temperature. Ideally, an isothermic insulating foam should surround the separator of flow to avoid the variations of heat on this level and condensation in the part of hygroscopy. For all the studies on bench, the number of measurements carried out for each studied condition must be preset (between three and six measurements). This bench can be used for the study of the filter humidifiers and the active filters [1, 29]

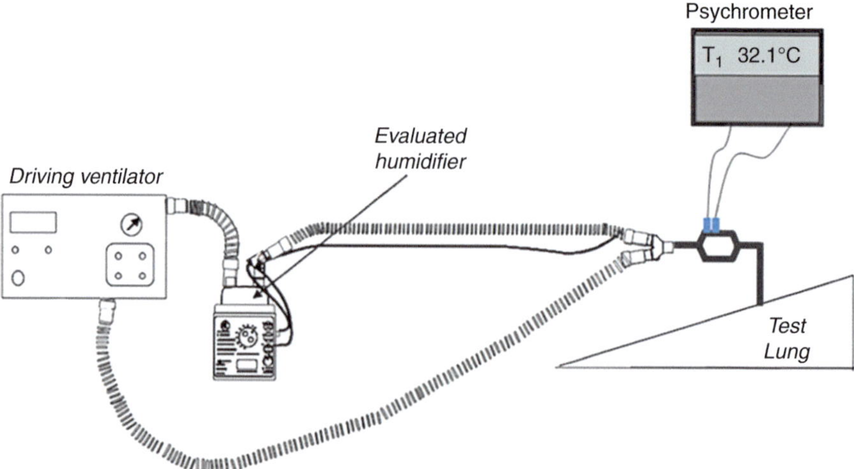

Fig. 3.9 Bench of psychometric measure used during different studies for the evaluation of the heating humidifiers

3.4   Use of the Heated Humidifier Heater Plate Temperature

It was previously demonstrated that humidity delivered to the patient was reduced when the temperature entering in the HH humidification chamber was high (mainly due to high ambient air or high outlet ventilator temperature) [6]. This can be explained by the regulation of HH that maintains a constant outlet chamber temperature (frequently around 37 °C in most heated wire humidifiers). This can be achieved by decreasing the heated plate energy, leading to reduced temperature in the humidification chamber when the inlet chamber temperature is high. We recently evaluated if heater plate temperature could be used as an accurate surrogate of humidity delivered with MR850 humidifier [50]. It turned out that there is a very strong correlation between the heater plate temperature and absolute humidity delivered at the Y-piece, which means that a precise hygrometer is integrated in the heated humidifier. This relationship is not affected by the ambient air temperature but is slightly modified by the minute ventilation. In this study, we found that monitoring of this parameter could be helpful to detect low humidification, especially when ambient temperature is high. Heater plate (HP) temperature above 62 °C could predict a humidity delivered above 30 mgH_2O/L with a good sensibility and specificity up to 12.5 L/min. Above this minute ventilation, heater plate temperature above 65 °C should be targeted. When HP temperature is below the target, specific settings should be used (increasing of chamber temperature by 1 to 3 °C or utilization of automated compensation function).

The heated humidifiers usually display the humidification chamber outlet temperature. However, this monitoring is useless and does not inform on humidity delivered [50]. Unfortunately, HP temperature is "hidden" and available only by accessing to the sub-menu as shown in the following video: https://www.youtube.com/watch?v=HImPXoIxLJw

The utilization of heater plate temperature monitoring was implemented in an ICU during the COVID-19 pandemic to avoid endotracheal tube occlusions [51]. After ICU rooms were equipped with negative pressure devices, the ambient temperature rose up to 28–30 °C leading to three episodes of ETO within few weeks, while humidification of the gases delivered to mechanically ventilated patients was performed with heated wire humidifiers. After implementation of measures to avoid under-humidification, including heater plate temperature monitoring, no more ETOs occurred [51]. This method has recently been described more in detail and confirms that when heater plate temperature is above 62 °C for minute ventilation below 12.5 L/min, the humidity delivered to the patients is above 30 mgH_2O/L [50].

Let us assume that a gas has a temperature of 25 °C with relative humidity of 80% (point A on the diagram). If the temperature is cooled down to 20 °C, the relative humidity will increase and attain the dew point (100% of relative humidity) (point B). Between points A and B, only relative humidity varies, while absolute humidity is constant. If the gas is further cooled, condensation appears: the relative humidity remains at 100%, but absolute humidity will be reduced (passage from point B toward point C).

References

1. Lellouche F, et al. Humidification performance of 48 passive airway humidifiers: comparison with manufacturer data. Chest. 2009;135(2):276–86.
2. Thiery G, et al. Heat and moisture exchangers in mechanically ventilated intensive care unit patients: a plea for an independent assessment of their performance. Crit Care Med. 2003;31(3):699–704.
3. Lellouche F, et al. How to avoid an epidemic of endotracheal tube occlusion. Lancet Respir Med. 2021;9(11):1215–6.
4. Beydon L, et al. Correlation between simple clinical parameters and the in vitro humidification characteristics of filter heat and moisture exchangers. Groupe de travail Sur les Respirateurs. Chest. 1997;112(3):739–44.
5. Ricard JD, et al. Bedside evaluation of efficient airway humidification during mechanical ventilation of the critically ill. Chest. 1999;115(6):1646–52.
6. Lellouche L, et al. Influence of ambient air and ventilator output temperature on performances of heated-wire humidifiers. Am J Respir Crit Care Med. 2004;170:1073–9.
7. Williams RB. The effects of excessive humidity. Respir Care Clin N Am. 1998;4(2):215–28.
8. Saussure H-BD. BARDE, editor. Défense de l'hygromètre à cheveu, pour servir de suite aux essais sur l'hygrométrie. Genève: MANGET. p. 1788.
9. Ingelstedt S. Studies on the conditioning of air in the respiratory tract. Acta Otolaryngol Suppl. 1956;131:1–80.
10. Sara C, Currie T. Humidification by nebulization. Med J Aust. 1965;191:174–9.
11. Sottiaux T, et al. Comparative evaluation of three heat and moisture exchangers during short-term postoperative mechanical ventilation. Chest. 1993;104(1):220–4.
12. Tsubota K, Harada J, Goto Y. Efficacy of nine heat and moisture exchangers for intraoperative airway heat conservation. J Aerosol Med. 1991;4(2):117–25.
13. Jackson C, Webb AR. An evaluation of the heat and moisture exchange performance of four ventilator circuit filters. Intensive Care Med. 1992;18(5):264–8.
14. Markowicz P, et al. Safety, efficacy, and cost-effectiveness of mechanical ventilation with humidifying filters changed every 48 hours: a prospective, randomized study. Crit Care Med. 2000;28(3):665–71.
15. Vanderbroucke-Grauls CM, et al. Bacterial and viral removal efficiency, heat and moisture exchange properties of four filtration devices. J Hosp Infect. 1995;29(1):45–56.
16. Chiumello D, et al. In vitro and in vivo evaluation of a new active heat moisture exchanger. Crit Care. 2004;8(5):R281–8.
17. Croci M, Elena A, Solca M. Performance of a hydrophobic heat and moisture exchanger at different ambient temperatures. Intensive Care Med. 1993;19(6):351–2.
18. Martin C, et al. Performance evaluation of three vaporizing humidifiers and two heat and moisture exchangers in patients with minute ventilation >10 L/min. Chest. 1992;102(5):1347–50.
19. Martin C, et al. Preservation of humidity and heat of respiratory gases in patients with a minute ventilation greater than 10 L/min. Crit Care Med. 1994;22(11):1871–6.
20. Martin C, et al. Comparing two heat and moisture exchangers with one vaporizing humidifier in patients with minute ventilation greater than 10 L/min. Chest. 1995;107(5):1411–5.
21. Miyao H, et al. Relative humidity, not absolute humidity, is of great importance when using a humidifier with a heating wire. Crit Care Med. 1992;20(5):674–9.
22. Ricard JD, et al. Efficiency and safety of mechanical ventilation with a heat and moisture exchanger changed only once a week. Am J Respir Crit Care Med. 2000;161(1):104–9.
23. Christiansen S, et al. Measurement of the humidity of inspired air in ventilated patients with various humidifier systems. Anasthesiol Intensivmed Notfallmed Schmerzther. 1998;33(5):300–5.
24. Fassassi M, et al. Airway humidification with a heat and moisture exchanger in mechanically ventilated neonates: a preliminary evaluation. Intensive Care Med. 2007;33(2):336–43.
25. Tontschev G, Lueder M, Bensow C. The efficiency of various humidifiers for respired gas. Resuscitation. 1980;8(3):167–79.

26. Walker AK, Bethune DW. A comparative study of condenser humidifiers. Anaesthesia. 1976;31(8):1086–93.
27. Condon E, Handbook of physics. New York. NY: Churchill Livingstone; 1967.
28. Lellouche F, Brochard L. Advanced closed loops during mechanical ventilation (PAV, NAVA, ASV, SmartCare). Best Pract Res Clin Anaesthesiol. 2009;23(1):81–93.
29. Lellouche F, et al. Impact of ambient air temperature on a new active HME and on standard HMES: bench evaluation. Intensive Care Med. 2003;29:S169.
30. Lellouche F, et al. Under-humidification and over-humidification during moderate induced hypothermia with usual devices. Intensive Care Med. 2006;32(7):1014–21.
31. Lellouche L, et al. Advantages and drawbacks of a heated humidifier with compensation of under-humidification. Am J Respir Crit Care Med. 2003;167(7):A909.
32. Standardization, I.O.f., Anesthetic and respiratory equipment. Heat and moisture exchangers for use in humidifying gases in humans 1st ed. ISO International Standard 9360, 1992.
33. Branson R, Davis J. Evaluation of 21 passive humidifiers according to the ISO 9360 standard: moisture output, dead space, and flow resistance. Respir Care. 1996;41:736–43.
34. Eckerbom B, Lindholm CE. Performance evaluation of six heat and moisture exchangers according to the draft international standard (ISO/DIS 9360). Acta Anaesthesiol Scand. 1990;34(5):404–9.
35. Mebius C. A comparative evaluation of disposable humidifiers. Acta Anaesthesiol Scand. 1983;27(5):403–9.
36. Mebius C. Heat and moisture exchangers with bacterial filters: a laboratory evaluation. Acta Anaesthesiol Scand. 1992;36(6):572–6.
37. Ogino M, Kopotic R, Mannino FL. Moisture-conserving efficiency of condenser humidifiers. Anaesthesia. 1985;40(10):990–5.
38. Shelly M, Bethune DW, Latimer RD. A comparison of five heat and moisture exchangers. Anaesthesia. 1986;41(5):527–32.
39. Tilling SE, Hancox AJ, Hayes B. An accurate method of measuring medical humidifier output. Clin Phys Physiol Meas. 1983;4(2):197–209.
40. Boisson C, et al. Changing a hydrophobic heat and moisture exchanger after 48 hours rather than 24 hours: a clinical and microbiological evaluation. Intensive Care Med. 1999;25(11):1237–43.
41. Davis K Jr, et al. Prolonged use of heat and moisture exchangers does not affect device efficiency or frequency rate of nosocomial pneumonia. Crit Care Med. 2000;28(5):1412–8.
42. Thomachot L, et al. Changing heat and moisture exchangers after 96 hours rather than after 24 hours: a clinical and microbiological evaluation. Crit Care Med. 2000;28(3):714–20.
43. Thomachot L, et al. Efficacy of heat and moisture exchangers after changing every 48 hours rather than 24 hours. Crit Care Med. 1998;26(3):477–81.
44. Dery R. Humidity in anesthesiology III. Heat and moisture patterns in the respiratory tract during anesthesia with the semi-closed system. Can Anaesth Soc J. 1967;14:287–98.
45. Dery R. The evolution of heat and moisture in the respiratory tract during anesthesia with a nonrebreathing system. Can Anaesth Soc J. 1973;20:296–309.
46. Chalon J, et al. The pall ultipor breathing circuit filter--an efficient heat and moisture exchanger. Anesth Analg. 1984;63(6):566–70.
47. Cigada M, et al. The efficiency of twelve heat and moisture exchangers: an in vitro evaluation. Int Care World. 1990;7:98–101.
48. Gedeon A, Mebius C. The hygroscopic condenser humidifier. A new device for general use in anaesthesia and intensive care. Anaesthesia. 1979;34(10):1043–7.
49. Unal N, et al. An experimental set-up to test heat-moisture exchangers. Intensive Care Med. 1995;21(2):142–8.
50. Lellouche F, Simard S, Bouchard PA. Monitoring of heated wire humidifier MR850 hygrometric performances with heater plate temperature. Respir Care. 2022;67(9):1147–53.
51. Lavoie-Berard CA, et al. Impact of airway humidification strategy in the mechanically ventilated COVID-19 patients. Respir Care. 2021;67(2):157–66.

Part II

Humidification and High-Flow Oxygen Therapy

Humidification During Conventional Oxygen Therapy: Physiology

4

Yoshinori Matsuoka, Kei Kurihara, Yoshitaka Nishiyama, and Takuma Sakai

4.1 Conventional Oxygen Therapy

Respiratory support is essential to maintain adequate oxygenation and alveolar ventilation and is the first-line treatment for hypoxemic respiratory failure using supplemental oxygen.

Devices for oxygen therapy include unassisted oxygen delivery and assisted ventilation devices [1]. Unassisted oxygen therapy, also known as conventional oxygen therapy, is the primary supportive treatment administered to patients with dyspnea and is usually delivered using nasal prongs or facemasks. Assisted ventilation devices, which are commonly used in hospitals, include noninvasive ventilation (e.g., continuous positive and biphasic positive airway pressures) and invasive mechanical ventilation.

4.2 Airway Humidification and Heating System

During spontaneous breathing, inspired air subsequently passes through the nose, pharynx, larynx, and trachea. Owing to the excellent ability of the human nose and upper airway to warm and humidify inspired gas on the way down to the alveoli, inspired air is warmed up to body temperature and fully saturated with water vapor by the time it reaches the alveoli. The nose and upper airway are also excellent radiators. Furthermore, during natural breathing, even when the ambient air is cold and dry, they can maintain the temperature in the oropharyngeal area [2, 3].

Y. Matsuoka (✉) · K. Kurihara · Y. Nishiyama · T. Sakai
Wide Area Medical Corporation EMS, Minami-Kyushu City, Kagoshima, Japan

© The Author(s), under exclusive license to Springer Nature Switzerland AG 2023
A. M. Esquinas (ed.), *Humidification in the Intensive Care Unit*,
https://doi.org/10.1007/978-3-031-23953-3_4

4.3   The Need for Warming and Humidification in Oxygen Therapy

During natural breathing, air is inhaled through the mouth and nose. The inhaled gas reaches the alveoli after being heated and humidified by water vapor from the mucous membrane while passing through the respiratory tract, such as the nasal and oral cavities. At the tracheal branch, it reaches approximately 37 °C and 100% relative humidity. However, since medical gas, such as compressed oxygen and air, does not contain humidity, high-flow oxygen administration tends to cause dryness of the oral cavity and nasal mucosa. Additionally, during tracheal intubation or tracheostomy, the artificial airway bypasses the upper airway, allowing cold and dry medical gas to enter the trachea directly.

Dry gas may have various adverse effects on the respiratory system. In dogs, breathing dry air causes a complete cessation of the flow of tracheal mucus, and in cultured human epithelial cells, it causes acute damage and inflammation [4, 5]. Moreover, in guinea pigs, it induces widespread loss of the cilia, associated with detachment or sloughing of the epithelium, subepithelial vascular congestion, edema, and cellular infiltration [6]. Cold air can also induce bronchoconstriction in patients with asthma [7]. The airway resistance increases to protect the lungs from the challenge of dry and cold gas by reducing the air flow in the upper airways and trachea. Thus, breathing dry air causes excessive water loss in the nasal mucosa [8], which may, in turn, reduce the nasal mucociliary clearance rate via changes in the rheological properties or adhesiveness of nasal mucus and/or slowing of ciliary pulses.

Cold and dry gases may have adverse effects in patients with respiratory failure. Conventional oxygen devices are associated with mask discomfort, nasal dryness, oral dryness, eye irritation, nasal and eye trauma, and gastric distention [9].

4.4   Humidification Effect

Humidifying and heating gases can aid in minimizing airway constriction, reduce the work of breathing, improve mucociliary function, facilitate clearance of secretions, and are associated with less atelectasis, resulting in a good ventilation/perfusion ratio and better oxygenation. Long-term humidification therapy statistically significantly reduces days of exacerbation, increases the time to first exacerbation, and generally improves lung function and quality of life in patients with chronic obstructive pulmonary disease and bronchiectasis [10].

4.5   Recommended Humidification Level

The recommended level of heating and humidification by the American Association for Respiratory Care is at a temperature of 34–41 °C and absolute humidity of 33–44 mgH$_2$O/L. For humidification with an artificial nose, we recommend an absolute humidity of 30 mgH$_2$O/L or higher [11].

Ventilation with an absolute humidity of ⟨25 mgH$_2$O/L for 1 h or more or an absolute humidity of ⟨30 mgH$_2$O/L for 24 h or more is associated with impaired ciliary motility of the airway mucosa. The humidification performed in the upper respiratory tract is considered to be about 75% of the total, and the theoretical value of humidification considered necessary when using an artificial airway is $44 \times 0.75 = 33$ mgH$_2$O/L. However, to avoid the loss of water vapor from the airway mucosa, an absolute humidity of 44 mgH$_2$O/L has been suggested as the ideal humidification level for inspiratory gas [11].

Low temperatures cause a decrease in absolute humidity and hypothermia, whereas high temperatures, above 41 °C, cause airway mucosal burns. Additionally, excessive humidification should be avoided because it causes condensation inside the airways, thereby decreasing ciliary motor function and increasing airway secretion [11].

References

1. Bell N, Hutchinson CL, Green TC, Rogan E, Bein KJ, Dinh MM. Randomised control trial of humidified high flow nasal cannulae versus standard oxygen in the emergency department. Emerg Med Australas. 2015;27(6):537–41. https://doi.org/10.1111/1742-6723.12490.
2. Rouadi P, Baroody FM, Abbott D, Naureckas E, Solway J, Naclerio RM. A technique to measure the ability of the human nose to warm and humidify air. J Appl Physiol. 1999;87(1):400–6. https://doi.org/10.1152/jappl.1999.87.1.400.
3. Nishimura M. High-flow nasal cannula oxygen therapy in adults: physiological benefits, indication, clinical benefits, and adverse effects. Respir Care. 2016;61(4):529–41. https://doi.org/10.4187/respcare.04577.
4. Hirsch JA, Tokayer JL, Robinson MJ, Sackner MA. Effects of dry air and subsequent humidification on tracheal mucous velocity in dogs. J Appl Physiol. 1975;39(2):242–6. https://doi.org/10.1152/jappl.1975.39.2.242.
5. Chidekel A, Zhu Y, Wang J, Mosko JJ, Rodriguez E, Shaffer TH. The effects of gas humidification with high-flow nasal cannula on cultured human airway epithelial cells. Pulm Med. 2012;2012:380686.
6. Barbet JP, Chauveau M, Labbé S, Lockhart A. Breathing dry air causes acute epithelial damage and inflammation of the Guinea pig trachea. J Appl Physiol. 1988;64(5):1851–7. https://doi.org/10.1152/jappl.1988.64.5.1851.
7. Berk JL, Lenner KA, McFadden ER Jr. Cold-induced bronchoconstriction: role of cutaneous reflexes vs. direct airway effects. J Appl Physiol. 1987;63(2):659–64. https://doi.org/10.1152/jappl.1987.63.2.659.
8. Van Oostdam JC, Walker DC, Knudson K, Dirks P, Dahlby RW, Hogg JC. Effect of breathing dry air on structure and function of airways. J Appl Physiol. 1986;61(1):312–7. https://doi.org/10.1152/jappl.1986.61.1.312.
9. Campbell EJ, Baker MD, Crites-Silver P. Subjective effects of humidification of oxygen for delivery by nasal cannula: a prospective study. Chest. 1988;93(2):289–93. https://doi.org/10.1378/chest.93.2.289.
10. Salah B, Dinh Xuan AT, Fouilladieu JL, Lockhart A, Regnard J. Nasal mucociliary transport in healthy subjects is slower when breathing dry air. Eur Respir J. 1988;1(9):852–5.
11. AARC, Restrepo RD, Walsh BK. Humidification during invasive and noninvasive mechanical ventilation: 2012. Resp Care. 2012;57:782–8. https://doi.org/10.4187/respcare.01766.

Humidification and High-Flow Oxygen Therapy in Critically Ill Patients: Devices and Humidification Technology and Clinical Implications

Avşar Zerman

5.1 Introduction

Acute respiratory failure followed by the need for respiratory support is a frequent reason for adults to apply to the intensive care unit (ICU) . Many pathological causes such as pneumonia, sepsis, acute exacerbations of chronic obstructive pulmonary disease (COPD), aspiration, and post-surgery can lead to this process.

Respiratory failure in critically unwell people can be considered due to hypoxemia, ventilatory failure, or both [1]. Oxygen is the most important supportive treatment for critically ill patients with respiratory failure. Oxygen is delivered to patients via low-flow systems (e.g., nasal cannulas or masks) or high-flow systems (e.g., Venturi masks, nonrebreathers). Such conventional oxygen systems may not provide a reliable fraction of oxygen depending on the patient's breathing pattern, peak inspiratory flow rate, delivery system, and mask characteristics. However, it may also not be enough to provide sufficient heating and humidification of the inhaled gas.

During spontaneous breathing, the gas is heated and humidified in the upper airways. Descending into the alveoli, it is heated to body temperature and is completely saturated with water vapor. It is known that the administration of dry and cold gases in the hospital environment has various negative effects, such as mucociliary dysfunction in the respiratory system, increased airway resistance, and decreased patient tolerance. Although clinical guidelines recommend humidification when the oxygen demand is above 4 L/min in the intensive care setting, it has also been shown that the absolute humidity of the resulting gas is low in humidification with bubble humidifiers [2, 3].

A. Zerman (✉)
Kırşehir Ahi Evran University Training and Research Hospital, Kırşehir, Turkey

© The Author(s), under exclusive license to Springer Nature Switzerland AG 2023

A. M. Esquinas (ed.), *Humidification in the Intensive Care Unit*, https://doi.org/10.1007/978-3-031-23953-3_5

The peak inspiratory flow rate during normal and calm breathing is about 30–40 L/min. For patients with respiratory failure, inspiratory flow is over a wide range from 30 to >120 L/min, with a mean flow rate above 70 L/min [4, 5]. The difference between the patient's inspiratory flow and the delivered flow is large at conventional oxygen devices. Therefore, a significant reduction in the oxygen fraction (FIO_2) reaching the alveoli can be observed.

The high-flow nasal cannula (HFNC) system is a noninvasive respiratory support device used to provide patients with high oxygen flow (up to 60–80 L/min) at a constant concentration (21–100%), temperature (31–37 °C), and humidity. It creates a low positive pressure in the upper airways due to the high flow of gas and prevents dead space ventilation in the upper airways and rebreathing of gas with high CO_2 and low O_2.

The HFNC system consists of a flow generator, an actively heated humidifier, a single-limb heated circuit, and a nasal cannula. Humidification systems contain active humidifiers, heat wire in the inspiratory limb, and temperature sensors.

Several nasal devices are currently available, including Vapotherm® and the Optiflow™ and AIRVO 2 devices from Fisher & Paykel Healthcare, Inc.

The HFNC system is increasingly used in patients with acute hypoxemic respiratory failure, such as pneumonia, acute respiratory distress syndrome (ARDS), and interstitial lung disease.

5.2 Devices and Humidification Technology

The gas flow in the humidification system should be warm (37 °C) and humidified [44 mg/L absolute humidity (AH), 100% relative humidity (RH)]. Unhumidified ambient gas heated in the upper airway during inspiration is humidified up to the isothermal saturation limit (ISB; 37 °C, AH 44 mg/L, RH 100%).

The composition of an HFNC system can differ between medical equipment manufacturers. The basic setup includes the same basic elements. These include a supply of pressurized oxygen and air regulated by a flow meter/mixer; a sterile water tank connected to an efficient heating humidifier; an insulated and/or heated circuit that maintains the temperature and relative humidity of the conditioned gas as it moves toward the patient; and a non-occlusive cannula interface.

5.3 Humidification Devices

The humidifier can be a pass-over heated humidification system or a filter-type humidification system. HFNC delivers the gas through a heated humidifier incorporated into the distribution system, usually at flows of 60 L/min.

Vapotherm provides a filter-type humidification system and delivers gas at flows of up to 40 L/min. Humidification is produced by passing the mixed gas through a narrow tube bundle (similar to a fluid heater for IV fluids) with a pore size of 0.005. Compared to pass-over heated humidification systems, filter systems require a large evaporation surface. Humidification performance may vary depending on the patients, the inhaled tidal volume, and changes in the inspiratory flow [6]. The humidification performance of pass-over and filter-type humidification devices is sufficient.

5.4 Flow Generator

There are three types of flow generators in HFNC system: air-oxygen blender devices, built-in flow generators (turbines), and entrainment systems (Venturi systems).

Air-oxygen mixers with flow meters titrate the oxygen concentration according to the amount of medical gas inhaled. It ensures stable transmission of FiO_2 and gas flow (Bird blender) and air-oxygen blender. It is the most popular.

Precision flow generators often use turbines and entrain room air to create high flow. High flow can also be created in the absence of air and high pressure oxygen wall sources. Precision flow generators are incorporated into devices manufactured by Fisher & Paykel Healthcare and Vapotherm.

When higher concentrations are necessary, a MaxVenturi generates high flow through using an air entrainment system: when equipped with a flow meter, it also titrates oxygen concentration.

In a number of critical care ventilators, an HFNC capability is integral to the machine. The ventilator allows control of FiO_2 and flow while using the heated humidifier commonly connected to the ventilator.

The Airvo 2 is an HFNC device that can deliver humidified gas with adjustable temperature (31, 34, or 37 °C) and gas flow (up to 60 L/min). It has a humidifier chamber standing on a plate heater, a digital console (gas flow and temperature control), and a breathing circuit with a double spiral heating element. Supplemental oxygen can be blended into the circuit and regulated through an external flow meter, while a built-in ultrasonic oxygen sensor analyzes the fraction of inspired oxygen (FiO_2).

The Precision Flow is a fully integrated device that uses a disposable high-efficiency hollow-fiber cartridge humidification system. Gas transits through the lumen of the hollow fibers, while heated water vapor is forced through its small particle (0.005 µm) pores. An intuitive single button interface controls gas temperature (33–43 °C, adjustable in 1 °C increments), FiO_2 (0.21–1, adjustable in 0.01 increments), and gas flow (1–40 L/min).

5.5 Inspiratory Limb

Inspiratory circuits with heated wires have been developed to minimize condensation in the inspiratory circuit in heated humidifiers. The electric current supplied to regulate the thermal output of the heating wire is servo controlled. Heating wire placement may differ depending on the manufacturer.

The AirSpiral (Fisher & Paykel) breathing tube uses heating wires embedded in the circuit wall to keep wall temperature high enough to avoid condensation.

In Vapotherm, instead of using a heating wire inside the circuit, warm water flows between the inner and outer lumens of the tubes where the medical gas is supplied. With this system, the amount of condensation in the inspiratory circuit is reduced.

5.6 Interface

HFNC nasal prongs are generally soft and pliable. In the Optiflow system (Fisher & Paykel), the nasal prongs and tubing between the nasal prong and inspiratory circuit are both large bore, and the flow to the prongs is delivered from one side only.

The high-velocity nasal insufflation system (Vapotherm) uses a slender nasal cannula similar in appearance to a regular nasal oxygen cannula. Both the internal diameter and nasal prong bore are narrow, and this results in high flow out of the nasal prongs. Moreover, via two connecting tubes, Hi-VNI delivers flow to each prong from either side.

5.7 Clinical Implications

The HFNC is a noninvasive respiratory support device used to provide a continuous humidified high oxygen flow (up to 60–80 L/min) at adjustable FiO_2 (21–100%) and temperature (31–37 °C). In this system, the gas flow is delivered through a cannula interface that does not obstruct the "open" system nostrils. The high flow of heated and humidified gas has a number of physiological effects.

5.7.1 Nasopharyngeal Dead Space Washout

The main mechanism of action of HFNC is through clearance of the nasopharyngeal anatomical dead space. During normal breathing, carbon dioxide-rich gas is present in the nasopharyngeal anatomical dead space at the end of the exhalation and is rebreathed during the respiratory cycle. This gas is rebreathed during the breathing cycle. Using the HFNC system clears CO_2 from the nasopharynx, reduces the inspired CO_2 fraction, and increases FiO_2 [7]. It allows the nasopharyngeal anatomical dead space to be used as a fresh gas reservoir. This results in a reduction in work of breathing and respiratory rate without reducing alveolar ventilation. Decreased dead space can result in increased alveolar ventilation. Spence et al. demonstrated that the flow pattern of gas in the nasopharynx was significantly altered by HFNC [8].

5.7.2 Mucociliary Clearance

The nasopharynx has a large surface area that provides humidification and heating of the inhaled gas. In addition, one of the important defense mechanisms against pathogens in the respiratory tract is the mucociliary transport mechanism. Moisture loss in this defense system can lead to serious problems. It is known that dry and cold gases given in the hospital environment have various adverse effects such as mucociliary dysfunction, decrease in patient tolerance, and increase in airway resistance. Maintaining optimum humidity with the HFNC system can prevent the airways from drying out, maintain the mucociliary transport system's function, and reduce the risk of respiratory tract infections [9]. Giving the humidified gas prevents the upper respiratory tract from drying out, as well as helping to prevent the bronchoconstriction effect of cold and dry gas [10].

The supply of humidified gas with HFNC prevents insensible fluid loss and reduces metabolic workload [11]. The HFNC system was associated with greater overall comfort, lower dyspnea scores, and lower dry mouth than conventional systems [12].

5.7.3 Reduction of Nasopharyngeal Resistance

Nasopharynx and nasopharyngeal gas volume may be responsible for a resistance to gas flow. Shepard and Burger showed that the nasopharynx has a distensibility that contributes to variable resistance [13]. When inspiratory gas is drawn across this large surface area, retraction of the nasopharyngeal boundaries results in a significant increase in inspiratory resistance compared to expiratory resistance. The HFNC system provides nasopharyngeal gas flows that match or exceed the patient's peak inspiratory flow, potentially minimizing nasopharyngeal-related inspiratory resistance. It causes a decrease in respiratory resistance and rate.

5.7.4 Positive Expiratory Pressure (PEEP Effect)

In the HFNC system, the high flow from the nasal cannula provides resistance to expiratory flow and increases airway pressure. The mean airway pressure generated is approximately 1 cmH_2O/10 L/min of flow [14]. The effect of positive airway pressure provides a certain level of pulmonary distention pressure and alveolar recruitment [15]. It can increase the functional residual capacity, reduce atelectasis, and improve oxygenation. Airway pressure recorded with HFNC correlates linearly with applied flow rate, producing a median pressure of 7.4 cmH_2O at 60 L/min with the mouth closed [15]. With an increase in flow rates, inspiratory effort decreases, while alveolar ventilation (minute ventilation – dead space ventilation) remains stable, and minute ventilation decreases. However, with constant flow, a rise in mean airway pressure occurs and increases with flow rate [14, 16].

5.8 Conclusion

The HFNC system provides respiratory support through continuous flow of humidified air and titratable FiO_2. The gas humidified by the active humidifier is delivered to the patient through a heated circuit. High flows of sufficiently heated and humidified gas have a number of physiological effects. It cleans the nasopharyngeal dead space, provides positive expiratory pressure, and reduces airway resistance.

The HFNC system is easy to implement and use. The clinician controls three main variables: gas temperature, FiO_2, and flow rate. It is increasingly used in various clinical conditions of patients with acute hypoxemic respiratory failure.

References

1. Shelly MP, Nightingale P. ABC of intensive care: respiratory support. BMJ. 1999; 318(7199):1674–7.
2. Kallstrom TJ. American Association for Respiratory C (2002) AARC clinical practice guideline: oxygen therapy for adults in the acute care facility—2002 revision and update. Respir Care. 2002;47:717–20.
3. Chanques G, Constantin JM, Sauter M, et al. Discomfort associated with underhumidified high-flow oxygen therapy in critically ill patients. Intensive Care Med. 2009;35(6):996–1003.
4. L'Her E, Deye N, Lellouche F, et al. Physiologic effects of noninvasive ventilation during acute lung injury. Am J Respir Crit Care Med. 2005;172(9):1112–8.
5. Anderson NJ, Cassidy PE, Janssen LL, et al. Peak inspiratory flows of adults exercising at light, moderate and heavy workloads. J Int Soc Respir Prot. 2006;23:53–63.
6. Tobin MJ, Mador MJ, Guenther SM, et al. Variability of resting respiratory drive and timing in healthy subjects. J Appl Physiol (1985). 1988;65(1):309–17.
7. Spence CJT, Buchmann NA, Jermy MC. Unsteady flow in the nasal cavity with high flow therapy measured by stereoscopic PIV. Exp Fluids. 2011;52:569–79.
8. Spence CJT, Buchmann NA, Jermy MC, et al. Stereoscopic PIV measurement of flow in the nasal cavity with high flow therapy. Exp Fluids. 2010;50:1005–7.
9. Restrepo RD, Walsh BK. Humidification during invasive and noninvasive mechanical ventilation: 2012. Respir Care. 2012;57(5):782–8.
10. Richards GN, Cistulli PA, Ungar RG, et al. Mouth leak with nasal continuous positive airway pressure increases nasal airway resistance. Am J Respir Crit Care Med. 1996;154:182–6.
11. Dysart K, Miller TL, Wolfson MR, et al. Research in high flow therapy: mechanisms of action. Respir Med. 2009;103:1400–5.
12. Roca O, Riera J, Torres F, et al. High-flow oxygen therapy in acute respiratory failure. Respir Care. 2010;55(4):408–13.
13. Shepard JW Jr, Burger CD. Nasal and oral flow-volume loops in normal subjects and patients with obstructive sleep apnea. Am Rev Respir Dis. 1990;142:1288–93.
14. Parke RL, Bloch A, McGuinness SP. Effect of very-high-flow nasal therapy on airway pressure and end-expiratory lung impedance in healthy volunteers. Respir Care. 2015;60(10):1397–403.
15. Groves N, Tobin A. High flow nasal oxygen generates positive airway pressure in adult volunteers. Aust Crit Care. 2007;20(4):126–31.
16. Ritchie JE, Williams AB, Gerard C, et al. Evaluation of a humidified nasal high-flow oxygen system, using oxygraphy, capnography and measurement of upper airway pressures. Anaesth Intensive Care. 2011;39(6):1103–10.

Part III

Humidification and Noninvasive Ventilation

Humidification and Noninvasive Ventilation

6

Meryem Merve Hasimoglu

Abbreviations

AH	Absolute humidity
CPAP	Continuous positive airway pressure
FiO_2	Fractional inspired oxygen
HH	Heated humidifier
HME	Heat and moisture exchanger
IMV	Invasive mechanical ventilation
IPAP	Inspiratory positive airway pressure
nCPAP	Nasal continuous positive airway pressure.
NIV	Noninvasive ventilation
OSA	Obstructive sleep apnea
RH	Relative humidity
WOB	Work of breathing

6.1 Introduction

During normal respiration, the respiratory tract is responsible for conditioning of inhaled air. It entraps the particulate matter, heats and moisturizes the inspired gas, completely saturates it with water vapor, and transmits it to the alveoli at core temperature [1]. Since the upper airway is bypassed during invasive mechanical ventilation (IMV) , artificial humidification is accepted as standard of care [1]. Lack of

M. M. Hasimoglu (✉)
Department of Intensive Care Medicine, Gazi University, Ankara, Turkey

A. M. Esquinas (ed.), *Humidification in the Intensive Care Unit*,
https://doi.org/10.1007/978-3-031-23953-3_6

required heating and humidification in patients who received IMV is associated with numerous adverse outcomes, including hypothermia, alterations in respiratory tract structure and functioning, ciliary dyskinesia and epithelial desquamation, bronchospasm, mucus viscosity and inspissation, mucosal obstruction of the respiratory tract, increased incidence of respiratory infections, atelectasis, and endotracheal tube obstruction [1–3]. Most clinicians agree that heating and humidification during IMV are necessary [1].

There is no clear consensus on the necessity of routine humidification as the upper airway is not bypassed during noninvasive mechanical ventilation (NIV) ; and therefore, in many centers, humidification is not a routine procedure during NIV [2, 4, 5]. Nevertheless, active humidification is strongly recommended to improve patient comfort and compliance [2]. Inadequate humidification during NIV procedures is associated with decreased patient comfort and compliance, resulting in impaired respiratory tract structure and functioning, increased nasal resistance, secretion retention, difficult intubation, increased dead space, increased work of breathing (WOB) , and respiratory symptoms [5, 6]. Here, in this chapter, we are going to summarize the effects of insufficient gas conditioning during the NIV procedure, the factors associated with worsening of those effects, and the recommendations for artificial humidification based on available data.

6.2 Effects of Insufficient Gas Conditioning During the NIV Procedure

The cold and dry gas inhaled during the NIV procedure may cause dryness of the mouth, nose, and respiratory tract and increase airway resistance [7]. Nasal symptoms, including dryness, nasal congestion, rhinorrhea, and nosebleeds, are prevalent in patients who receive NIV [8, 9]. These side effects may lead to reduced patient comfort and compliance, ultimately resulting in NIV failure [6]. The NIV success rate may increase upon improvement or prevention of the above complications using correct humidification. Compared to spontaneous breathing, there was a significant decrease in the relative humidity (RH) of inspired air during NIV. A study on patients with obstructive sleep apnea (OSA) syndrome who received long-term nasal continuous positive airway pressure (nCPAP) and complained about nasal discomfort found that the use of nCPAP alone caused a significant decrease in the RH of the inspired air compared to spontaneous breathing. Furthermore, RH reached spontaneous respiratory levels upon the addition of heated humidity to the circuit [10]. A study on the nasal symptomatology in patients with OSA reported a significant decrease in upper respiratory tract symptoms upon application of heated humidification compared to placebo humidification and the continuous positive airway pressure (CPAP) procedure [8]. Patients with OSA who underwent CPAP with heated humidification reported fewer upper respiratory symptoms, felt more refreshed when they woke up in the morning, and were more compliant with their treatment [9].

The nasal mucosa secretes vasoactive amines and leukotrienes when exposed to cooling and drying. These mediators have the potential to cause nasal resistance by increasing both superficial mucosal blood flow and vascular congestion at deeper capacitance [11]. According to a study, nCPAP increased nasal resistance in healthy subjects, which could be significantly reduced by heated humidification [12]. Metaplastic changes and keratinization in the nasal epithelium and submucosa were reported in patients who received NIV at home for prolonged periods without adequate humidification [5]. A study on patients with OSA who were treated with CPAP due to nasal obstruction symptoms suggested that adding heated humidification to the circuit during the CPAP treatment reduced nasal resistance and the levels of nasal lavage inflammatory mediators. Histopathological examination revealed a significant decrease in inflammation and fibrosis of the nasal mucosa [8].

Insufficient humidification may be associated with mucosal drying, increased mucus viscosity, and retention of secretion, resulting in endotracheal intubation difficulty in the case of NIV failure [3, 7]. Life-threatening complications, including the obstruction of the upper airway by inspissated secretions, were also reported in cases of prolonged NIV [7]. Furthermore, obstruction of the airways by mucus may lead to a likely increase in the respiratory workload [2]. Oral flora may be altered due to dry mouth, thus increasing the risk of aspiration pneumonia [7].

6.3 Factors Contributing to Insufficient Gas Conditioning During NIV

Factors affecting the airway conditioning during NIV procedures include the type of ventilator, inspiratory positive airway pressure (IPAP), inspiratory flow, fractional inspired oxygen (FiO$_2$), air leaks, interface, temperature of the inhaled gas, and type of humidifier [5].

Ventilator type is an important factor because the intensive care unit ventilators that use dry medical gas directly from the hospital outlet have a lower humidity level than home ventilators that use compressed ambient air. A high initial IPAP reduces RH. High flow speeds may cause inadequate humidification even when certain humidifiers are in use, causing less contact of dry gas with the humidification process [5]. An increase in the expiratory positive airway pressure was also shown to be associated with lower absolute humidity (AH) levels [7]. It was also reported that the increased FiO$_2$ (especially at >60%) application was linked to a proportional reduction in the RH of the air due to the dehydrated composition of medical oxygen [5].

The one-third of the water transmitted during inspiration is regained during expiration by the nasal mucosa [10]. In patients who receive NIV, air leaks in the mouth and/or peripheral mask (around the mask) may cause unidirectional nasal airflow [10, 12]. Because of one-way air leakage, the mucosa regains less heat and moisture during expiration [5]. This may result in a continuous decrease in the AH of the air in the airways and progressive drying of the nasal mucosa [5, 10]. This could be due to the release of inflammatory mediators, increased mucosal blood flow, or increased nasal airway resistance [5]. Exposure of the nasal mucosa to cold and dry air is also associated with increased nasal resistance [11]. Increased nasal resistance may cause oral leaks due to mouth breathing, which creates a vicious circle. This cycle can be broken, and the patient's compatibility with NIV can be increased as the RH of the air is increased by humidification, leading to a reduced nasal resistance [4, 12]. During the nCPAP procedure in healthy subjects, oral leaks contributed to progressive dryness in the nasal mucosa and increased nasal resistance [10, 12]. It was reported that the relative reduction in the humidity of inhaled air could be significantly, albeit not completely, prevented by heating and humidification of the air, even in the presence of oral leaks [10]. It was also observed that the duration of oral leaks had shortened by 50%. The breakage of the vicious circle may account for the said improvement [10]. In healthy subjects who receive nCPAP, an increased nasal mucosal blood flow in the presence of oral leaks was observed. Furthermore, there was no change in nasal mucosal blood flow even in the presence of oral leaks when heated moisturization accompanied the nCPAP procedure [11]. In addition, air leaks would affect the performance of heat and moisture exchangers (HMEs) as there would be less moisture and heat recovery during expirium due to air leaks [2, 5].

Several interfaces can be used during the NIV procedure for the patients. Many interfaces have been developed to improve the NIV's success rates. Facemask use is associated with a more suitable airway moisture gradient by preserving the saturated gas that returns during expiration. CPAP treatment with a facemask prevented RH decrease in the inhaled air in patients with OSAS when compared to the ones who received nCPAP [10]. The large interior space inside the helmet masks can serve as a "mixing room," where humidity in the expired air humidifies the dry medical gases, thereby eliminating the need for active humidification. Application of NIV with helmet masks allowed adequate conditioning of the inhaled gas, optimized comfort, and improved patient–ventilator interaction without additional humidification in patients with hypoxemic respiratory failure. Due to an excessive increase in heat and humidity, adding heated humidifiers (HHs) or HMEs to the circuit was associated with more intense dyspnea [13]. An unacceptable decrease in AH and RH levels may occur, and additional humidification should be considered when high FiO_2 (>50%) and high flow rates (up to 80 L/min) are applied during the transmission of NIV by a helmet [6].

6.4   Types of Humidifiers

Active humidification via heated humidifiers and passive humidification via heat and moisture exchangers can be used to heat and humidify gases administered to ventilated patients [2]. As HME is inexpensive and easier to apply, it is widely used in invasively ventilated patients. Significant disadvantages were reported regarding HME compared to HH in the NIV setting [5]. Compared to HH, HME use in NIV was associated with a substantial increase in dead space and higher $PaCO_2$ values. An increase in the dead space reduces the alveolar ventilation in terms of ventilation per minute. Ventilation per minute is increased by increasing the respiratory rate as there can be no meaningful change in the tidal volume under constant pressure support to overcome decreasing alveolar ventilation. HME may also lead to a significant increase in $PaCO_2$ despite the increase in ventilation per minute [14]. Alveolar ventilation can only be maintained at the expense of greater WOB with HME compared to a heated humidifier [2]. The aforementioned effects of humidifiers on physiological parameters and respiratory mechanics should be considered in the use of NIV, although the aim of NIV use is to increase the alveolar ventilation and relieve the patient's respiratory workload. A long-term (12-month) randomized cross-pilot study in patients with chronic hypercarbic respiratory failure who received NIV reported that HHs and HMEs were associated with similar tolerance, airway symptoms (excluding dry throat), and side effects. Nevertheless, the number of patients who chose to continue with HHs for home use was higher at the end of the study [6].

In HMEs, heat and humidity are captured when the patient exhales and are given back to the patient in the next inspirium. These devices may provide up to 30–32 mgH_2O/L AH at 27–30 °C under optimum conditions. The ambient temperature, inspiratory and expiratory flow rates, surface area of the medium, and water vapor content affect its performance since no active energy is used in the system. A study that investigated the performance of many HMEs in adults indicated that, similar to previous studies, a number of HMEs were inadequate for the humidification task [3].

The accumulation of condensate in the tubes during humidification and the subsequent colonization thereof with microorganisms are important risk factors for ventilator-associated pneumonia. By retaining heat and moisture during the expirium, HMEs reduce the accumulation of condensate and bacterial colonization in the circuit. HMEs also feature bacterial and/or viral filtration capacities [15]. Cross-infection may especially limit the use of HH. HHs may be associated with the risk of spreading respiratory viral infections (severe acute respiratory syndrome (SARS), H1N1) or aerosols of *Mycobacterium tuberculosis*. A potential risk of colonization and infection was identified in patients with OSA due to prolonged NIV use at home [4].

6.5 Humidifier Settings During Noninvasive Ventilation

There is no clear consensus regarding humidification use during NIV, humidification settings in acute and chronic uses, timing, and the type of humidifier [5]. Humidification requirements, patient characteristics, the type of mechanical ventilator and the interface, and the mechanical ventilator settings in use should be taken into consideration and personalized for the patients. There is no clear recommendation concerning the extent of humidification and its settings during NIV [7]. It was reported that exposure to 25 mgH_2O/L for 1 h or <30 mgH_2O/L for ≥24 h was associated with mucosal dysfunction [2]. It should be noted that an AH level of <5 mgH_2O/L is the "critical" threshold for the likelihood of complications associated with inadequate gas conditioning of the inhaled air [5]. The American

Association for Respiratory Care recommends that the AH level of inhaled gas in invasive patients should be >30 mg/L, whereas the International Organization for Standardization recommends >33 mg/L [2].

6.6 Conclusion

Humidification during NIV should be considered, particularly in patients associated with inadequate conditioning of inhaled air and in symptomatic patients. NIV accompanied by humidification may increase patient compliance and comfort, thus ensuring more effective treatment. NIV success rates can also be increased; thereby, patients can be protected from the extra complications of IMV.

> **Key Major Recommendations**
>
> Humidification during NIV primarily can prevent patient's respiratory symptoms and might improve patient compliance, comfort, and adherence. This in turn can increase NIV success.
>
> The use of humidification in NIV should be considered, particularly in patients with risk factors for inadequate conditioning of inspired air (e.g., dry gas inhalation by ICU ventilators; high IPAP, inspiratory flow, or FiO_2; mouth leaks; nasal mask use) and who are symptomatic.
>
> Although the disadvantages of HME such as increasing dead space and WOB, CO_2 retention, and increased nasal airway resistance during NIV have been shown compared to HH, there are not enough data to support one humidification system over the other.
>
> Humidification requirements, patient characteristics, the type of mechanical ventilator and the interface, and the mechanical ventilator settings in use should be taken into consideration and personalized for the patients.

References

1. Branson RD, Gentile MA. Is humidification always necessary during noninvasive ventilation in the hospital? Respir Care. 2010;55(2):209–16.
2. Restrepo RD, Walsh BK. Humidification during invasive and noninvasive mechanical ventilation: 2012. Respir Care. 2012;57(5):782–8. https://doi.org/10.4187/respcare.01766.
3. Gross J, Park G. Humidification of inspired gases during mechanical ventilation. Minerva Anestesiol. 2012;78(4):496–502.
4. Esquinas AM, Al-Jawder SE, BaHammam AS. Practice of Humidification During Noninvasive Mechanical Ventilation (NIV): Determinants of Humidification Strategies. Humid Intensive Care Unit. 2012:93–102.

5. Esquinas Rodriguez AM, Scala R, Soroksky A, BaHammam A, de Klerk A, Valipour A, et al. Clinical review: humidifiers during non-invasive ventilation - key topics and practical implications. Crit Care. 2012;16(1):203. https://doi.org/10.1186/cc10534.

6. Ozsancak AU, Esquinas AM. Humidification for noninvasive ventilation: key technical determinants and clinical evidence. In: Esquinas AM, editor. Noninvasive mechanical ventilation: theory, equipment, and clinical applications. Cham: Springer International Publishing; 2016. p. 183–90.

7. Oto J, Imanaka H, Nishimura M. Clinical factors affecting inspired gas humidification and oral dryness during noninvasive ventilation. J Crit Care. 2011;26(5):535. e9-e15

8. Koutsourelakis I, Vagiakis E, Perraki E, Karatza M, Magkou C, Kopaka M, et al. Nasal inflammation in sleep apnoea patients using CPAP and effect of heated humidification. Eur Respir J. 2011;37(3):587–94. https://doi.org/10.1183/09031936.00036910.

9. Massie CA, Hart RW, Peralez K, Richards GN. Effects of humidification on nasal symptoms and compliance in sleep apnea patients using continuous positive airway pressure. Chest. 1999;116(2):403–8. https://doi.org/10.1378/chest.116.2.403.

10. Martins de Araújo MT, Vieira SB, Vasquez EC, Fleury B. Heated humidification or face mask to prevent upper airway dryness during continuous positive airway pressure therapy. Chest. 2000;117(1):142–7. https://doi.org/10.1378/chest.117.1.142.

11. Hayes MJ, McGregor FB, Roberts DN, Schroter RC, Pride NB. Continuous nasal positive airway pressure with a mouth leak: effect on nasal mucosal blood flux and nasal geometry. Thorax. 1995;50(11):1179–82.

12. Richards GN, Cistulli PA, Ungar R, Berthon-Jones M, Sullivan CE. Mouth leak with nasal continuous positive airway pressure increases nasal airway resistance. Am J Respir Crit Care Med. 1996;154(1):182–6.

13. Bongiovanni F, Grieco DL, Anzellotti GM, Menga LS, Michi T, Cesarano M, et al. Gas conditioning during helmet noninvasive ventilation: effect on comfort, gas exchange, inspiratory effort, transpulmonary pressure and patient–ventilator interaction. Ann Intensive Care. 2021;11(1):1–12.

14. Jaber S, Chanques G, Matecki S, Ramonatxo M, Souche B, Perrigault P-F, et al. Comparison of the effects of heat and moisture exchangers and heated humidifiers on ventilation and gas exchange during non-invasive ventilation. Intensive Care Med. 2002;28(11):1590–4.

15. Alp E, Voss A. Ventilator associated pneumonia and infection control. Ann Clin Microbiol Antimicrob. 2006;5(1):1–11.

Humidification in Mechanically Ventilated Patients and Selection of Devices

Carvalho Catarina and Carvalho João

7.1   Introduction

Humidification during invasive mechanical ventilation is currently accepted as a standard of care. Under normal conditions, the upper airway and respiratory tract are responsible for humidifying and heating inspired air [1]. The connective tissue of the nose is characterized by a rich vascular system which is responsible for warming the inspired air. As the inspired air goes down the respiratory tract, it reaches a point at which its temperature is 37 °C and is fully saturated with 44 mgH$_2$O/L, with a relative humidity of 100%, usually located 5 cm below the carina [2, 3].

Humidity is the amount of water vapor contained in a gas and is generally characterized in terms of absolute (AH) or relative humidity (RH) . AH corresponds to the total amount of water vapor contained in a gas, expressed in milligrams of water suspended in liters of gas (mg/L), and the RH is the percentage (%) of water vapor contained in a gas relative to its maximum carrying capacity [1, 2].

Humidifiers are devices that add molecules of water to gas, and this can be done through a process of active humidification, using a heated humidifier (HH) , or passive humidification, through a heat and moisture exchanger (HME) . It is still unknown which is most beneficial, and one reason for that lies on the fact that the optimal levels of humidity and temperature are also unknown. The ideal humidifier should provide optimal temperature and humidification with minimal risk of adverse events and be simple to use and inexpensive [2].

C. Catarina (✉) · C. João
Department of Intensive Care, Centro Hospitalar de Trás-os-Montes e Alto Douro,
Vila Real, Portugal

A. M. Esquinas (ed.), *Humidification in the Intensive Care Unit*,
https://doi.org/10.1007/978-3-031-23953-3_7

7.2   Effects of Inadequate Humidification

After endotracheal intubation, as the upper airway is bypassed, it loses its capacity to heat and moisture the inhaled gas, which imposes a burden to the lower respiratory tract, as it is not prepared to do this kind of process. Consequently, the delivery of partially cold and dry medical gases leads to potential damage to the respiratory epithelium, manifested by thick and dehydrated secretions, atelectasis, cough, bronchospasm, and increased work of breathing [3].

Currently, there are no criteria for over-humidification. In some reports, it has been suggested that over-humidification occurs when the delivered inspired gas is above BTPS body temperature and pressure satured is a physical condition, wich presumes the combined environmental circunstances --> warmed to 37° C and fully satured with water vapor (=100 % relative humidity). Over-humidification reduces mucus viscosity, increases the periciliary layer, dilutes surfactant, and causes neutrophilic infiltration of lungs and bronchioles. Delivering inspired over-humidification gas may cause water to condense on the walls of the breathing circuit resulting in increased airflow resistance [2].

7.3   Passive Humidification

HMEs operate passively by storing heat and moisture from the patient's exhaled gas and releasing it to the inhaled gas. There are three types of HME, also recognized as artificial noses: hydrophobic, hygroscopic, and a filtered HME [4]. These humidifiers are composed of material of high thermal capacity and conductivity that is arranged in a spun and pleated fashion to allow gas to cool and condense on expiration and warm and evaporate on inspiration. HMEs are placed between the patient and the Y connector of the inspiratory and expiratory limbs. The main advantages of these systems are their simplicity and low cost. However, they are contraindicated in patients with thick or copious secretions and when there is loss in expired tidal volume (e.g., large bronchopleurocutaneous fistulas, presence of endotracheal tube cuff leak, in difficult to wean patients and those with limited respiratory reserve, and in hypothermic patients with body temperature of <32 °C), because they contribute to additional dead space, increasing the ventilation requirements and arterial partial pressure of carbon dioxide [3, 4].

When providing passive humidification to patients under invasive mechanical ventilation, the HME should provide a minimum humidity level of 30 mgH$_2$O/L, but their ultimate performance is dependent on certain factors such as ambiance temperature, inspiratory and expiratory flow rates, surface area, and water vapor content of the medium [2].

7.4   Hydrophobic HMEs

In hydrophobic HMEs, the condenser is made of water-repelling element, with low thermal conductivity, that maintains higher temperature gradients than in the case of hygroscopic HMEs. This type of devices causes more narrowing in endotracheal tube diameter compared to hygroscopic ones, which is one of the reasons why it is less used [3].

7.5   Hygroscopic HMEs

They have only the hygroscopic compartment. During exhalation, vapor condenses in the element (synthetic fiber), as well as in the hygroscopic salts (calcium or lithium chloride). These salts have a chemical affinity to attract water particles and thus increase the humidification capacity of the HME. During inspiration, water vapor is obtained from the salts, reaching an absolute humidity ranging between 22 and 24 mgH$_2$O/L. It is possible to combine hydrophobic with hygroscopic HMEs, adding a hygroscopic salt inside the hydrophobic HME. The synthetic fiber also helps to decrease the accumulation of condensation in a device-dependent position [1, 7].

7.6   Pleated or Electrostatic Filters

Filters can be added to either hydrophobic or hygroscopic HMEs resulting in a heat and moisture exchanger filter (HMEF). These filters operate based on the predominant incorporated mechanism—electrostatic or pleated filters.

The pleated filters (PF): have more dense fibers and less electrostatic charges. PF function better as barriers to bacterial and viral pathogens than electrostatic filters. However, they confer higher airflow resistance and have a small impact on the humidification process [3].

The electrostatic filters: have more electrostatic charges and less dense fibers [3].

7.7   Active Humidification

Heated humidifiers (HHs) have traditionally been the gold standard in providing humidification, as they theoretically deliver gas temperature of 33 ± 2 °C with an AH of 44 mgH$_2$O/L and RH 100%. Nonetheless, its use in clinical practice may only deliver AH levels between 35 and 40 mgH$_2$O/L. They have a heating element, which warms up the water inside a chamber—dry gas flows through this compartment, over the hot liquid surface, or through the bubbled water to become humidified. The chamber temperature is thermostatically controlled. The water level in the humidification chamber can be maintained manually or by using an automatic feeding system, with an integrated float valve inside the water chamber, which regulates and maintains a constant level of water. Automatic methods eliminate the risk of contamination and overfilling. HHs are more efficient in providing humidification when compared to HMEs, but the risks and costs are greater. Risks include overheating, causing inhalation burns, and the possibility of water condensing within the inspiratory limb of ventilator tubing, which may lead to bacterial colonization [2, 3].

HHs have distinctive designs and different techniques for humidification. Accordingly, these devices are classified as bubble (BH), pass-over (POH), and counter-flow humidifiers (CFH) [2, 3].

7.8 Bubble Humidifiers

In bubble humidifiers (BH) , the gas is forced down a tube into the bottom of a water container. The gas escapes from the distal end of the tube, under the water surface, forming bubbles, which gain humidity as they rise to the surface. These humidifiers generally use diffusers to increase the liquid-air interface. A problem with BH is that they exhibit high resistance to airflow, imposing higher work of breathing than in POH. The use of BH during mechanical ventilation has fallen in favor of pass-over humidifiers [3].

7.9 Pass-Over Humidifiers

In pass-over humidifiers (POH) , the gas passes over a heated water reservoir carrying water vapor to the patient. It is important to consider that the water temperature in the enclosure will be a determining factor for humidity. In comparison to the previously described device, POH have lower resistance [1].

7.10 Counter-Flow Humidifiers

In the counter-flow humidifiers (CFH) , the water is heated outside the vaporizer and then is pumped to the top of the humidifier, through small-diameter pores, and runs down a large surface area—gas flows in counter direction. During its passage through the humidification chamber, the air is moisturized and warmed up to the body temperature. The performance of the CFH is independent of the flow and respiratory rate, and for this reason, it imposes less work of breathing compared to the other devices [3, 4].

7.11 Monitoring on Humidification Systems

As stated by the American Association for Respiratory Care (AARC) guidelines, HH should provide an absolute humidity level between 33 and 44 mgH$_2$O/L and an inspiratory gas temperature between 34 °C and 41 °C (measured at the Y-piece). Regarding HMEs, these should provide a minimum of 30 mgH$_2$O/L of absolute humidity, 100% of relative humidity, and 34 °C of temperature [3].

The most reliable method to measure humidity is by using a hygrometer-thermometer system; however, the most used is the clinical evaluation of certain parameters such as respiratory secretion characteristics, requirement for saline instillation to fluidize them, and visual inspection of condensate in the tubing system. In general, the volume of secretions is directly proportional to the degree of humidification – excessive humidification will increase their volume, and suboptimal humidification will lead to thick secretions and a decrease in their volume [3].

The humidification performance is an area of evolving research. Most manufacturers recommend changing HMEs every 24 or 48 h to secure adequate AH levels and mean airway pressures. Despite this, regular inspections should be made, and HMEs must always be replaced if there are secretions contaminating the insert or the filter or if the flow resistance has increased, causing an increase in the work of breathing [3]. When using an active humidifier, the following parameters should be frequently monitored: water and temperature level (the low temperature should be set no lower than 2 °C below the desired temperature at the circuit Y-piece) and the presence of condensation [1].

7.12 Selecting the Appropriate Humidifier

The selection of the appropriate humidifier system should have in consideration the different clinical scenario of each patient since each device features properties that can affect their clinical situation.

HMEs are easy to use and lighter than HHs; therefore, they facilitate transportation of mechanically ventilated patients and do not carry the same thermal hazards. One major disadvantage of this system is that they confer worst humidity levels when compared to HHs. When considering its use, there are some contraindications that must be analyzed, namely, hemoptysis, thick or copious secretions, and patients who present an expired tidal volume less than 70% of the inspired volume (e.g., large bronchopleurocutaneous fistulas, tracheal tube cuff malfunction, or presence of uncuffed endotracheal tube). The use of an HME is also contraindicated for patients with body temperature less than 32 °C and dehydration of the airway if temperature is set to body temperature, yet the RH is low [5, 6].

When providing humidification to patients with low tidal volumes, such as when lung-protective ventilation strategies are used, HMEs are not recommended because they contribute additional dead space (PaCO$_2$), which can increase the ventilation requirements: increased minute ventilation, ventilatory drive, and work of breathing. $PaCO_2$ and minute ventilation were found to be higher with HMEs suggesting that HHs could be better options in patients with limited respiratory reserve [8, 9].

HHs are preferred when long-term ventilation is sought, in patients with viscid secretions or in those who exhibit contraindications for HME. This system has demonstrated better gas humidification than the HMEs, but they have some drawbacks, such as cost, condensation of water vapor in the ventilatory circuit and reservoir, need for a power supply and a constant water feeding system (with risk of an airway thermal injury), and patient-ventilator asynchrony, due to pooled condensation in the circuit. A characteristic disadvantage of HHs is the condensate formation in the circuit—although some earlier studies reported an increased risk of nosocomial infections, recent meta-analyses revealed that there is no significant difference regarding the incidence of ventilator-associated pneumonia in patients humidified with HMEs versus HHs [3, 8, 9].

7.13 Conclusion

Airway humidification represents a key intervention in mechanically ventilated patients. Inappropriate selection of devices or humidifier settings may negatively impact on clinical outcomes by damaging airway mucosa, increasing work of breathing, and prolonging mechanical ventilation. Humidification devices may function passively or actively, depending on the source of the heat and humidity. According to the clinical scenario, humidifier selection may change over time; therefore, knowledge of the technical specifications and the advantages and disadvantages of each type of system is crucial for professionals who provide care to patients in the intensive care unit.

Finally, there is little evidence demonstrating advantage of one humidifying system over the other, even in what preventing mortality and other complications is concerned [2].

References

1. Plotnikow GA, Accoce M, Navarro E, Tiribelli N. Humidification and heating of inhaled gas in Patients with artificial airway. A narrative review. Rev Bras Ter Intensiva. 2018;30(1):86–97. https://doi.org/10.5935/0103-507X.20180015.6.
2. Gross JL, Park GR. Humidification of inspired gases during mechanical ventilation. Minerva Anestesiol. 2012;78:496–502.
3. Al Ashry HS, Modrykamien AM. Humidification during mechanical ventilation in the adult patient. Biomed Res Int. 2014;2014:715434. https://doi.org/10.1155/2014/715434.2.
4. Priebe H, Guttmann J. Moisturizing and mechanical characteristics of a new counter-flow type heated humidifier. Br J Anaesth. 2007;98(4):531–8. https://doi.org/10.1093/bja/aem006.32.

5. Lellouche F, Qader S, Taille S, et al. Under-humidification and over-humidification during moderate induced hypothermia with usual devices. Intensive Care Med. 2006;32:1014–21. https://doi.org/10.1007/s00134-006-0192-8.
6. Sottiaux TM. Consequences of under- and over-humidification. Respir Care Clin N Am. 2006;12(2):233–52. https://doi.org/10.1016/j.rcc.2006.03.010.
7. Branson RD, Davis K Jr, Campbell RS, Johnson DJ, Porembka DT. Humidification in the intensive care unit. Prospective study of a new protocol utilizing heated humidification and a hygroscopic condenser humidifier. Chest. 1993;104(6):1800–5. https://doi.org/10.1378/chest.104.6.1800.
8. Nava S, Cirio S, Fanfulla F, Carlucci A, Navarra A, Negri A, Ceriana P. Comparison of two humidification systems for long-term noninvasive mechanical ventilation. Eur Respir J. 2008;32(2):460–4. https://doi.org/10.1183/09031936.00000208.
9. American Association for Respiratory Care, Restrepo RD, Walsh BK. AARC clinical practice guideline humidification during invasive and noninvasive mechanical ventilation: 2012. Respir Care. 2012;57:782–8. https://doi.org/10.4187/respcare.01766.

Impact of Humidification Strategy During Lung (and Heart)-Protective Ventilation

8

François Lellouche

8.1 Lung-Protective Ventilation Is Not Only Tidal Volume Reduction

Lung-protective ventilation (LPV) strategies refer to the ventilator settings that allow a protection of the lungs from injuries related to high volumes and consequently high alveolar and transpulmonary pressures that occur during invasive mechanical ventilation [1]. Lung-protective ventilation proved benefits on mortality and is recommended in ARDS patients [2–5] and in patients without ARDS [6–8]. The first component of LPV is the reduction of the tidal volume, but this is not the only parameter involved in LPV. There are other important ventilator settings to consider as well as airway management to optimize.

To ensure adequate carbon dioxide removal, the reduction in tidal volume should be associated with increasing of the respiratory rate. The tidal volumes have progressively been decreased over time in the operating room and in critically ill patients [9]. Similarly, respiratory rates have been progressively increased, up to 30–35 breath/min in most severe patients [10], and low or very low tidal volumes (below 6 ml/kg PBW) must be associated with high or very high respiratory rates (25 breaths/min or even higher) (Fig. 8.1). In those situations, the impact of dead space on CO_2 removal is critical [10].

FiO_2 and positive end-expiratory pressure (PEEP) settings are mainly focusing on oxygenation control but may also have an impact on CO_2 removal. High PEEP levels and low compliance may lead to alveolar distention and alveolar capillaries compression that may be responsible for an increase in alveolar dead space, a

F. Lellouche (✉)
Centre de recherche de l'Institut Universitaire de Cardiologie et de Pneumologie de Québec, Département d'Anesthésiologie et de Soins Intensifs. Faculté de médecine, Université Laval, Québec, Canada
e-mail: francois.lellouche@criucpq.ulaval.ca

A. M. Esquinas (ed.), *Humidification in the Intensive Care Unit*, https://doi.org/10.1007/978-3-031-23953-3_8

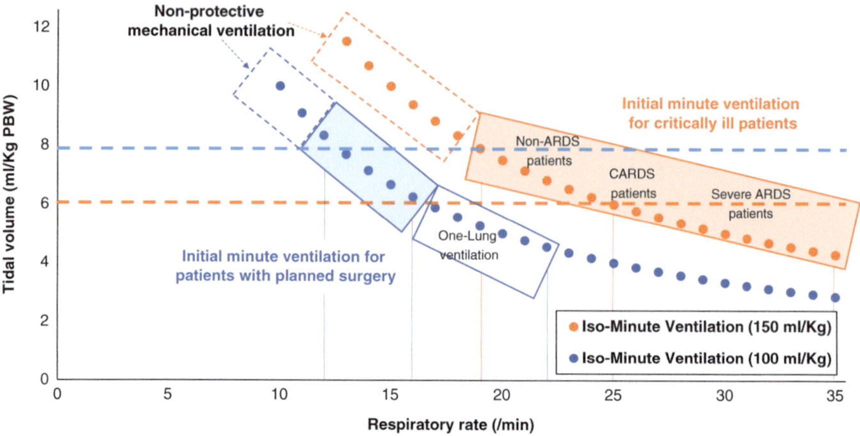

Fig. 8.1 This figure is a schematic representation of the findings based on the analysis of more than 30 studies providing respiratory rate and tidal volumes in different settings (intensive care units and operating room) for more than 40,000 patients [10]. Usual respiratory rates and tidal volumes are represented for surgical patients (planned surgery and one-lung surgery with protective ventilation) and critically ill patients (non-ARDS, ARDS with protective and ultra-protective ventilation and CARDS (COVID-19 ARDS) patients). The targeted minute ventilations are very different as well as the tidal volume and respiratory rate based on the category of patients. **In the operating room for planned surgery,** the patient's metabolism is usually low, and the body temperature is frequently below or equal to 36 °C. The CO_2 production is therefore low, and minute ventilation around 100 ml/kg/min PBW as shown by Radford in 1955 and used for a long time, is still adequate [10, 44, 67]. In addition, the recommended target tidal volume has progressively been reduced and is now around 8 ml/kg PBW or below; consequently, respiratory rate should be set between 12 and 16 breaths/min. In patients with one-lung ventilation (targeted tidal volume 4–6 ml/kg PBW), the respiratory rate should be set between 16 and 22 breaths/min. **In critically ill patients**, the metabolism is high and body temperature may be elevated. The CO_2 production is high, the dead space is high (including instrumental dead space), and ventilation needs to allow CO_2 elimination are higher than normal. In our study, we showed that in mechanically ventilated patients in ICU, minute ventilation was around 150 ml/kg/min PBW (25 studies conducted in ICUs) [10]. The respiratory rate must be frequently set above 20 breaths/min in critically ill patients. It is logical to use high respiratory rate after intubation of septic patients (with pneumonia or other cause of SIRS) breathing above 30/min before intubation. Some patients are ventilated after intubation with both reduced tidal volume and low respiratory rates (15 or below), which can result in severe acidosis

marker of ARDS severity [11, 12]. High FiO_2, when associated with hyperoxaemia, will be responsible for the Haldane effect, the reduction in haemoglobin affinity for CO_2 leading to increased $PaCO_2$ [13]. PEEP and FiO_2 settings are part of LPV and may have a role to explain severe hypercapnia during LPV but will not be discussed here.

The other frequently overlooked parameter involved in the CO_2 control is the total dead space that is part of the formula of the alveolar ventilation (Valv) that

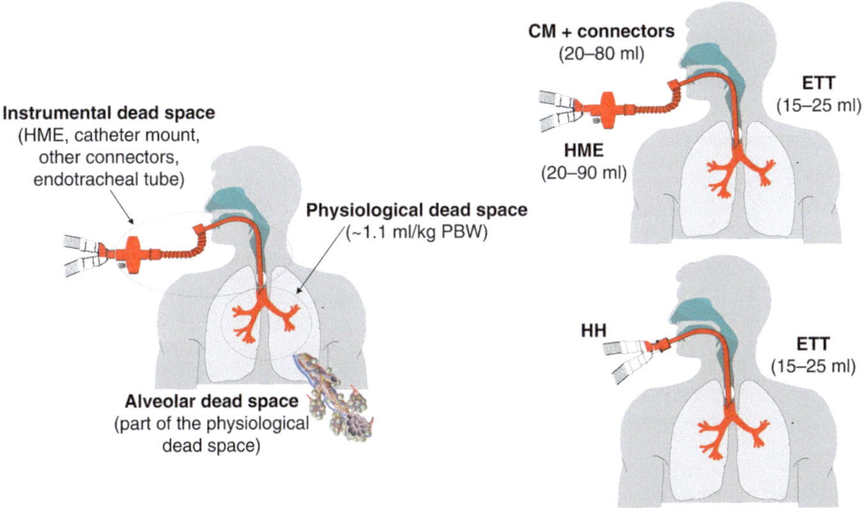

Fig. 8.2 Different portions of the dead space in the intubated patient. Dead space may be divided into instrumental dead space and physiological dead space (including airway and alveolar dead space). Part of the instrumental dead space may be easily limited by reducing the number of useless connections and by using a heated humidifier instead of a heat and moisture exchanger (HME) for gas humidification. Part of the instrumental dead space is not easily reduced: the endotracheal tube (ETT) may be changed for a tracheostomy tube to reduce the dead space by 10–12 ml, or ETT may be cut but the gain is very limited (2–4 ml)

reflects the part of the effective ventilation for CO_2 clearance. Noteworthy, dead space is frequently described as physiological and alveolar dead space, and instrumental dead space is usually neglected [14, 15], while it may represent the main dead space volume [16, 17].

The different parts of the total dead space (alveolar dead space, anatomic dead space and instrumental dead space) must be known to optimize mechanical ventilation during lung-protective ventilation (Fig. 8.2) [18]. This is particularly true in most severe patients when tidal volumes are low or very low and respiratory rate is high (Fig. 8.1). Consequently, the humidification strategy is critical through the limitation of instrumental dead space that is mainly related to connectors after the Y-piece and frequently to heat and moisture exchangers [18–20]. The current management in most ICU patients with or without ARDS must include lung-protective ventilation and should also incorporate heart-protective ventilation with optimization of CO_2 removal (Fig. 8.3).

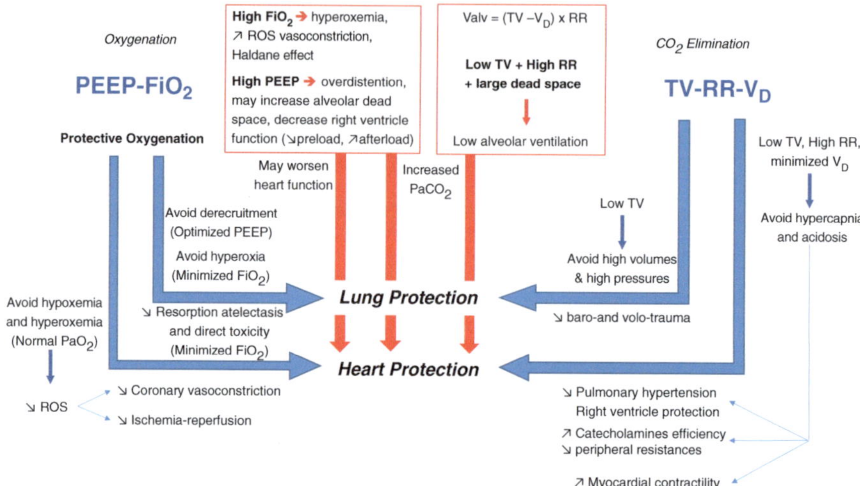

Fig. 8.3 Concept of heart- and lung-protective mechanical ventilation. Respiratory parameters to manage oxygenation (PEEP, FiO₂) and the parameters involved in carbon dioxide clearance (tidal volume (TV), respiratory rate (RR) and total dead space (VD)) may all have an impact both on lung and heart protection by different mechanisms. *PEEP* positive end-expiratory pressure, *FiO₂* fraction of inspired oxygen, *TV* tidal volume, *RR* respiratory rate, *VD* total dead space, *Valv* alveolar ventilation, *ROS* reactive oxygen species

8.2 From Lung-Protective Ventilation to Lung- and Heart-Protective Ventilation

The concept of heart-protective ventilation, and especially right ventricle-protective ventilation, is derived from an abundant literature that describes the impact of mechanical ventilation, acidosis and hypercapnia on heart function [21] (Fig. 8.3). There was a gradual shift from tolerance of severe acidosis associated with promotion of lung-protective ventilation and "permissive hypercapnia" to more cautious management and recommendations to avoid severe respiratory acidosis, especially in the case of right ventricular dysfunction.

While "permissive hypercapnia" has been the first name of lung-protective ventilation [22, 23], high levels of hypercapnia have been accepted and encouraged with associated respiratory or mixed acidosis in ICU patients [24]. In addition to the beneficial impact of reduced tidal volumes, hypercapnia could have additional benefits in experimental studies [25]. The questions regarding the haemodynamic impact of metabolic and respiratory acidosis have been debated for a long time [26–28]. Although hypercapnic acidosis reduces myocardial contractility and reduces the effect of epinephrine on contractility [26] and reduces systemic vascular resistance [29–31], the net impact of hypercapnia is an increase in cardiac output [28, 31] through sympatho-adrenal mechanisms. Oxygen delivery is further increased in hypercapnic acidosis as a result of a rightward shift in the oxyhaemoglobin dissociation curve [32].

However, recent data have highlighted the deleterious effects of excessively high $PaCO_2$ leading to increased arterial pulmonary hypertension [31, 33, 34], right ventricle failure and possibly increased mortality [31, 35–37]. Other unfavourable effects of hypercapnia have been described [15], and the current trend is to be more cautious with excessively high $PaCO_2$. "Too little of a good thing" [24] progressively shifted to "too much or too little of a good thing" [15], and it may be now discouraged to keep the $PaCO_2$ above 50 mmHg [35, 36]. There is a strong physiological rationale to avoid severe hypercapnia, leading to increased pulmonary hypertension, right ventricle dysfunction and peripheral vasodilatation [17, 21, 31]. However, the maximum $PaCO_2$ or minimum pH that may be tolerated is still debated. The values of 48 or 50 mmHg above which there is an increase in mortality came from observational studies that showed an association between severe hypercapnia with acidosis [35, 36, 38, 39] and mortality, but the direct causal effect remains unclear [40]. The severity of the acidosis and hypercapnia are certainly related in part to the severity of the patients.

In this regard, the negative impacts of hypocapnia are very well described [41], and the clinical impact may be at least as relevant [38, 42] and must be kept in mind when setting the ventilator. In conclusion, both severe hypocapnia and severe hypercapnia should be avoided. Therefore, optimized ventilator settings immediately after intubation and throughout the duration of invasive mechanical ventilation are required. For this, in addition to the reduced tidal volume, optimal settings of the respiratory rate, taking into account the dead space, must be put in place.

8.3 How to Set the Initial Respiratory Rate in Critically Ill Patients with Low or Very Low Tidal Volumes?

To ensure adequate CO_2 removal and to target moderately increased (below 50 mmHg) or normal $PaCO_2$, several actions are possible. The main ones are the increase in the respiratory rate and the minimization of the instrumental dead space [10].

It is easy to provide charts for the tidal volume based on gender and height and predicted body weight (PBW) to provide 6 or 8 ml/kg PBW to the patients. However, there are no clear recommendation and clues for the initial setting of the respiratory rate and therefore minute ventilation. This may be more a habit or intuitions and by experience: RR is set around 10 breaths/min in the operating room and around 20 breaths/min in newly intubated critically ill patients and sometimes increased to 25 or 30 in ARDS patients. A classical recommendation for minute ventilation is 100 ml/kg PBW/min (for instance, used to set the ASV mode [43] and recommended since 1955 [44]). However, in order to get a reasonable level of $PaCO_2$, 100 ml/kg PBW/min is not appropriate for most critically ill patients [10]. Ventilator settings in the operating room or in critically ill patients (in the emergency department and in the ICU) are very different, leading to minute ventilation around 100 ml/kg/min PBW in the operating room and at least 150 ml/kg/min PBW in critically ill patients. To reach 100 ml/kg PBW/min with 8 ml/kg PBW, a respiratory rate around

12 breaths/min should be used. In most severe patients, such as ARDS patients, a tidal volume of 6 ml/kg PBW associated with a respiratory rate of 25 breaths/min allows to get a minute ventilation of 150 ml/kg PBW/minute. These are two different worlds in terms of minute ventilation to match with patient's needs (Fig. 8.1). It should be noted that in case of high respiratory rate (greater than 20 breaths/min), the inspiratory flow must be kept high (greater than 40 l/min and up to 80 l/min) to promote low inspiratory time and sufficient expiratory time to avoid intrinsic PEEP [45].

Other measures to reduce $PaCO_2$ such as the use of an inspiratory pause have been proposed [46–48], but the effects are marginal compared to the increase in respiratory rate and the decrease in dead space and contradictory with the use of a high respiratory rate. The risk of an end-inspiratory pause prolonging the inspiratory time and reducing the expiratory time is to promote intrinsic PEEP in the case of high respiratory rate [45]. The utilization of ECMO or $ECCO_2R$ has been proposed to manage severe hypercapnia or to implement ultra-protective ventilation [49–52]. However, these complex and expensive techniques, associated with significant complications, should only be used if the simple measures described here (increase in respiratory rate and optimization of instrumental dead space) have been implemented [18, 53, 54].

In addition to the tidal volume and respiratory rate, the other major parameter to consider when initiating mechanical ventilation is the total dead space, including instrumental dead space. For this last parameter, the humidification strategy has a major impact.

8.4   What Is the Dead Space During Invasive Mechanical Ventilation?

The instrumental dead space is frequently overlooked during mechanical ventilation. Yet, many studies showed its large impact on the work of breathing during assisted ventilation [55–57] and on alveolar ventilation (CO_2 elimination) during controlled ventilation [16, 58–61]. Surprisingly, however, in many studies evaluating respiratory mechanics in ARDS or in COVID-19 patients, the instrumental dead space is not provided nor mentioned, even when V_D/V_T is evaluated.

The different parts of the dead space in mechanically ventilated patients are shown in Fig. 8.2. From the lungs to the Y-piece, this volume represents the "volume with CO_2 rebreathing" and the "wasted part of the respiration", which makes the gas exchanges less efficient [14, 62]. The alveolar dead space is the part of the lung that is ventilated but not perfused (capillary micro-thrombosis, capillary compression by overdistention), and it may be reduced by limiting overdistention; the dead space of the airways is difficult to modify and is mildly increased by PEEP and bronchodilation; the instrumental dead space is the easiest to modify and may account for almost half of the total dead space [16, 17]. The instrumental dead space includes the heat and moisture exchanger at the Y-piece, the CO_2 sensor, the connections, the catheter mount, the flex tube, etc. Using a heated humidifier instead of a heat and moisture exchanger is a very efficient way to reduce this dead space [16, 58–61]. This is recommended in the most recent guidelines to manage ARDS patients [5].

8.5 Impact of the Instrumental Dead Space on V_D/V_T and Alveolar Ventilation During Lung-Protective Ventilation

Alveolar ventilation (Valv) is the efficient part of the minute ventilation for gas exchange and CO_2 elimination [62].

$$Valv = RR \times \left(V_T - V_D\right) = RR \times V_T - RR \times V_D$$

The utilization of small tidal volumes (V_T) and high respiratory rates (RR) has several consequences in terms of alveolar ventilation and impact of the dead space. Firstly, it is easy to understand that **V_D/V_T increases as tidal volume decreases** if V_D remains constant (Fig. 8.4a). The weight of dead space increases in proportion of tidal volume decrease for a constant minute ventilation. Secondly, the dead space which is the "wasted part of the breath" intervenes more frequently when respiratory rate increases.

Consequently, for a steady minute ventilation, when the respiratory rate or the dead space is increased, **alveolar ventilation is reduced** (Fig. 8.4b). If the respiratory rate is increased in proportion of the decrease in tidal volume, the alveolar ventilation will be reduced, and $PaCO_2$ will be increased. For example, if the settings are modified from 6 ml/kg PBW × 25 (150 ml/kg/min of minute ventilation) to 5 ml/kg PBW × 30 (150 ml/kg/min of minute ventilation), the alveolar ventilation will be lower. With an average instrumental dead space, to keep Valv constant with 5 ml/kg PBW of tidal volume, the respiratory rate should be 34/min (with 170 ml/kg PBW/min). This explains why reduction of the instrumental dead space is recommended in the situations of lung-protective ventilation [5] (i) by removing useless connectors (only closed-suction connector is really necessary) and (ii) by using HH instead of HME to humidify gases. This is also why ultra-protective lung ventilation may be implemented without ECMO or ECCOR, only when the instrumental dead space is minimized [53, 54].

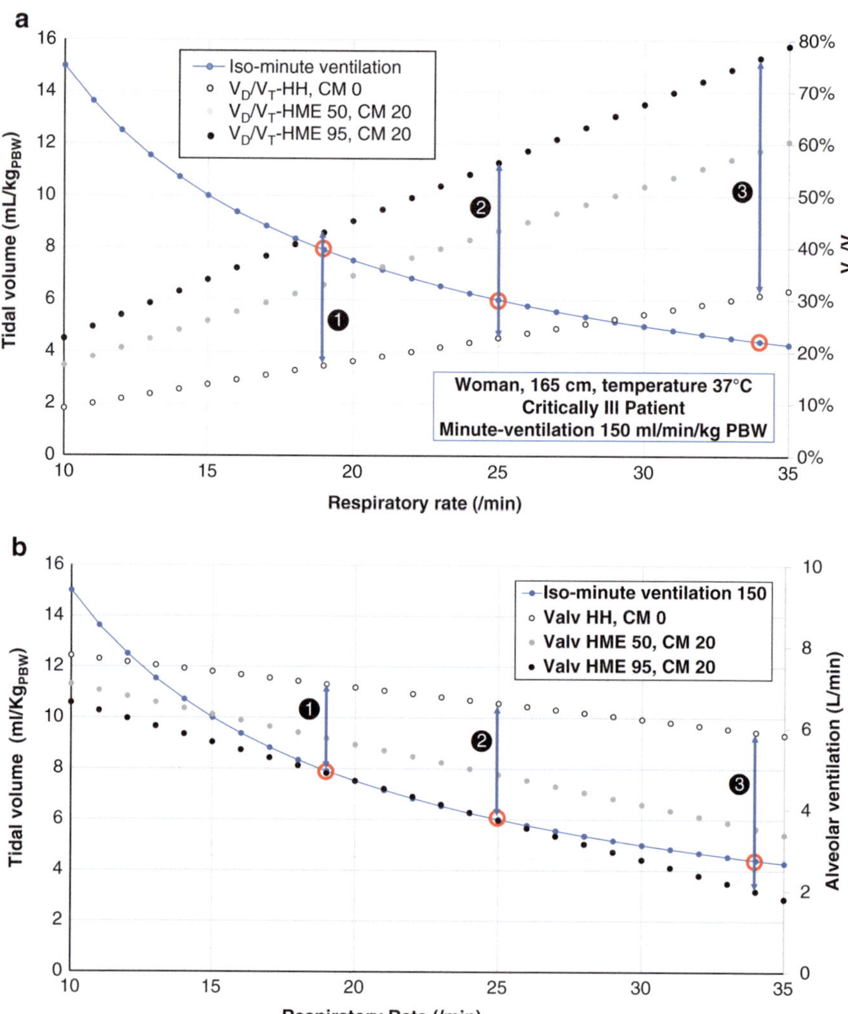

Fig. 8.4 Impact of instrumental dead space on V_D/V_T (**a**) and on alveolar ventilation (**b**) in critically ill patients with different instrumental dead spaces. The example used for the calculations is the case of a woman of 165 cm, PBW 57 kg. The blue line represents the iso-minute ventilation for 150 ml/kg PBW/min (8.5 l/min with PBW of 57 kg). In setting ❶, with a V_T of 8 ml/kg and a RR of 19 breaths/min, V_D/V_T is 17% with the lowest instrumental dead space and 43% with a higher dead space; alveolar ventilation went from 4.9 l/min to 7.1 l/min. When increasing the respiratory rate and decreasing the tidal volume (settings ❷ and ❸), the difference is even more striking. In the most severe situation, reflecting a low compliance requiring ultra-protective ventilation (case ❸) with a TV of 4.4 ml/kg and a RR of 34 breaths/min, V_D/V_T is 31% with the lowest instrumental dead space and 77% with a higher dead space. In this situation, alveolar ventilation goes from 6.0 to 2.0 l/min. *HH* heated humidifiers *HME* heat and moisture exchangers, *CM* catheter mount

8.6   Impact of Dead Space Reduction on Respiratory Parameters with Constant Alveolar Ventilation

The previous figures showed the impact of the dead space on alveolar ventilation (CO_2 clearance). Figure 8.5a and b shows that with a constant alveolar ventilation, it is possible to substantially decrease the respiratory rate (with constant tidal volume) (Fig. 8.5a) or the tidal volume (with constant respiratory rate) (Fig. 8.5b) when decreasing the dead space.

If the $PaCO_2$ is maintained within reasonable values (<50 mmHg based on several authors [35, 36]), the reduction of the instrumental dead space will allow a reduction of the respiratory rate (Fig. 8.5a) or a reduction of the tidal volumes (and plateau pressures [16, 59]) (Fig. 8.5b) while maintaining constant the alveolar ventilation (and $PaCO_2$). Both reduction of the respiratory rate and tidal volume associated with reduced instrumental dead space would also reduce mechanical power [19]. In addition, the reduction of the instrumental dead space reduces the ventilatory ratio [19, 63]. In the same patient, after reduction of the dead space, the ventilatory ratio would drop significantly, as the $PaCO_2$ will decrease. Similarly, the mechanical power which is associated with mortality in patients with ARDS will decrease just by decreasing the instrumental dead space if the $PaCO_2$ is maintained constant with reducing the respiratory rates. High mechanical power likely reflects a more severe disease with higher pressures, lower compliance requiring lower tidal volumes and higher respiratory rates. There is no evidence that the reduction of this parameter would decrease mortality, more than a decrease of the plateau pressure or driving pressure would decrease mortality. Ventilatory ratio [64] and mechanical power [65] are new markers of severity of ARDS but cannot be determined without taking into account the instrumental dead space (and mainly the humidification strategy used).

We have developed a free educational application, VentilO, to facilitate the initial management of protective mechanical ventilation (tidal volume, respiratory rate and dead space optimization). This tool evaluates the alveolar ventilation required based on the height, the gender (providing the predicted body weight), the actual weight, the temperature, the type of patient and the estimated dead space. Based on these data, it provides recommendations for tidal volume and respiratory rates.

In summary, in critically ill patients, the minute ventilation necessary to maintain $PaCO_2$ within a reasonable range is frequently at or above 150 ml/kg PBW/min. In non-ARDS patients if 8 ml/kg PBW is the targeted volume, a respiratory rate around 20 breaths/min may be adequate; with a tidal volume of 6 ml/kg PBW, respiratory rate around 25 breaths/min may be necessary (e.g., COVID patients). In severe ARDS with low compliance, requiring tidal volumes of 6 ml/kg PBW or lower to maintain plateau pressure below 30 cmH_2O, respiratory rate should be set at 25–30 breaths/min or even higher. The utilization of a heated humidifier in these situations to humidify and warm gases delivered to intubated patients allows minimizing the instrumental dead space and a better control of the $PaCO_2$. In most severe patients, with tidal volumes equal or below 6 ml/kg PBW, the minimization of the dead space is mandatory [54]. In CARDS patients (COVID-19 ARDS) , the same principles apply [20, 66].

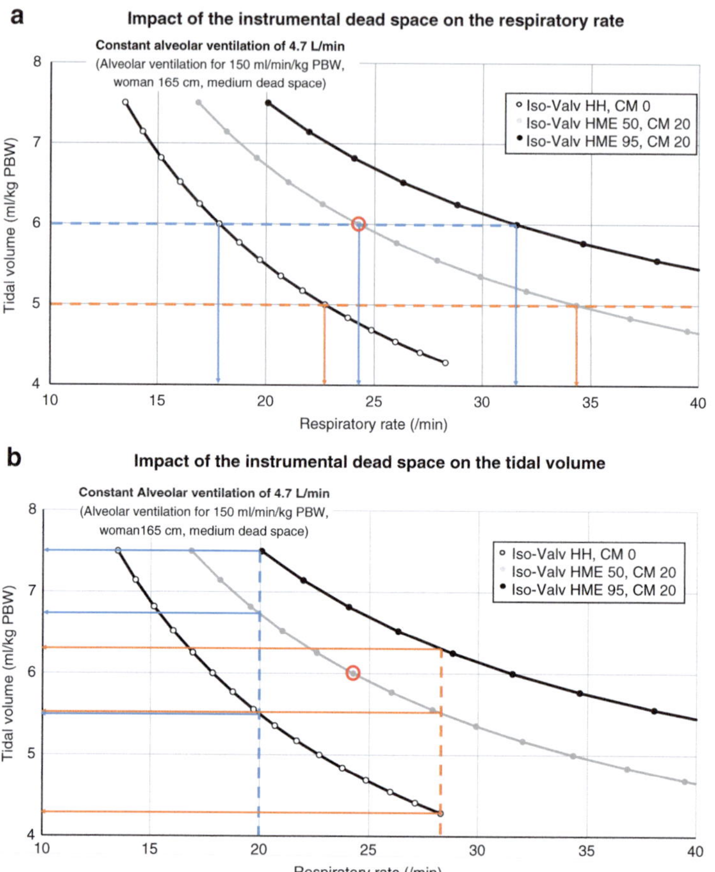

Fig. 8.5 Impact of different instrumental dead space on the respiratory rate (**a**) and the tidal volume (**b**) to maintain a constant alveolar ventilation in critically ill patients. The example used for the calculations is the case of a woman of 165 cm, PBW 57 kg. The target alveolar ventilation is 4.7 l/min which is the alveolar ventilation in this patient with a minute ventilation of 150 ml/kg/min PBW and with a medium instrumental dead space (HME 50 ml, catheter mount and connections 20 ml). The different lines represent the iso-alveolar ventilation lines (4.7 l/min) and the different combinations of respiratory rate and tidal volumes to attain this alveolar ventilation. Based on the application VentilO calculations. (**a**) This figure shows the potential reduction of respiratory rate when reducing the instrumental dead space to keep constant alveolar ventilation (4.7 l/min) for a constant tidal volume. For example, for a tidal volume of 6 ml/kg PBW (blue lines), the respiratory rate required is 32 breaths/min with the highest dead space and 18 breaths/min with the lowest dead space. For a tidal volume of 5 ml/kg PBW (orange lines), the respiratory rate required is very high (above 40 breaths/min) with the highest dead space, 34 breaths/min with intermediate dead space and 23 breaths/min with the lowest dead space. *HH* heated humidifiers, *HME* heat and moisture exchangers, *CM* catheter mount. (**b**) This figure shows the potential tidal volume reduction when reducing the instrumental dead space to keep constant alveolar ventilation (4.7 l/min) for a constant respiratory rate. For example, for a respiratory rate of 20 breaths/min (blue lines), the tidal volume required is 7.5 ml/kg PBW with the highest dead space and 5.5 ml/kg with the lowest dead space. This will translate in a gain in plateau pressure or driving pressure related to the pulmonary compliance. For a respiratory rate of 28 breaths/min (orange lines), the tidal volume required is 6.3 ml/kg with the highest dead space and 4.2 ml/kg with the lowest dead space. Ultra-protective ventilation with tidal volumes around 4 ml/kg cannot be achieved with excessive dead space as previously shown [54]. *HH heated humidifiers, HME* heat and moisture exchangers, *CM* catheter mount

Instrumental dead space may be very high (above 100 ml) when counting HME, catheter mount, connectors and endotracheal tube. Most efficient HMEs have usually a volume above 50 ml (up to 90 ml) [68], catheter mount may have a volume of 20–60 ml, and many connectors may be used in patients (CO_2 cuvette, closed suction and other adaptors for inhalation therapies) and may represent an important additional dead space.

References

1. Slutsky AS, Ranieri VM. Ventilator-induced lung injury. N Engl J Med. 2014;370(10):980.
2. Acute Respiratory Distress Syndrome Network, Brower RG, Matthay MA, Morris A, Schoenfeld D, Thompson BT, Wheeler A. Ventilation with lower tidal volumes as compared with traditional tidal volumes for acute lung injury and the acute respiratory distress syndrome. The acute respiratory distress syndrome network. N Engl J Med. 2000;342(18):1301–8.
3. Fan E, Brodie D, Slutsky AS. Acute respiratory distress syndrome: advances in diagnosis and treatment. JAMA. 2018;319(7):698–710.
4. Fan E, Del Sorbo L, Goligher EC, et al. An official American Thoracic Society/European Society of Intensive Care Medicine/Society of Critical Care Medicine clinical practice guideline: mechanical ventilation in adult patients with acute respiratory distress syndrome. Am J Respir Crit Care Med. 2017;195(9):1253–63.
5. Papazian L, Aubron C, Brochard L, et al. Formal guidelines: management of acute respiratory distress syndrome. Ann Intensive Care. 2019;9(1):69.
6. Serpa Neto A, Cardoso SO, Manetta JA, et al. Association between use of lung-protective ventilation with lower tidal volumes and clinical outcomes among patients without acute respiratory distress syndrome: a meta-analysis. JAMA. 2012;308(16):1651–9.
7. Lellouche F, Lipes J. Prophylactic protective ventilation: lower tidal volumes for all critically ill patients? Intensive Care Med. 2013;39(1):6–15.
8. Rubenfeld GD, Shankar-Hari M. Lessons from ARDS for non-ARDS research: remembrance of trials past. JAMA. 2018;320(18):1863–5.
9. Schaefer MS, Serpa Neto A, Pelosi P, et al. Temporal changes in ventilator settings in patients with uninjured lungs: a systematic review. Anesth Analg. 2019;129(1):129–40.
10. Lellouche F, Delorme M, Brochard L. Impact of respiratory rate and dead space in the current era of lung protective mechanical ventilation. Chest. 2020;158(1):45–7.
11. Matamis D, Lemaire F, Harf A, Teisseire B, Brun-Buisson C. Redistribution of pulmonary blood flow induced by positive end-expiratory pressure and dopamine infusion in acute respiratory failure. Am Rev Respir Dis. 1984;129(1):39–44.
12. Nuckton TJ, Alonso JA, Kallet RH, et al. Pulmonary dead-space fraction as a risk factor for death in the acute respiratory distress syndrome. N Engl J Med. 2002;346(17):1281–6.
13. Haldane J. The relation of the action of carbonic oxide to oxygen tension. J Physiol. 1895;18(3):201–17.
14. Sinha P, Flower O, Soni N. Deadspace ventilation: a waste of breath! Intensive Care Med. 2011;37(5):735–46.
15. Marhong J, Fan E. Carbon dioxide in the critically ill: too much or too little of a good thing? Respir Care. 2014;59(10):1597–605.
16. Pitoni S, D'Arrigo S, Grieco DL, et al. Tidal volume lowering by instrumental dead space reduction in brain-injured ARDS patients: effects on respiratory mechanics, gas exchange, and cerebral hemodynamics. Neurocrit Care. 2021;34(1):21–30.
17. Mekontso Dessap A, Charron C, Devaquet J, et al. Impact of acute hypercapnia and augmented positive end-expiratory pressure on right ventricle function in severe acute respiratory distress syndrome. Intensive Care Med. 2009;35(11):1850–8.
18. Lellouche F. Decrease dead space prior to calling the ECMO! Chest. 2021;159(4):1682–3.

19. Lavoie-Bérard CA, Lefebvre JC, Bouchard PA, Simon M, Lellouche F. Impact of the airway humidification strategy in mechanically ventilated COVID-19 patient. Retrospective analysis and literature review. Respir Care. 2021;67(2):157–66. https://pubmed.ncbi.nlm.nih.gov/34670857/.
20. Lellouche F, Grieco DL, Maggiore SM, Antonelli M. Instrumental dead space in ventilator management. Lancet Respir Med. 2021;9(3):e22.
21. Paternot A, Repesse X, Vieillard-Baron A. Rationale and description of right ventricle-protective ventilation in ARDS. Respir Care. 2016;61(10):1391–6.
22. Hickling KG, Henderson SJ, Jackson R. Low mortality associated with low volume pressure limited ventilation with permissive hypercapnia in severe adult respiratory distress syndrome. Intensive Care Med. 1990;16(6):372–7.
23. Hickling KG, Walsh J, Henderson S, Jackson R. Low mortality rate in adult respiratory distress syndrome using low-volume, pressure-limited ventilation with permissive hypercapnia: a prospective study. Crit Care Med. 1994;22(10):1568–78.
24. Laffey JG, Kavanagh BP. Carbon dioxide and the critically ill--too little of a good thing? Lancet. 1999;354(9186):1283–6.
25. Curley GF, Laffey JG, Kavanagh BP. CrossTalk proposal: there is added benefit to providing permissive hypercapnia in the treatment of ARDS. J Physiol. 2013;591(11):2763–5.
26. Bendixen HH, Laver MB, Flacke WE. Influence of respiratory acidosis on circulatory effect of epinephrine in dogs. Circ Res. 1963;13:64–70.
27. Viitanen A, Salmenpera M, Heinonen J. Right ventricular response to hypercarbia after cardiac surgery. Anesthesiology. 1990;73(3):393–400.
28. Andersen MN, Mouritzen C. Effect of acute respiratory and metabolic acidosis on cardiac output and peripheral resistance. Ann Surg. 1966;163(2):161–8.
29. McIntyre RC Jr, Haenel JB, Moore FA, Read RR, Burch JM, Moore EE. Cardiopulmonary effects of permissive hypercapnia in the management of adult respiratory distress syndrome. J Trauma. 1994;37(3):433–8.
30. Pfeiffer B, Hachenberg T, Wendt M, Marshall B. Mechanical ventilation with permissive hypercapnia increases intrapulmonary shunt in septic and nonseptic patients with acute respiratory distress syndrome. Crit Care Med. 2002;30(2):285–9.
31. Gendreau S, Geri G, Pham T, Vieillard-Baron A, Mekontso DA. The role of acute hypercapnia on mortality and short-term physiology in patients mechanically ventilated for ARDS: a systematic review and meta-analysis. Intensive Care Med. 2022;48(5):517–34.
32. Severinghaus JW. Oxyhemoglobin dissociation curve correction for temperature and pH variation in human blood. J Appl Physiol. 1958;12(3):485–6.
33. Feihl F, Eckert P, Brimioulle S, et al. Permissive hypercapnia impairs pulmonary gas exchange in the acute respiratory distress syndrome. Am J Respir Crit Care Med. 2000;162(1):209–15.
34. Amato MB, Barbas CS, Medeiros DM, et al. Beneficial effects of the "open lung approach" with low distending pressures in acute respiratory distress syndrome. A prospective randomized study on mechanical ventilation. Am J Respir Crit Care Med. 1995;152(6 Pt 1):1835–46.
35. Nin N, Muriel A, Penuelas O, et al. Severe hypercapnia and outcome of mechanically ventilated patients with moderate or severe acute respiratory distress syndrome. Intensive Care Med. 2017;43(2):200–8.
36. Mekontso Dessap A, Boissier F, Charron C, et al. Acute cor pulmonale during protective ventilation for acute respiratory distress syndrome: prevalence, predictors, and clinical impact. Intensive Care Med. 2016;42(5):862–70.
37. Repesse X, Charron C, Vieillard-Baron A. Acute cor pulmonale in ARDS: rationale for protecting the right ventricle. Chest. 2015;147(1):259–65.
38. Tiruvoipati R, Serpa Neto A, Young M, et al. An exploratory analysis of the association between hypercapnia and hospital mortality in critically ill patients with sepsis. Ann Am Thorac Soc. 2022;19(2):245–54.
39. Tiruvoipati R, Pilcher D, Botha J, Buscher H, Simister R, Bailey M. Association of Hypercapnia and Hypercapnic Acidosis with Clinical Outcomes in mechanically ventilated patients with cerebral injury. JAMA Neurol. 2018;75(7):818–26.

40. Tiruvoipati R, Gupta S, Pilcher D, Bailey M. Hypercapnia and hypercapnic acidosis in sepsis: harmful, beneficial or unclear? Crit Care Resusc. 2018;20(2):94–100.
41. Laffey JG, Kavanagh BP. Hypocapnia. N Engl J Med. 2002;347(1):43–53.
42. Madotto F, Rezoagli E, McNicholas BA, et al. Patterns and impact of arterial CO_2 Management in Patients with Acute Respiratory Distress Syndrome: insights from the LUNG SAFE study. Chest. 2020;158(5):1967–82.
43. Arnal JM, Wysocki M, Nafati C, et al. Automatic selection of breathing pattern using adaptive support ventilation. Intensive Care Med. 2008;34(1):75–81.
44. Radford EP Jr. Ventilation standards for use in artificial respiration. J Appl Physiol. 1955;7(4):451–60.
45. Brochard L. Intrinsic (or auto-) PEEP during controlled mechanical ventilation. Intensive Care Med. 2002;28(10):1376–8.
46. Devaquet J, Jonson B, Niklason L, et al. Effects of inspiratory pause on CO_2 elimination and arterial PCO_2 in acute lung injury. J Appl Physiol (1985). 2008;105(6):1944–9.
47. Aboab J, Niklason L, Uttman L, Brochard L, Jonson B. Dead space and CO(2) elimination related to pattern of inspiratory gas delivery in ARDS patients. Crit Care. 2012;16(2):R39.
48. Aguirre-Bermeo H, Moran I, Bottiroli M, et al. End-inspiratory pause prolongation in acute respiratory distress syndrome patients: effects on gas exchange and mechanics. Ann Intensive Care. 2016;6(1):81.
49. Combes A, Auzinger G, Capellier G, et al. ECCO2R therapy in the ICU: consensus of a European round table meeting. Crit Care. 2020;24(1):490.
50. Combes A, Hajage D, Capellier G, et al. Extracorporeal membrane oxygenation for severe acute respiratory distress syndrome. N Engl J Med. 2018;378(21):1965–75.
51. Combes A, Peek GJ, Hajage D, et al. ECMO for severe ARDS: systematic review and individual patient data meta-analysis. Intensive Care Med. 2020;46(11):2048–57.
52. Combes A, Tonetti T, Fanelli V, et al. Efficacy and safety of lower versus higher CO_2 extraction devices to allow ultraprotective ventilation: secondary analysis of the SUPERNOVA study. Thorax. 2019;74(12):1179–81.
53. Retamal J, Libuy J, Jimenez M, et al. Preliminary study of ventilation with 4 ml/kg tidal volume in acute respiratory distress syndrome: feasibility and effects on cyclic recruitment—derecruitment and hyperinflation. Crit Care. 2013;17(1):R16.
54. Richard JC, Marque S, Gros A, et al. Feasibility and safety of ultra-low tidal volume ventilation without extracorporeal circulation in moderately severe and severe ARDS patients. Intensive Care Med. 2019;45(11):1590–8.
55. Girault C, Breton L, Richard JC, et al. Mechanical effects of airway humidification devices in difficult to wean patients. Crit Care Med. 2003;31:1306–11.
56. Jaber S, Chanques G, Matecki S, et al. Comparison of the effects of heat and moisture exchangers and heated humidifiers on ventilation and gas exchange during non-invasive ventilation. Intensive Care Med. 2002;28(11):1590–4.
57. Lellouche F, Maggiore SM, Deye N, et al. Effect of the humidification device on the work of breathing during noninvasive ventilation. Intensive Care Med. 2002;28(11):1582–9.
58. Hinkson CR, Benson MS, Stephens LM, Deem S. The effects of apparatus dead space on P(aCO2) in patients receiving lung-protective ventilation. Respir Care. 2006;51(10):1140–4.
59. Moran I, Bellapart J, Vari A, Mancebo J. Heat and moisture exchangers and heated humidifiers in acute lung injury/acute respiratory distress syndrome patients. Effects on respiratory mechanics and gas exchange. Intensive Care Med. 2006;32(4):524–31.
60. Prat G, Renault A, Tonnelier JM, et al. Influence of the humidification device during acute respiratory distress syndrome. Intensive Care Med. 2003;29:2211–5.
61. Prin S, Chergui K, Augarde R, Page B, Jardin F, Veillard-Baron A. Ability and safety of a heated humidifier to control hypercapnic acidosis in severe ARDS. Intensive Care Med. 2002;28:1756–60.
62. Lucangelo U, Blanch L. Dead space. Intensive Care Med. 2004;30(4):576–9.

63. Beloncle F, Studer A, Seegers V, et al. Longitudinal changes in compliance, oxygenation and ventilatory ratio in COVID-19 versus non-COVID-19 pulmonary acute respiratory distress syndrome. Crit Care. 2021;25(1):248.
64. Sinha P, Fauvel NJ, Singh S, Soni N. Ventilatory ratio: a simple bedside measure of ventilation. Br J Anaesth. 2009;102(5):692–7.
65. Gattinoni L, Tonetti T, Cressoni M, et al. Ventilator-related causes of lung injury: the mechanical power. Intensive Care Med. 2016;42(10):1567–75.
66. Lavoie-Berard CA, Lefebvre JC, Bouchard PA, Simon M, Lellouche F. Impact of airway humidification strategy in the mechanically ventilated COVID-19 patients. Respir Care. 2022;67(2):157–66.
67. Kenny S. The Adelaide ventilation guide. Br J Anaesth. 1967;39(1):21–3.
68. Lellouche F, Taille S, Lefrancois F, et al. Humidification performance of 48 passive airway humidifiers: comparison with manufacturer data. Chest. 2009;135(2):276–86.

Effect of Airway Humidification Devices in Lung Mechanics (Volume/Airflow)

Nicola Launaro and Monica Giordanengo

9.1 Introduction

Patients undergoing oral-tracheal intubation or with tracheal cannula have a problem of humidification and heating of the inhaled gas as a result of the exclusion of the nose and upper airways from the flow of inhaled air.

In fact, it is known that about 75% of the heat and humidity content of the inhaled air in the inspiratory phase is supplied in the nasopharyngeal and oropharyngeal tract. The remaining 25% is added into the trachea [1–3].

Humidity refers to the amount of water vapor in a gaseous environment. It depends on the gas temperature and can be expressed in two ways, as absolute humidity and relative humidity. Absolute humidity (AH) is the amount of water in a given gas volume usually expressed in mg H_2O/L volume. Relative humidity (RH) is the amount of water vapor in a volume of gas, expressed as a percentage of the amount of water vapor required to completely saturate the same volume of gas at the same temperature and pressure.

By the time the inhaled gas reaches the lungs, it will have reached base body temperature (37 °C) and saturated state (44 mg/L). The level at which this occurs is also called the isothermal saturation point.

This process occurs through contact with the nasal mucosa which is moist and highly vascularized. The geometry of the nasal cavity is effective in dividing the flow which initially laminar becomes a slower turbulent flow. This slow and turbulent flow allows the inhaled air to have maximum contact with the warmer nasal mucosa, and, therefore, the ambient air is heated to about 34 °C at rest.

N. Launaro (✉) · M. Giordanengo
Intensive Care Unit, Saluzzo Hospital, Saluzzo, Italy

© The Author(s), under exclusive license to Springer Nature Switzerland AG 2023
A. M. Esquinas (ed.), *Humidification in the Intensive Care Unit*,
https://doi.org/10.1007/978-3-031-23953-3_9

The respiratory mucosa is lined with ciliated columnar pseudostratified epithelium and numerous goblet cells, and these submucosal cells and glands are responsible for maintaining the mucous layer that acts as a trap for pathogens and as an interface for the exchange of moisture.

As the air moves through the airways, it will be humidified and heated. When it reaches the middle trachea, the temperature and AH reach approximately 34 °C and 34–38 mgH$_2$O/L, respectively.

The point where the gas stabilizes at 37 °C with a relative humidity of 100% (which corresponds to an absolute humidity of 44 mgH$_2$O/L) is known as the isothermal saturation limit and is approximately 5 cm below of the keel during resting breath, between the fourth and fifth generation of the bronchial tree. Humidity and temperature are constant below the isothermal saturation limit. This provides the optimal conditions for gas exchange in the alveolo-capillary membrane and avoids damage to the mucosa and ciliary epithelium.

During exhalation: about 20–30% of the heat and humidity added during inspiration are recovered through the exhaled gases. Most of these are recovered in the nasopharyngeal and oropharyngeal tract. About 70–80% of heat and humidity are lost from the body.

In the patient intubated via orotracheal route or wearing a tracheal cannula with cuff, the upper airways are excluded from the flow of inhaled air (Fig. 9.1), and therefore, the function is lost with serious damage to the mucociliary epithelium, loss of bacterial and viral filter function, and loss of motility of the cilia with stagnation of mucus which facilitates bacterial proliferation. The isothermal saturation limit, under these conditions, can be reached at a much lower level or even not be reached. This induces a deficit in gas exchanges.

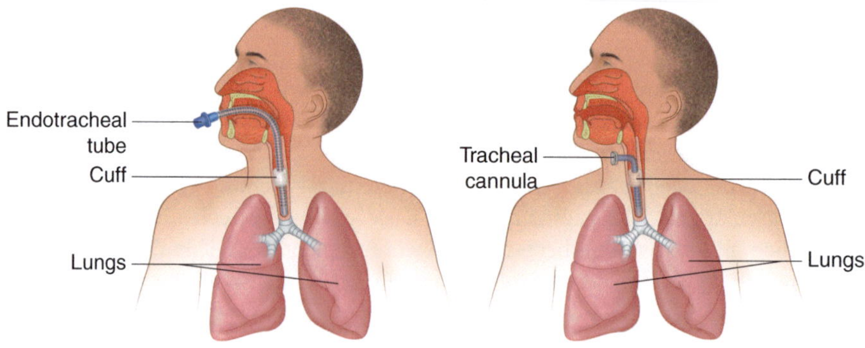

Fig. 9.1 Airflow in ventilated patient

9.2   Humidification Techniques [4–12]

We believe it is necessary to humidify the gases administered during ventilation, whether invasive or non-invasive, in order to avoid the inhalation of dry gas in the airways with the following associated risks:

1. Damage to the ciliated epithelium with loss of ciliary motility [13].
2. Thickening of secretions and risk of formation of mucus plugs that can occlude the airways or the cannula with reduction of compliance and residual functional capacity of the lungs, atelectasis, and shunts.
3. Increased risk of infections, also linked to the loss of the nasal filter.

Humidification of gases inspired during ventilation has become an effective and accepted practice in intensive care units and during narcosis in the operating room as well as in patients undergoing treatment with home ventilation [14].

Currently, it is possible to humidify the inspiratory gas flow in two different ways:

1. Active humidification.
2. Passive humidification.

9.3   Active Humidification

It is carried out with tools commonly called heated humidifiers. All systems of this type exploit the contact of the blown gas with water or water vapor. Different models are recognized:

1. Passover.

    They use a heating plate and a container placed above the plate filled with water. Heating the plate increases the temperature of the water until it evaporates. The water vapor saturates with moisture and heats the gas flow from the fan (Fig. 9.2a).

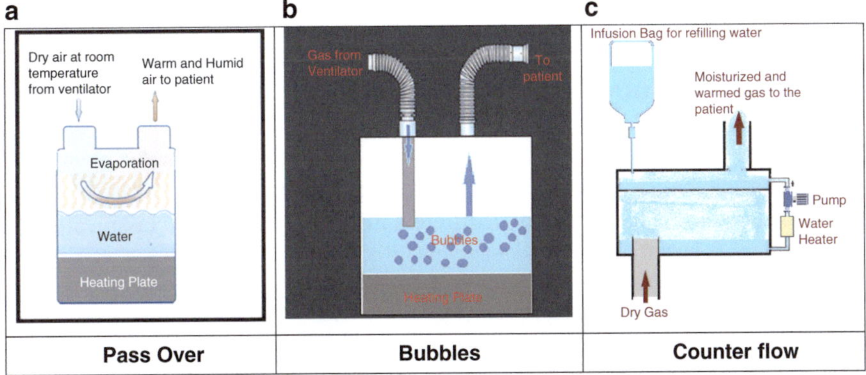

Fig. 9.2 Active humidifiers. (**a**) Pass over (**b**) Bubbles (**c**) Counter flow

Fig. 9.3 Unheated bubble
humidifier

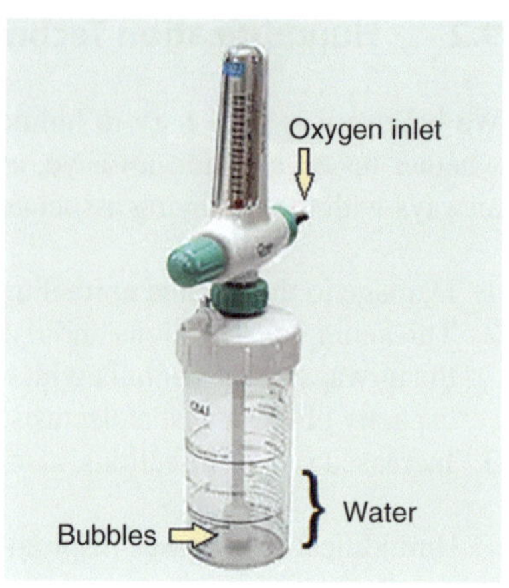

2. Bubble

   The gaseous mixture from the ventilator escapes from the distal end of a tube placed under the surface of the water, forming bubbles that gain moisture as they rise to the surface of the water. Most models feature a diffuser at the distal end of the tube that splits the gas into smaller bubbles to increase the gas-water interface and therefore water vapor content. The level of gas humidification also depends on the height of the water column and the gas flow. In fact, the higher the column, the greater the gas/water interface, and the slower the flow, the longer the time to humidify the gaseous mixture. These humidifiers can also be used with water at room temperature (Fig. 9.3) and therefore not heated. The increase in water temperature is directly proportional to the increase in relative humidity of the gaseous mixture supplied to the patient (Fig. 9.2b).

3. Counter-flow [15]

   In this case, the heated water is dropped into suspension through a membrane that produces small bubbles that fall toward the dry gas mixture coming from the fan. The contact between the gas that proceeds upward and the particles of liquid that fall downward humidifies the gas itself. The liquid that falls on the bottom of the humidifier is recovered and pushed back upward by a pump. In this path, the liquid is heated (Fig. 9.2c).

9.4 Passive Humidification [16–19]

These devices retain the heat and humidity eliminated by the patient during exhalation and enrich the gas inhaled during subsequent inspiration (Fig. 9.4). The "passive" function can be performed with different mechanisms, and the classification of these devices is based on their mechanisms [20].

1. Heat and moisture exchangers (HMEs)

   Heat and humidity exchangers are simple condensers built with elements of disposable foam, synthetic fiber, or paper, with a large exchange surface. In hydrophobic HMEs, the paper or polypropylene membrane is coated with a mix-

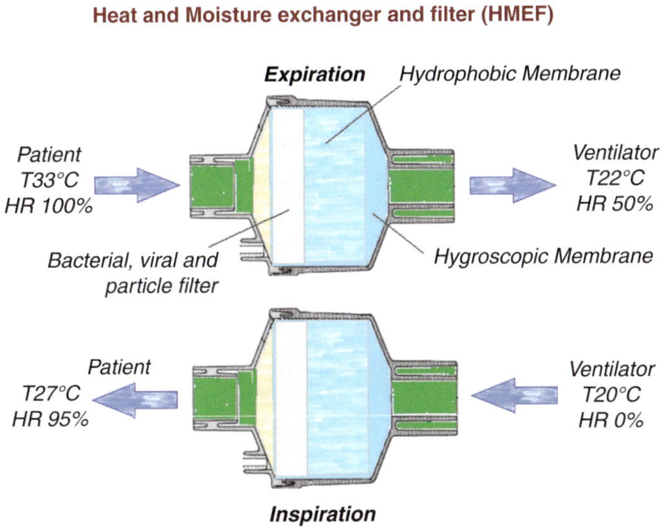

Heat and Moisture exchanger and filter (HMEF)

Fig. 9.4 Passive humidifier operation

ture of calcium or lithium chloride to prevent moisture absorption and retain the heat of the exhaled gas, delivering it in the subsequent inhalation.

2. Hygroscopic condenser humidifiers (HCHs)

The term indicates a chemical substance that absorbs moisture from the air. Hygroscopic substances have the ability to attract and retain the water molecules exhaled by the patient. During the expiratory phase of breathing, the hot exhaled gas cools as it passes through the membrane, releasing heat to the membrane. During inhalation, cold and dry gases pass through the membrane, and the absorbed heat evaporates the condensate.

Passive humidification devices are increasingly assembled with filters whose function is to prevent viruses and bacteria from being carried into the bronchial tree with the flow of gas from the ventilator. These filters work by removing viruses and bacteria from the gas stream by various mechanisms [21, 22]:

1. Diffusion

The smallest particles (<0.1 μm) have Brownian movements due to impacts with the gas molecules. These movements can take them out of the gas flow into contact with the filter fibers to which they will adhere.

2. Interception

Medium-sized particles (0.1–0.5 μm) that follow the flow, if they find themselves passing at a certain distance from the filter fibers, can adhere to the latter.

3. Inertial impact

The largest particles (0.5–1 μm) due to their inertia are unable to follow the rapid changes in the direction of the gas flow inside the filter and therefore impact the fibers to which they adhere.

4. <u>Gravitational sedimentation</u>

Larger particles (>1 μm) as a function of the gravitational force fall inside the filter.

5. <u>Electrostatic attraction</u>

The filter can be electrically charged, and therefore electrically charged particles are attracted to the opposite charged fibers. Neutral particles can also be attracted because the electric field generates a dipole in the particle which is therefore attracted to the regions with opposite charge.

6. <u>Sieving</u>

The pores of the filter prevent the passage of particles according to their size.

Once the operating mechanisms of the filters have been defined, we can classify them into two broad categories:

1. <u>Mechanical filters</u>

They act by sieving. They consist of glass fibers packed and assembled with a resin. This material induces a significant increase in flow resistance. To reduce the increase in resistance, the exchange surface is increased by creating pleated panels. It is evident that the smaller the pores through which the gas flow must pass, the greater the filtering capacity and therefore also the resistance to flow.

2. *Electrostatic filters*

The mechanism of action is electrostatic attraction. They can be tribocharged, i.e., made up of monoacrylic and polypropylene fibers that form an electrically charged non-woven fabric, or fibrillated, i.e., an electrically charged propylene sheet and then reduced into fibrils which are assembled to form a wad.

In clinical practice, heat and humidity exchangers with filters are increasingly used. These devices are made of materials necessary for hydration and heating according to their principle of operation (hydrophobic or hygroscopic). They also contain an electrostatic filter.

Finally, it is possible to use combined heat and humidity exchangers. Hygroscopic and hydrophobic elements are used to create a combined HME. The performance in terms of absolute humidity is better in HCHs than in HMEs. However, the performance is similar between HCH and HME combined.

9.5   Humidifier Filters and Respiratory Mechanics [23–26]

A filter inserted on the breathing circuit can somehow modify the flow of gases, increase the resistance of the circuit, and generate dead space within the circuit.

9.6   Dead Space [27, 28]

The dead space generated by a HME filter varies between the various models from a minimum of approximately 40 ml to a maximum of 90 ml (Fig. 9.5). Active humidifiers generate a dead space share of approximately 20–25 ml.

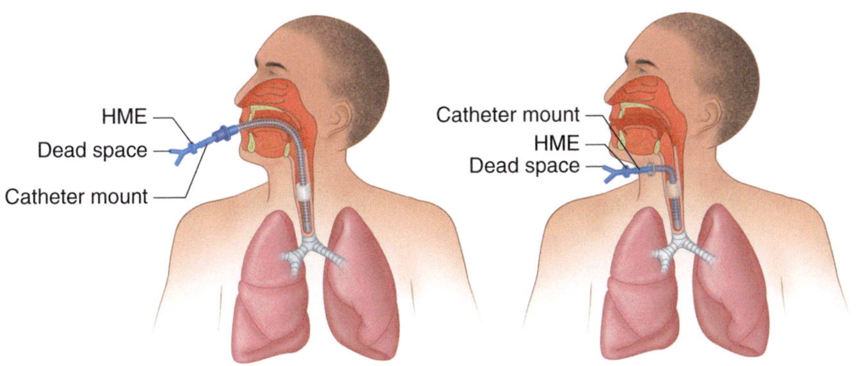

Fig. 9.5 Dead space

Alveolar ventilation is the amount of air per unit time that is involved in gas exchange. It is known that alveolar ventilation (V_A) is determined by the product of the effective tidal volume (tidal volume [V_t] − total dead space volume [V_D]) and respiratory rate (RR).

$$V_A = (V_t - V_D) \times RR$$

The alveolar ventilation equation therefore defines that the greater the volume of dead space, the lower the volume of gas that will reach the alveoli and participate in gas exchanges.

The volume of total dead space can be divided into various components:

1. Physiological dead space (V_{Dphys}).
   (a) In the spontaneously breathing patient, V_{Dphys} is due to the anatomical dead space (conduction airways: trachea, bronchi, bronchioles [V_{Daw}]) plus alveolar dead space (V_{Dalv}).
   (b) Alveolar dead space is an expression of the perfusion ventilation mismatch. Physiologically there are three different compartments, i.e., areas of perfect coupling between ventilation and perfusion, areas where perfusion is greater than ventilation (shunt), and finally areas where the alveoli are ventilated but not perfused (alveolar dead space). This "physiological" alteration is not measurable, but various formulas can be used to know the alveolar dead space.

$$V_{Dphys} = V_{Dan} + V_{Dalv}$$

   (c) In ventilated patients, dead space resulting from the ventilation circuit (humidifier filter, catheter holder, and tubing or cannula) is added to the anatomical dead space. In addition to the increase in circuit-induced dead space in many patients, especially in intensive care, there is a significant increase in alveolar dead space that occurs as an effect of the V/Q mismatch caused by the pathology that produced respiratory failure.

$$V_{Dtot} = V_{Dphys.} + V_{Dcirc.} + V_{Dmis}$$

Alveolar ventilation must therefore be understood as that fraction of ventilation that actually participates in gas exchanges. This concept is of fundamental importance in the presence of pathologies that significantly alter the coupling between ventilation and perfusion.

In clinical practice, it is possible to calculate the volume of dead space using the Bohr-Enghoff equation. This method calculates the volume of dead space by measuring the arterial pressure of CO_2, and the partial pressure of CO_2 in the average exhaled air remains the most commonly used method to calculate dead space.

Enghoff Modification of Bohr's Method.

$$\frac{V_D}{V_t} = \frac{PaCO_2 - PeCO_2}{PaCO_2} = 0.20 - 0.40$$

$PeCO_2$ is the partial pressure of carbon dioxide and can be accurately calculated with volumetric capnography measurements.

Under these conditions, the compensation mechanisms for an increase in dead space can be:

1. Respiratory rate increase
   (a) In fact, this represents a compensation mechanism if $V_t - V_D > 0$.
2. Increase in Vt
   (a) From the equation of motion of the respiratory system, we know that the increase in V_t can obtained by increasing the pressure applied to the system.
3. Improvement of the ventilation/perfusion ratio.
   (a) Application of PEEP, alveolar recruitment maneuvers.

$$P_{musc} = V_t \times E + \tilde{V} R + PEEP_i \left(during\ spontaneous\ breathing \right)$$

$$P_{musc} + P_{vent} = V_t \times E + \tilde{V} R + PEEP_i \left(during\ ventilation \right)$$

P_{musc} = pressure generated by the respiratory muscles
P_{vent} = pressure applied by the fan
E = elastance
$\tilde{V}$ = flow
R = airway and system resistance when ventilated
$PEEP_i$ = intrinsic positive end-expiratory pressure.

The increase in pressure requires an increase in respiratory work of breathing (WoB). In physics, work is determined by the force applied to the system for the displacement it generates. In the respiratory field, the force is represented by the applied pressure multiplied by the volume variation that is generated at each inspiratory act

$$\text{WoB} = P \times \Delta V$$

$$P = V_t \times E + \tilde{V} R + \text{PEEP}_i$$

Combining the two equations

$$\text{WoB} = \left(V_t \times E + \tilde{V} R + \text{PEEP}_i \right) \times \Delta V$$

Normal WOB is 0.3–0.7 J/L.

As can be seen from the above formula, respiratory work depends on:

1. Resistive forces applied to the system.
   (a) Airway resistance.
2. Elastic forces.
   (a) Elastic recall forces of the lung and thoracic cage.

During assisted mechanical ventilation, the increased work of breathing required to increase tidal volume can be achieved by correcting the support pressure. If this correction is not established, it is possible to find an increase in respiratory rate due to greater stimulation of the respiratory drive highlighted by the increase in $P_{0\text{-}1}$ from 60% to 100% of the basal value depending on the size of the filter.

In spontaneously breathing patients, the greater demand for minute volume and the consequent increase in WoB can be crucial if they have a reduced respiratory reserve.

From what has been said in mechanical ventilation, the application of the filter in the ventilation circuit can cause an increase in dead space which will affect the mechanics of our patient's breathing.

These considerations, given the small increase in dead space due to the humidifier filter, represent a simple theoretical disquisition in most ventilated patients but become of crucial importance whenever ventilation with small volumes is performed or in the presence of increases in alveolar dead space as in the case of ALI/ARDS [29].

Example	
65 kg patient with ARDS $V_t = 390$ ml	$V_t = 6$ ml × 65 kg =
$PaCO_2 = 49$ mmHg $PeCO_2 = 21$ mmHg	
$V_D/V_t = 0.57$	$\dfrac{V_D}{V_t} = \dfrac{PaCO_2 - PeCO_2}{PaCO_2}$
$V_D = 222$ ml (V_D filter 60 ml)	$V_D = V_t \times 0.57$
Effective $V_t = 168$ ml	Effective $V_t = V_t - V_D$

| If the filter is not inserted, actual $V_t = 228$ ml
In this case, the filter worsens the efficiency of ventilation by over 30% | |

In patients with ARDS, a small variation in dead space can generate a significant increase in $PaCO_2$ which we know is inversely proportional to the VA.

$$PaCO_2 = k \times \frac{\tilde{V}CO_2}{V_A}$$

K is a constant value (0.863)

$\tilde{V}CO_2$ is metabolic production of CO_2

V_A is alveolar ventilation

The simple measurement of the total dead space that can be calculated using Enghoff modification of Bohr's method should be carried out before inserting the filter into the respiratory circuit and after inserting the filter. As is known, this measure has numerous limiting factors, but in the specific case, it will allow us to differentiate the increase in $PaCO_2$ that derives from an expansion of the alveolar dead space consequent to the V/Q mismatch compared to that following the insertion of the filter and therefore correct the ventilation to compensate for this loss.

The use of heated humidifier does not add any instrumental dead space.

These can be an alternative solution in patients with high $PaCO_2$ levels. Dead space reduction by HH decreases $PaCO_2$ allowing a reduction of V_t with improvement of lung compliance and reduction of plateau pressure.

9.7 Resistance and Flow [30–35]

The resistance expresses the opposition to the flow of gases within the airways and, during mechanical ventilation, within the various components of the respiratory circuit.

Resistance then defines the pressure difference required to produce one unit of gas flow through the airways.

$$Resistance = \Delta P / \tilde{V}$$

$$\Delta P = P_{peak} - P_{plat}$$

ΔP = pressure difference between the ventilator and the alveoli ($P_{insp} - P_{alv}$ = driving pressure)

$\tilde{V}$ = flow in the airways.

The unit of measurement is cmH$_2$O/L/s.

During mechanical ventilation, it is therefore necessary to add to the resistances of the patient's respiratory system those of the respiratory circuit.

In turn, the resistances of the respiratory system are composed of two elements:

1. Frictional.
   (a) They depend on the forces of friction opposing the flow. Mainly determined by the airways.
2. Viscoelastic.
   (a) Due to deformation of the chest tissues (lung and chest wall).

Respiratory circuit resistances are mainly determined by the prosthesis used (endotracheal tube, tracheal cannula) and to a lesser extent by circuits and filters.

In the presence of laminar flow, the frictional resistances respond to Poiseuille's law.

$$\tilde{V} = \frac{\Delta P \times \pi \times r^4}{8 \times \eta \times l}$$

$$R = \Delta P / \tilde{V}$$

By combining the two equations, we obtain.

$$R = \frac{8 \times \eta \times l}{\pi \times r^4}$$

$\tilde{V}$ = flow in the airways
ΔP = pressure difference
r = radius
η = viscosity
l = length
R = resistance

The equation highlights the radius as the determining factor because it is raised to the fourth power.

During ventilation, especially in relation to the alterations caused by the disease in progress, the flow is more often turbulent. In this case, the driving pressure will be determined by the square of the gas flow multiplied by a constant.

In summary, therefore, the pressure difference will be defined by the sum of the laminar flow and the turbulent flow (Fig. 9.6).

$$\text{Driving pressure} = K_1 \tilde{V} + K_2 \tilde{V}^2$$

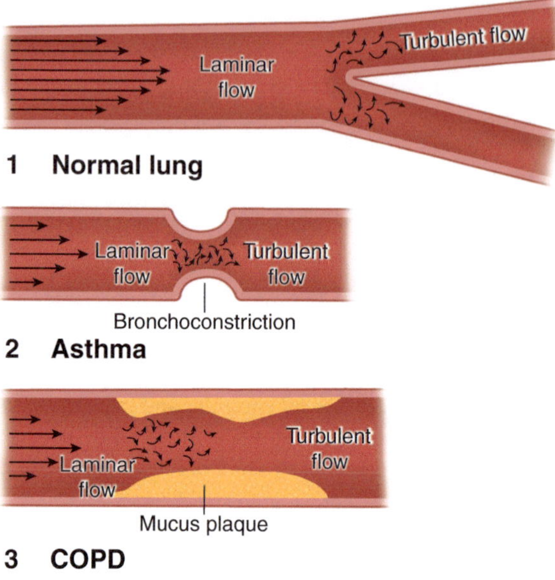

Fig. 9.6 Laminar and turbulent flow

$K_1 \tilde{V}$ = laminar flow component
$K_2 \tilde{V}^2$ = turbulent flow component

In a spontaneously breathing adult, normal airway resistance is estimated at 2 to 3 cmH$_2$O/L/s.

During mechanical ventilation, the resistance is determined by the difference between the peak pressure and the plateau pressure divided by the flow. The peak pressure in turn is a consequence of numerous factors such as the tidal volume, the respiratory rate, the flow rate, and the diameter of the endotracheal tube. Plateau pressure is measured with an inspiratory pause in a patient who has no respiratory muscle activity and is equal to the alveolar pressure. This depends on the tidal volume and the compliance of the respiratory system.

In subjects without respiratory diseases during controlled mechanical ventilation, the resistance value varies between 15 and 20 cmH$_2$O/L/s.

All humidifier filters on the market have an intrinsic resistance to flow which can be considered negligible according to the limits stipulated by the international standard for the HME (International Standards Organization Draft International Standard 9360-2).

This limit was set at 5 cmH$_2$O for a flow of 1 L/min when the filter did not collect the patient's moisture.

The resistance produced by HME filters varies in relation to the following factors:

1. Level of humidity saturation.
2. Deposition of secretions in the filter.
3. Variations in the ventilation parameters.

The hygroscopic filters appear to be those burdened by a minor increase in resistances when they reach the maximum level of humidity saturation.

Secretions can clog the filters and thus raise the resistance to a level that makes ventilation ineffective [36].

The increase in the flow speed leads to an increase in the resistance value offered by the filter.

Changes in tidal volume do not significantly affect resistance.

There are currently no studies showing an increase in WoB and consequent alterations of the blood gas analytical parameters with the use of HME filters during NIV.

The use of active humidifiers generates an increase in resistance and therefore an increase in respiratory work if condensation collects inside the circuit. It is possible to overcome this complication by using heated circuits that keep the water vapor in suspension, avoiding the formation of condensation liquid.

9.8 Conclusions

Bacterial humidifying filters (HME) modify to a small extent the respiratory mechanics during mechanical ventilation.

In some specific conditions (ALI/ARDS), these variations can have a significant impact on ventilation. It is therefore of fundamental importance [37, 38]:

1. To know the effects in terms of dead space and increase of the characteristic resistances of the filter we are using.
2. To measure the changes in respiratory mechanics over time, bearing in mind that the use of the filter may be the cause in whole or in part.

Heated humidifiers develop a lower impact on respiratory mechanics resulting in a lower increase in WoB in PSV [39].

It is therefore necessary if you want to use a humidifier filter to evaluate the possible increase in dead space, respiratory work, and ultimately $PaCO_2$.

References

1. Sahin-Yilmaz A, Naclerio RM. Anatomy and physiology of the upper airway. Proc Am Thorac Soc. 2011;8:31–9.
2. Doorly D, Taylor DJ, Franke P, Schroter RC. Experimental investigation of nasal airflow. Proc Inst Mech Eng H. 2008;222:439–53.

3. Lindemann J, Leiacker R, Rettinger G, Keck T. Nasal mucosal temperature during respiration. Clin Otolaryngol Allied Sci. 2002;27(3):135–9.
4. McNulty G, Eyre L. Humidification in anaesthesia and critical care. Br J Anaesth Ed. 2015;15(3):131–5.
5. Al Ashry HS, Modrykamien AM. Humidification during mechanical ventilation in the adult patient. BioMed Res Int. 2014;2014:715434, 12 pages
6. Branson RD, Campbell RS, Davis K, Porembka DT. Anaesthesia circuits, humidity output, and mucociliary structure and function. Anaesth Intensive Care. 1998;26(2):178–83.
7. Plotnikow GA, Accoce M, Navarro E, Tiribelli N. Humidification and heating of inhaled gas in patients with artificial airway. A narrative review. Rev Bras Ter Intensiva. 2018;30(1):86–97.
8. Cerpa F, Cáceres D, Romero-Dapueto C, Giugliano-Jaramillo C, Pérez R, Budini H, Hidalgo V, Gutiérrez T, Molina J, Keyme J. Humidification on ventilated patients: heated Humidifications or heat and moisture exchangers? Open Respir Med J. 2015;9(Suppl 2: M5):104–11.
9. American Association for Respiratory Care, Restrepo RD, Walsh BK. Humidification during invasive and noninvasive mechanical ventilation: 2012. Respir Care. 2012;57(5):782–8.
10. Shelly MP. The humidification and filtration functions of the airways. Respir Care Clinics N Am. 2006;12:139–48.
11. Boyer A, Vargas F, Hilbert G, Gruson D, Mousset-Hovaere M, Castaing Y, Dreyfuss D, Ricard JD. Small dead space heat and moisture exchangers do not impede gas exchange during noninvasive ventilation: a comparison with a heated humidifier. Intensive Care Med. 2010;36(8):1348–54. https://doi.org/10.1007/s00134-010-1894-5. Epub 2010 Apr 27
12. Esquinas Rodriguez AM, Scala R, Soroksky A, BaHammam A, de Klerk A, Valipour A, et al. Clinical review: humidifiers during non-invasive ventilation: key topics and practical implications. Crit Care. 2012;16(1):203.
13. Kilgour E, Rankin N, Ryan S, Pack R. Mucociliary function deteriorates in the clinical range of inspired air temperature and humidity. Intensive Care Med. 2004;30:1491–4.
14. Williams R, Rankin N, Smith T, Galler D, Seakins P. Relationship between the humidity and temperature of inspired gas and the function of the airway mucosa. Crit Care Med. 1996;24:1920–9.
15. Schumann S, Stahl CA, Möller K, Priebe H-J, Guttmann J. Moisturizing and mechanical characteristics of a new counter-flow type heated humidifier. Br J Anaesth. 2007;98(4):531–8.
16. Wilkes AR. Heat and moisture exchanges and breathing system filters: their use in anaesthesia and intensive care. Part 1 - history, principles and efficiency. Anaesthesia. 2011;66:31–9.
17. Wilkes AR. Heat and moisture exchanges and breathing system filters: their use in anaesthesia and intensive care. Part 2—practical use, including problems, and their use with paediatric patients. Anaesthesia. 2011;66:40–51.
18. Lucato JJ, Adams AB, Souza R, Torquato JA, Carvalho CR, Marini JJ. Evaluating humidity recovery efficiency of currently available heat and moisture exchangers: a respiratory system model study. Clinics (Sao Paulo). 2009;64(6):585–90.
19. Schreiber AF, Ceriana P, Ambrosino N, Piran M, Malovini A, A. Carlucci short-term effects of an active heat-and-moisture exchanger during invasive ventilation. Respir Care. 2019;64(10):1215–21.
20. Branson R, Davis K Jr. Evaluation of 21 passive humidifiers according to the ISO 9360 standard: moisture output, dead space, and flow resistance. Respir Care. 1996;41:736–43.
21. Lee MG, Ford JL, Hunt PB, et al. Bacterial retention properties of heat and moisture exchange filters. Br J Anaesth. 1992;69:522–5.
22. Vanderbroucke-Grauls CM, Teeuw KB, Ballemans K, Lavooij C, Cornelisse PB, Verhoef J. Bacterial and viral removal efficiency, heat and moisture exchange properties of four filtration devices. J Hosp Infect. 1995;29(1):45–56.
23. Iotti GA, Olivei MC, Braschi A. Mechanical effects of heat–moisture exchangers in ventilated patients. Crit Care. 1999;3:R77–82.
24. Iotti GA, Olivei MC, Palo A, et al. Unfavorable mechanical effects of heat and moisture exchangers in ventilated patients. Intensive Care Med. 1997;23:399–405.

25. Dellamonica J, Boisseau N, Goubaux B, Raucoules-Aime M. Comparison of manufacturers' specifications for 44 types of heat and moisture exchanging filters. Br J Anaesth. 2004;93(4):532–9. https://doi.org/10.1093/bja/aeh239.
26. Le Bourdelles G, Mier L, Fiquet B, Djedaini K, Saumon G, Coste F, Dreyfuss D. Comparison of the effects of heat and moisture exchangers and heated humidifiers on ventilation and gas exchange during weaning trials from mechanical ventilation. Chest. 1996;110(5):1294–8.
27. Hinkson CR, Benson MS, Stephens LM, Deem S. The effects of apparatus dead space on $P(aCO_2)$ in patients receiving lung-protective ventilation. Respir Care. 2006;51(10):1140–4.
28. Campbell RS, Davis K Jr, Johannigman JA, Branson RD. The effects of passive humidifier dead space on Respiratory variables in paralyzed and spontaneously breathing patients. Respir Care. 2000;45(3):306–12.
29. Prat G, Renault A, Tonnelier JM, et al. Influence of the humidification device during acute respiratory distress syndrome. Intensive Care Med. 2003;29:2211–5.
30. Pelosi P, Solca M, Ravagnan I, Tubiolo D, Ferrario L, Gattinoni L. Effects of heat and moisture exchangers on minute ventilation, ventilatory drive, and work of breathing during pressure-support ventilation in acute respiratory failure. Crit Care Med. 1996;24(7):1184–8.
31. Oh TE, Lin ES, Bhatt S. Resistance of humidifiers, and inspiratory work imposed by a ventilator-humidifier circuit. Br J Anaesth. 1991;66(2):258–63.
32. Lucato JJJ, Tucci MR, Schettino GPP, Adams AB, Carolina Fu GF Jr, de Carvalho CRR, de Souza R. Evaluation of resistance in 8 different heat-and-moisture exchangers: effects of saturation and flow rate/profile. Respir Care. 2005;50(5):6.
33. Johnson PA, Raper RF, Fisher MM. The impact of heat and moisture exchanging humidifiers on work of breathing. Anaesth Intensive Care. 1995;23(6):697–701.
34. Pelosi P, Severgnini P, Selmo G, Corradini M, Chiaranda M, Novario R, Park GR. In vitro evaluation of an active heat-and-moisture exchanger: the hygrovent gold. Respir Care. 2010;55(4):460–6.
35. Morgan-Hughes NJ, Mills GH, Northwood D. Air flow resistance of three heat and moisture exchanging filter designs under wet conditions: implications for patient safety. Br J Anaesth. 2001;87(2):289–91.
36. Chung MY, et al. Airway obstruction in HMEF. Anesth Pain Med. 2011;6:96–9.
37. Prat G, Renault A, Tonnelier J-M, Goetghebeur D, Oger E, Boles J-M, L'Her E. Influence of the humidification device during acute respiratory distress syndrome. Intensive Care Med. 2003;29:2211–5.
38. Morán I, Bellapart J, Vari A, Mancebo J. Heat and moisture exchangers and heated humidifiers in acute lung injury/acute respiratory distress syndrome patients: effects on respiratory mechanics and gas exchange. Intensive Care Med. 2006;32:524–31.
39. Jaber S, et al. Comparison of the effects of heat and moisture exchangers and heated humidifiers on ventilation and gas exchange during non-invasive ventilation. Intensive Care Med. 2002;28:1590–4.

Humidification During Invasive Mechanical Ventilation

10

François Lellouche

10.1 Introduction

Humidification of gases delivered to patients on invasive mechanical ventilation has been recommended since the early days of mechanical ventilation in intensive care units [1]. The deleterious impact of dry gases on airway mucosa was described very early [2]. Abundant human and animal literature is available demonstrating a relationship between airway mucosal dysfunction, inflammation, and atelectasis and (i) the level of gas humidity delivered during invasive mechanical ventilation and (ii) the duration of exposure to this gas [3]. There is still an ongoing debate around the optimal level of inspiratory gas humidity. There are several recommendations published on this optimal level of humidification required during invasive mechanical ventilation. Most of these publications are not recent. In general, it is recommended that the humidification systems should provide at least 30 mgH_2O/L for the inspiratory gases [4–8]. Many studies were published that allow us to better determine what a safe level of humidification is. If we consider as a minimum clinical requirement to avoid obstruction of endotracheal tube, slightly lower levels of humidity may be sufficient [9]. However, tube occlusion is a late marker, and impacts on tracheal tube diameter, on mucociliary transport system, and on bronchial inflammation probably occur before tube occlusions. Few authors recommend to use levels of humidity of gas corresponding to the water content in the alveoli or 44 mgH_2O/L which corresponds to 100% of relative humidity at 37 °C [10]. These latter requirements are not usually attained with humidification systems used so far [9, 11]. Until now, no study really did compare stable systems delivering 40 mgH_2O/L

F. Lellouche (✉)
Institut Universitaire de Cardiologie et de Pneumologie de Québec-Université Laval, Centre de recherche, Québec, QC, Canada
e-mail: francois.lellouche@criucpq.ulaval.ca

A. M. Esquinas (ed.), *Humidification in the Intensive Care Unit*,
https://doi.org/10.1007/978-3-031-23953-3_10

with stable systems delivering 30 mgH$_2$O/L. In some clinical situations, such as patients ventilated with ARDS or severe asthma, other criteria than the level of humidification should be considered, in particular, to take into account the mechanical characteristics of the different humidification systems (especially the dead space) [12]. Finally, the issue of the humidification systems' cost cannot be set aside at the time of the choice.

Recently, the SARS-CoV-2 pandemic has shown that both aspects of humidification devices (dead space and humidification properties) may have a relevant impact on the management of ARDS patients [13].

10.2 Hygrometric Performances of the Main Humidification Systems

10.2.1 What Is the Optimal Level of Humidification During Invasive Mechanical Ventilation?

This difficult question has been debated for a long time, and if the answer is more accurate, it has not changed much since 50 years. Chamney in 1969 defined the targets that were required by the humidification systems used in patients intubated or tracheostomized [14]. Among these conditions, the author recommended that the gases reaching the trachea should be between 30 and 36 °C in the range of 30 to 40 mgH$_2$O/L. In an editorial in 1987, "A rational basis for humidity therapy," Chatburn proposed to provide saturated gas at 32–34 °C (33.9–37.7 mgH$_2$O/L), which is the humidity level of the gas at the trachea in healthy subjects [15]. He also concluded in the same editorial that there was no rationale for proposing to issue gas saturated at 37 °C.

Several different organizations have provided recommendations for humidifying gases during invasive mechanical ventilation. The British Standards Institution has recommended providing an absolute humidity of 33 mgH$_2$O/L in 1970 [4]. In 1979, ANSI (American National Standards Institute) has recommended a minimum level of moisture delivered of 30 °C at 100% of relative humidity (i.e., 30.4 mgH$_2$O/L of absolute humidity) with the heated humidifier [5]. In addition, the AARC (American Association for Respiratory Care) recommended a minimum humidity delivered of 30 mgH$_2$O/L with HMEs and between 33 and 44 mgH$_2$O/L with active humidification [8]. ISO 8185 also recommended 30 mg/L for humidification systems in 1988 [6]. Finally, the ISO 8185 standards recommended 33 mgH$_2$O/L, but this standard "does not apply to heat and moisture exchangers" (1.1) [16].

10.2.2 Effects of Under-Humidification of Delivered Gases

There is an abundant literature that describes the impact of under-humidification on airway mucosal and mucociliary transport dysfunction and bronchial inflammation [3]. Epithelial dysfunction modifies the properties of the mucus, leading to intraluminal depositions of viscous mucus, reduction of endotracheal diameter [17, 18], increased tube resistance [19], or endotracheal tube occlusions [9] in a few hours. This may require an emergent change of the endotracheal tube, cardiac arrest, or even death [20]. More frequently, sub-occlusions result in increased resistance of the endotracheal tube [19] and increased respiratory drive and work of breathing, potentially aggravating the lung injuries or delaying weaning.

However, it may not be easy for the clinicians to recognize early signals of under-humidification. On the other hand, endotracheal tube occlusion is a late marker but easy to recognize as it is frequently associated with emergent need to change ETT and is half of the cases associated with cardiac arrest [20, 21]. This potentially fatal complication was very rare and usually below 1% [20, 21].

During the recent pandemic, very high rates of occlusions have been described with COVID-19, up to 72% [22–27]. Some authors had questionable recommendations such as the systematic change of endotracheal tube every week in these patients [25] or the systematic use of ETT cleaning devices [24], procedures at high risk of viral contamination for healthcare workers. The main reason that explained these high rates of ETO was probably the under-humidification of the gases delivered to the patients [28].

Recently, Al Dorzi et al. provided additional evidence that optimization of humidification during mechanical ventilation had a major impact on the rate of endotracheal tube occlusions and other clinical endpoints [29]. After modification of the humidification strategies, the authors report that the rate of endotracheal tube occlusions was strikingly reduced (8.1 vs. 1.0 tube occlusion per 1000 ventilator day). Interestingly, ETO were not suspected in 94.4% of the cases. When compared with 51 matched controls, ETT occlusion cases had significantly longer duration of mechanical ventilation (13.5 vs. 4.0 days; $P = 0.002$) and ICU stay (26.5 vs. 11.0 days; $P = 0.006$) and more tracheostomy (55.6% vs. 9.8%; $P < 0.001$) [29].

10.2.3 Risk Scale for Endotracheal Tube Occlusion

The hygrometric performance of the humidification devices is the first parameter to consider when assessing such systems. There are several hygrometric techniques that make difficult the comparison of the humidification devices. We had the opportunity to measure with the same technique (psychrometric method) the hygrometric performances of a wide variety of humidification systems currently available on the market, the majority of heated humidifiers of previous generations as well as the most recent ones, many heat and moisture exchangers (HME), and the majority of active HME available on the market [9]. Comparing our results with those of the literature (Table 10.1) [17, 30–46], we have designed a risk scale for endotracheal tube occlusion according to the humidification systems used and their conditions of use (Fig. 10.1). Above 28 mgH$_2$O/L of humidity delivered (measured with the psychrometric method), the risk of endotracheal tube occlusion seems to be low [9, 47], when other risk factors of tube obstruction (such as bloody secretions) are not present. We discuss in this chapter the main characteristics of the currently available humidification devices.

Table 10.1 Summary of published studies comparing HME and heated humidifiers (upper table) or evaluating only HMEs (lower table) for which the frequency of catheter occlusion is reported [17, 30–46]. The humidification systems are reported. For HMEs, performance measured by the psychrometric method is reported [9]

	Heated humidifiers			Heat and moisture exchangers			
First author [reference]	Device	Included patients/ occlusions	Percentage of endotracheal tube occlusions	Device	Included patients/ occlusions	Percentage of endotracheal tube occlusions	Absolute humidity (psychrometry) in mgH$_2$O/L
Cohen [30]	Cascade	81/1	1.2	BB2215	170/15	8.8	21.8
Martin [31]	HHBW (32 °C)	42/0	0.0	BB2215	31/6	19.4	21.8
Misset [32]	MR 450 (32–34 °C)	26/2	7.7	BB2215	30/4	13.3	21.8
Roustan [33]	Aquapor (31–32 °C)	61/0	0.0	BB2215	55/9	16.4	21.8
Branson [41]	ConchaTherm III (32–34 °C)	32/0	0.0	Aqua+	88/0	0.0	ND
Dreyfuss [36]	MR 450	70/0	0.0	Hygrobac	61/1	1.6	31.7
Villafane [17]	MR 310 (32 °C)	7/1	14.3	BB2215	8/3	37.5	21.8
				Hygrobac	8/0	0.0	31.7
Boots [35]	MR 730 (37/35)	41/0	0.0	Humid-vent light	75/0	0.0	30.8
Hurni [37]	F&P (32 °C)	56/1	1.8	Hygroster	59/0	0.0	30.7
Kirton [39]	Marquest	140/1	0.7	BB100	140/0	0.0	26.8
Kollef [46]	MR 730 (35–36)	147/0	0.0	Duration	163/0	0.0	NA
Thomachot [40]	Cascade 2 (32 °C)	20/0	0.0	Humid-vent light	9/0	0.0	30.8
Jaber [42]	MR 730 (37/40)	34/2	5.9	Hygrobac	26/1	3.8	31.7
Lacherade [38]	MR 730 (37/40)	185/5	2.7	Hygrobac	185/1	0.5	31.7
Boots [34]	MR 730 (37/40 or 37/35*)	191/0	0.0	Humid-vent light	190/0	0.0	30.8
	Total HH	**1133/13**	**1.1%**	**Total HME 1**	**1298/40**	**3.1%**	

Study						
			Total HME 1 (excluding BB2215)	**814/3**	**0.4%**	
Thomachot [45]			Humid-vent light	66/1	1.5	30.8
			BB100	70/1	1.4	26.8
Thomachot [44]			Humid-vent	77/1	1.3	30.8
			Clear-Therm	63/0	0.0	26.2
Boisson [68]			MaxiPleat	12/0	0.0	20.1
Davis [78]			Aqua+ (24 h)	100/0	0.0	NA
			Duration (120 h)	60/0	0.0	NA
			Aqua+ (120 h)	60/0	0.0	NA
Markowicz [103]			Hygrobac	21/0	0.0	31.7
			Humid-vent	20/0	0.0	30.8
			Clear-Therm	20/0	0.0	26.2
Ricard [77]			Hygrobac	33/0	0.0	31.7
Thomachot [43]			Thermovent Hepa+ (1j)	84/0	0.0	27.8
			Thermovent Hepa+ (7 days)	71/0	0.0	27.8
Boyer [111]			EdithFlex	22/0	0.0	NA
			Hygrolife	21/0	0.0	NA
			Total HME 2	**800/0**	**0.4%**	
			Total HME 1 + 2	**2098/43**	**2.0%**	
Total HH	**1133/13**	**1.1%**	**Total HME 1 + 2 (excluding BB2215)**	**1614/6**	**0.4%**	

NA not available

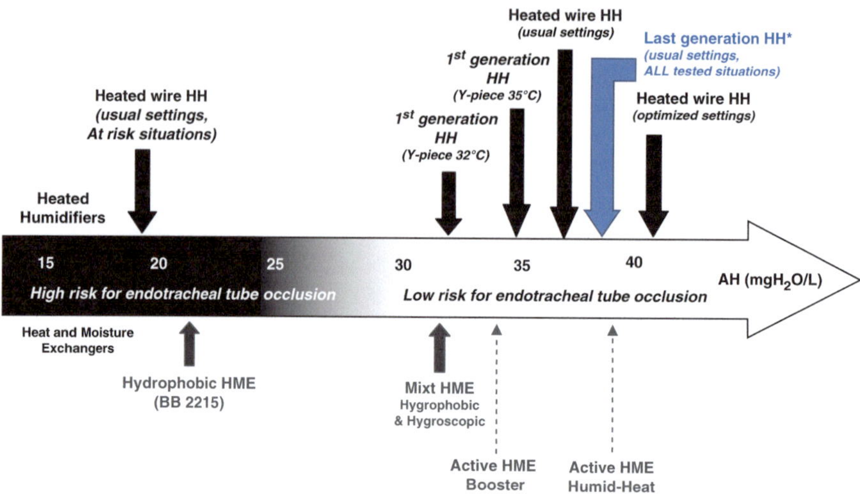

Fig. 10.1 Psychrometric risk scale. Position of different humidification systems in connection with their humidification performance based on the same technique of measurement (psychrometric method) (personal data combined with the literature data) [9, 11, 23, 28, 51, 52, 69, 71, 118]. Between 25 and 30 mgH$_2$O/L of absolute humidity is a gray zone where the risk of occlusion exists but is less known. Under 25 mgH$_2$O/L, that risk is probably important [17, 30–33], and above 30 mgH$_2$O/L, the risk is low [36, 38, 77, 102]. Furthermore, there is a potential risk of over-humidification with systems with the highest performances in terms of hygrometry [114]. However, this risk is currently difficult to estimate. The "at-risk situations" is high ambient or ventilator temperature which are associated with low humidification performances with these devices. The last-generation HH stands for recent HH with advanced closed-loop regulations (that incorporate ambient temperature, inlet temperature, heater plate temperature, humidity sensor, etc.). *Heated humidifiers FP950 (Fisher & Paykel) and VHB20 (Vincent Medical) were tested on bench with ambient temperature from 20 to 30 °C and minute ventilation at 10 and 15 L/min and provide highly humidified gases (between 31 and 39 mgH$_2$O/L) under all tested conditions. *HH* heated humidifiers, *HME* heat and moisture exchangers

10.2.4 Heated Humidifiers' Humidification Performances

Heated humidifiers are usually considered as the most efficient systems in terms of humidification performances. This conviction must be qualified. It has been shown that the performances of heated humidifiers with heated wires vary widely, from 20 to 40 mgH$_2$O/L, and are influenced by external conditions, particularly ambient and ventilator outlet temperatures [11]. When these temperatures are high, inlet chamber temperature is high leading to the reduction of the heater plate temperature. Indeed, with these humidifiers, the regulation of the heater plate temperature aims at maintaining a constant humidification chamber temperature (usually set at 37 °C). The temperature of the water in the humidification chamber is related to the heater plate temperature. Water with a low temperature will not produce moisture. Consequently, there is a strong inverse relationship between the inlet chamber temperature and the humidification performances (Fig. 10.2) [11]. Thus, the very low

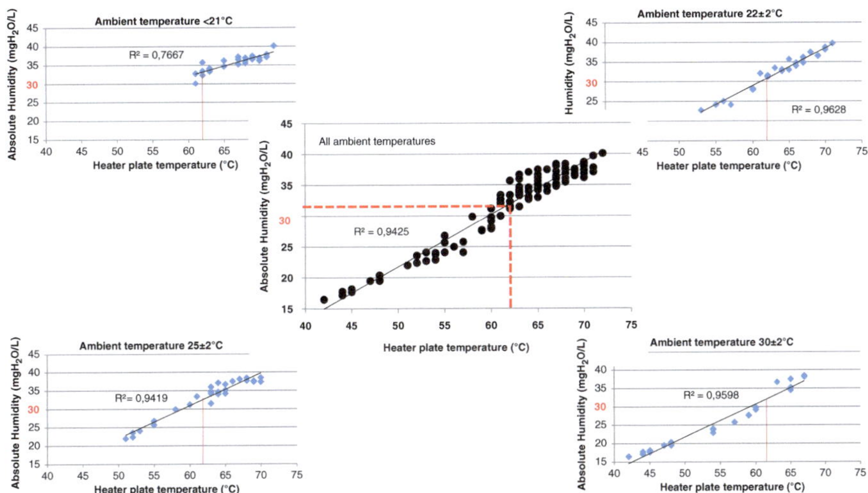

Fig. 10.2 Correlation between heated wire humidifier performance and heater plate temperature. A very close correlation was found between humidifier performance (absolute humidity [mgH₂O/L] of inspiratory gas) and heater plate temperature (°C). This correlation was hardly modified by ambient temperature. The monitoring of this parameter should be promoted in the case of sticky secretions or situations at risk (from reference 23). Above heater plate temperature of 62°C, the absolute humidity delivered is most frequently above 30 mgH O/L. In a recent study we showed that this relation is influenced by minute ventilation (reference 60)

humidity levels (around 20 mgH₂O/L and even lower), described as being likely to cause endotracheal tube obstruction, are delivered by these systems in the most adverse conditions (high ambient temperature, turbine ventilators delivering high temperatures, and high minute ventilation) [48]. These humidity levels are comparable to or even lower than those measured with the HME BB2215, with which the incidence of endotracheal tube occlusions ranged from 10 to 20% [17, 30–33]. Furthermore, even in favorable situations (normal ambient and ventilator temperatures), measured performances are below what is advertised by manufacturers (44 mgH₂O/L) [11, 49]. This again argues for an independent evaluation of humidification systems [9, 50].

In another study, we evaluated the influence of ambient temperature and ventilator output temperature for many heated humidifiers, particularly those of previous generations without heated wire (requiring water traps in the ventilator circuits) [51]. This study showed that for settings equivalent to heated humidifiers with heated wire (35 and 37 °C at the Y-piece), the heated humidifiers without heated wire (i) have more stable hygrometric performances with little influence from external conditions and (ii) deliver gases with inspiratory absolute humidity levels above 30 mgH₂O/L. In contrast, (iii) for more traditional settings (32 °C), the performances of these systems were near the limit of 30 mgH₂O/L and sometimes below.

We also evaluated heated humidifiers with different technologies (counter-flow heated humidifier) and devices incorporating an algorithm to reduce the risk of under-humidification [52]. We found significant improvements with the algorithm that compensates for low humidity with the MR 850 (Fisher & Paykel) and good performances with the humidifier HC 200 (Hamilton Medical) to obtain inspiratory water content between 35 and 40 mgH$_2$O/L, with moderate influence of ambient and ventilator temperatures, flows, and tidal volumes used [52]. Similar data have been published for counter-flow heated humidifiers [53]. In addition to compensation algorithm, specific settings that increase the temperature of the humidification chamber (and reduce the gap with the Y-piece temperature) can be used to prevent from under-humidification on most several models of heated wire humidifier.

Recently, several new heated humidifiers with advanced algorithm have been launched. The new FP950 (Fisher & Paykel) has been evaluated on bench, and it was shown that whatever the conditions of ambient temperature (from 20 to 30 °C), the mean absolute humidity delivered was around 35 mgH$_2$O/L [54]. We also evaluated the new humidifier VHB20 (Vincent Medical) on bench and found that humidity delivered was above 35 mgH$_2$O/L, even when ambient temperature was above 25 °C [55].

Even if the humidification performance improves with most recent heated humidifiers (with new algorithms and specific settings), the problem of condensation in the circuit remains in spite of heated wires in certain circumstances. This question has been raised since a long time with the heated humidifiers [56], and the objective of heated wires was to limit this risk. Yet, the frequency of condensation in the inspiratory circuit is high [57], especially with the turbine ventilators and in case of low or variable ambient temperatures [58]. New "porous" expiratory circuits limit the problem in the expiratory circuit, while in the inspiratory circuit, this issue is still there. The interest of the "porous" circuits is to reduce the water content in the expiratory limb, which could limit the risk of condensation of gases that carries potential interference with measures of expiratory flow with some pneumotachograph [59].

Clinicians must be aware of these technical issues to interpret specific clinical situations (i.e., thick secretions or endotracheal tube occlusion or sub-occlusion in spite of heated humidifier use). When used in normal conditions, heated humidifiers are performing systems. Normal conditions mean (i) stable and moderate ambient temperature (south-facing rooms with sun on the humidifier may be a problematic situation!) and (ii) moderate output ventilator temperature with a specific precaution in case of turbine ventilator use.

Based on new data that demonstrate an excellent correlation between heater plate temperature and humidity delivered (with MR 850) [60], this parameter should be used to monitor the performances of the humidifiers when under-humidification is suspected (high ambient temperature, thick secretions, endotracheal tube occlusions or sub-occlusions).

During the COVID-19 pandemic, endotracheal tube occlusions have been described even with heated humidifiers [13, 24, 26]. In one US center, it was recommended to switch off the humidifier to avoid aerosolization [26]. We measured humidity delivered of 7.8 mgH$_2$O/L with such condition (corresponding to cold humidification) which is not acceptable even for few hours [28]. There are several studies that reported ETO even when heated humidifiers were used. In the largest cohort of patients, 11 endotracheal tube occlusions occurred out of 187 patients managed for COVID-19 [24]. Seven cases were related to poor-performing HME [28], while four were related to HH [24]. In a study comparing two humidification strategies to manage this population, three endotracheal tube occlusions occurred within few weeks, while HH were used, due to high ambient air in the rooms with recently installed negative pressure devices [23]. A strategy to avoid under-humidification stopped the epidemic of tube occlusions: heated humidifier performances were regularly evaluated with heater plate temperature monitoring, the air conditioning system was changed to control the ambient temperature, and compensation algorithm of the HH was activated [61].

10.2.5 Heat and Moisture Exchangers' Humidification Performances

10.2.5.1 Comparison with the Literature on the Risk of Tracheal Occlusion (Fig. 10.3)

Heat and moisture exchangers (HMEs) are the most commonly used humidification devices in Europe [62] and are being increasingly used in North America [63].

As for heated humidifiers, many technological improvements have led to the emergence of new models of performing HME on the market. The very first

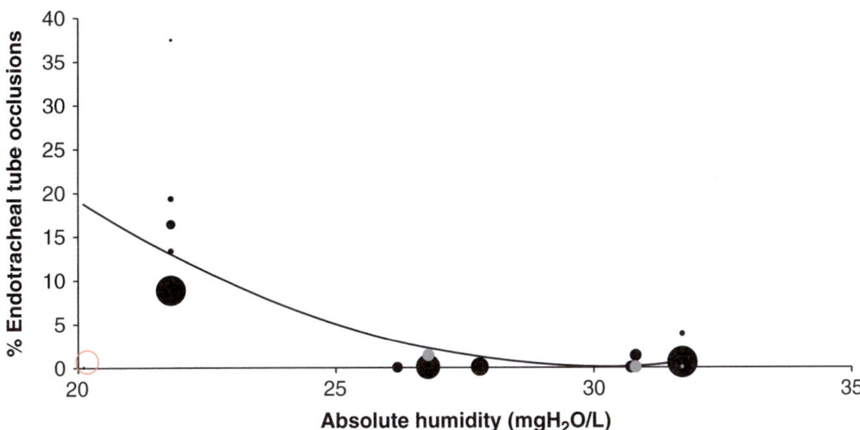

Fig. 10.3 Frequency of endotracheal tube occlusions reported in the literature with heat and moisture exchangers [17, 30–46, 77] in relation with the absolute humidity delivered by the HMEs measured using the bench test apparatus (see Table 10.1) (from reference 9). One study (red circle) is an outlier [68] with no endotracheal occlusions despite very poor humidification. However, this study only included 12 patients, which is not enough to reach a conclusion about the safety of the device tested. A hydrophobic HME (Pall BB2215), which delivered a measured absolute humidity of 21.8 ± 1.5 mgH₂O/L, has been associated with high rates of endotracheal tube occlusions in five previously published studies [17, 30–33] (Table 10.1). A number of studies are represented by gray dots to make them stand out. The sizes of the dots are proportional to the number of patients in the studies

metallic HMEs were not disposable and generated significant resistance [64–66]. The first disposable HME was available in 1976 and was used during anesthesia [67]. The first HMEs proposed for ICU patients (hygroscopic HME) had insufficient humidification performances, responsible for their poor reputation [17, 30–33]. This poor reputation is not justified anymore. Improved materials have reduced the size of HMEs and improved their performances. We conducted a large-scale evaluation of the humidification performances of 48 devices (HME, HMEF, antibacterial filters) [9]. The main result was the heterogeneous performances of these systems. Antibacterial filters should not be used to humidify gases. However, some of the filters have fairly similar appearance compared with HME or HMEF, but water contents are very different, with the possibility of confusion. The most efficient HMEs provide humidity of inspired gases slightly above 30 mgH_2O/L, but some systems proposed for airway humidification provide water contents below 25 and sometimes below 20 mgH_2O/L. Moreover, comparing with data from manufacturers, we have observed some significant differences, which again call for independent evaluations.

We used data from this study and from the literature to try to assess the humidification level associated with a risk of endotracheal tube occlusions. The BB2215 device with performance of about 22 mgH_2O/L resulted in a significant increased risk of occlusions [17, 30–33]. HMEs providing absolute humidity above 25 mgH_2O/L seem to be at lower risk. But there is little data with humidification systems with intermediate performance (between 25 and 30 mgH_2O/L); the few studies available show that the risk of catheter occlusion is also low in that zone [39, 43, 45]. However, it is likely that this risk is directly linked to the hygrometric performances. Although no formal data exist on the risk of occlusion around 25 mgH_2O/L, caution is warranted and it is recommended to approach or exceed 30 mgH_2O/L to minimize these risks.

In the literature, there are several conflicting studies with the previous results. In the study of Boisson et al. [68], no occlusion occurred while a low-performing hydrophobic HME was used (absolute humidity just above 20 mgH_2O/L). But this study had included only 12 patients. While the main issue is safety, we cannot conclude positively considering the small number of patients. Moreover, Kapadia et al. [20, 21] reported the incidence of endotracheal tube occlusions over a series of nearly 8000 patients during a period of 5 years. While the HMEs used were BB2215 (22 mgH_2O/L) and Cleartherm (26 mgH_2O/L), the frequency of occlusions was "only" 0.16%. In analyzing the results, it appears that the average duration of mechanical ventilation was less than 2 days, which probably explains the low rate of occlusion in this study. The duration of ventilation must obviously be taken into consideration when analyzing the risk of endotracheal tube occlusion. Thus, these discordant publications should not be reassuring. During the COVID-19 pandemic, several studies reported endotracheal tube occlusions in patients on invasive mechanical ventilation (Table 10.2). The high rate of tube occlusion may be explained by several factors including prolonged durations of intubation in this population, reduction of suctioning frequency, and utilization of low-performing HME [28]. In a recent study, the ISO 9360 standard used to ensure ECH

Table 10.2 Studies reporting endotracheal tube occlusions in COVID-19 patients. Rate of endotracheal tube occlusions, type of humidification device, and absolute humidity according to the manufacturer and measured on bench with the psychrometric method

Authors (reference)	No. of patients with COVID-19	Rate of ETO	Humidification device used	AH (mgH$_2$O/L) according to the manufacturer (ISO)	AH (mgH$_2$O/L) measured with psychrometric method
Lavoie-Bérard et al. [23]	6 HME 14 HH	HME: 0 (0%) HH: 3 (21%)	HME[a] HH (MR 850)	Hygrobac S: 33.6	Hygrobac S: 28.9 ± 1.1 MR 850 (normal AT): 35.2 ± 1.8 MR 850 (high AT): 23.4 ± 2.4
Wiles et al. [24]	187	12 (6.4%)	HME (7 ETO)[b] HH (4 ETO)	Medline: 31.0 SunMed: 33.4	Medline: 25.1 ± 0.6 SunMed: 25.4 ± 0.4
Rubano et al. [25]	110	28 (25%)	?	NA	NA
Perez Acosta et al. [22]	22	16 (72%)	?	NA	NA
Panchamian et al. [115]	48	14 (29%)	HME[c] (anesthesia machines)	Aero-pro (not reported) AirLife Edith 1000: 30.0	Aero-pro: NA AirLife Edith 1000: NA
Zaidi and Narasimhan [26]	?	"Frequent ETO"	HH turned off	NA	MR 850 off: 7.8 ± 0.2
Bottirolli et al. [27]	17	3 (18%), 1 death	HME (anesthesia machines)	NA	NA
Sugimoto et al. [116]	Case report	1	HME[d]	Inter-Therm: 32.3	Inter-Therm: 26.9 ± 0.6
Van Boven et al. [117]	Case reports	2	HME[e]	Hydro-guard: 23.0	NA

[a] DAR™ Adult – pediatric electrostatic filter HME (small) (previously Hygrobac S)
[b] Sunmed FH603008 and the Medline DYNJAAHME1B
[c] Aero-Pro™ HEPA Light Machine and AirLife® Edith 1000
[d] Inter-Therm, Intersurgical
[e] Hydro-Guard, Intersurgical
ETO Endotracheal Tube Occlusion, *HME* Heat and Moisture Exchanger, *HH* Heated Humidifier, *AH* Absolute Humidity, *AT* Ambient Temperature

manufacturers' market devices that provide minimal humidity to intubated patients has been called into question. Indeed, this method and standard failed to detect poor-performing HMEs that were responsible for ETO [28]. All HMEs responsible for ETO during the pandemic passed the ISO 9360 test (mean ± SD delivered absolute humidity with ISO = 32.2 ± 1.2 mgH$_2$O/L), while they all performed very poorly on the hygrometric test bench (mean ± SD delivered absolute humidity with psychrometric method to evaluate humidity = 25.8 ± 1.0 mgH$_2$O/L).The main message is the heterogeneity of the performances of the HME on the market and that the data provided by the manufacturers may not be helpful in choosing the right device based on the current ISO standards [9].

10.2.5.2   Impact of External Conditions on HME's Hygrometric Performances

HMEs are more stable and less influenced by environmental conditions but may be influenced by patient's core temperature. We studied the impact of ambient temperature on HME and showed that high ambient temperature did not affect HME performances [69]. Croci et al. showed with hydrophobic HMEs that low ambient temperature (20 °C vs. 26 °C) slightly reduces their efficiency (21 vs. 23 mgH$_2$O/L) [70].

HME's performances may be significantly influenced by the patient's core temperature. Indeed, with these devices, the quantity of water delivered to the patient during inspiration is highly dependent on the amount of water present in the exhaled gas (Fig. 10.4). In patients with induced hypothermia to 32 °C [71], the expiratory water content is about 27 mgH$_2$O/L, while it is about 35 mgH$_2$O/L in patients with a normal core temperature [71, 72]. Therefore, even best-performing HMEs can

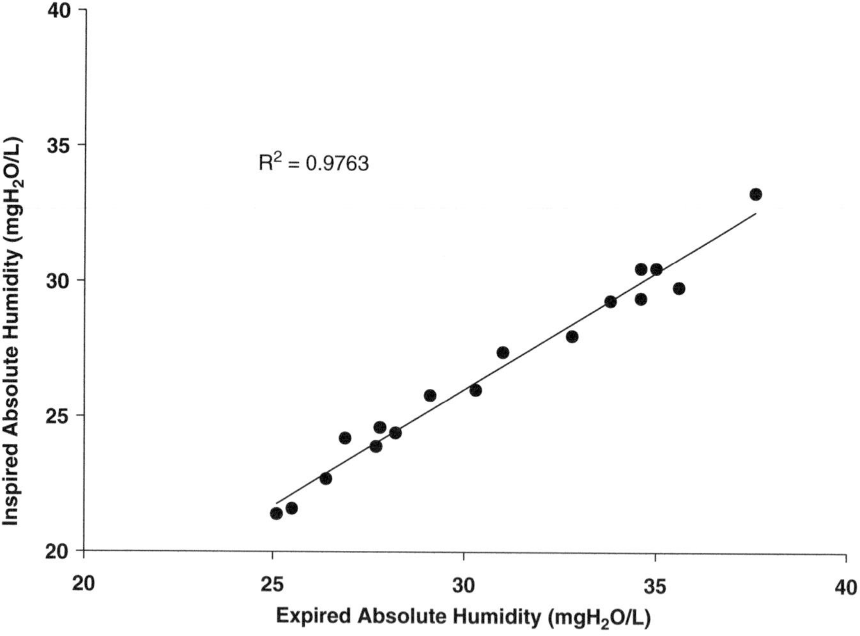

Fig. 10.4 Correlation between inspired and expired absolute humidity of the gas (expressed in mgH$_2$O/L) with heat and moisture exchangers. A strong correlation exists between inspired and expired gas hygrometry with heat and moisture exchangers. With the high-performing heat and moisture exchangers used in this study, the rate of inspired humidity corresponded to 87% of expired humidity [71]

only deliver inspiratory gases with water content around 25 mgH₂O/L during hypothermia. In this situation, even heated humidifiers provided non-optimal levels, and the moisture target is uncertain during hypothermia.

HME's performances can be reduced in case of high minute ventilation [73, 74]. This has been described with hydrophobic HMEs, but most recent hydrophobic and hygroscopic HMEs do not seem to be influenced by the level of minute ventilation [69].

10.2.5.3 Other Parameters to Evaluate Airway Humidification Impact

Furthermore, we must wonder about the value of this clinical parameter, that is, the occlusion of endotracheal tube, used in most studies. This parameter is easy to detect, but it represents only the easily visible part of the problem. Studies using other parameters are difficult to interpret because they compare humidification systems with close performances and few provide humidification measurements to better understand what is effectively compared. Studies from Hurni et al. [37] and Nakagawa et al. [75] used original techniques (cytology of bronchial cells in one case and rheological properties of secretions in another) and compared HME with first-generation heated humidifiers. But the performances of these systems are very similar (probably within 5 mgH₂O/L), which does not allow demonstrating significant difference. Moreover, the study of Jaber et al. [42] using the acoustic method to evaluate the resistance of endotracheal tube with HME and HH (with heated wire) did not provide humidity data. Again, this makes it difficult to interpret these results, especially as humidifiers used in this study had no compensation system and that their humidification performances are highly variable [11]. To note, during the same time, a study showed a non-significant increased risk of endotracheal tube occlusion with heated wire heated humidifiers compared to HME (2.7% vs. 0.5%, $P = 0.12$) [38]. In these studies comparing the HME to HH and more generally in the literature, there is an implicit starting premise that HH outperform HME. We have shown that it cannot be used as a given, especially with humidifiers with heated wire [76].

Another issue with HMEs is their obstruction or occlusion with plugged secretions. In the study by Ricard et al. with HME elevated above the endotracheal tube to limit the passage of secretions in the device, this risk was 10% despite a period of prolonged use of HMEs up to 7 days [77]. Replacement of HMEs secondary to obstruction was 15% in the study of Kollef et al. [46]; again HME could be used up to 7 days. In the study by Davis et al. where there were no specific precautions, the frequency of partial occlusion was 3% when the HMEs were changed every 24 h and 9% when the HMEs were changed every 5 days [78]. In the same study, resistances of 12 partially occluded HMEs were measured [78]. The devices' resistances increased from a mean of 1.1 before use to 2.8 cmH₂O/L/s. The highest resistance involved two cases of partial occlusion by hemorrhagic secretions where the resistance went from 0.85 before use to 5.8 cmH₂O/L/s. This increase in resistance of the HME or of the endotracheal tube associated with inadequate humidification or thick secretions may delay weaning patients and remains a real problem.

10.2.5.4 Active HME

The place of active HME is probably very limited. This type of device was first described in 1992 by Kapadia et al. [79] The Booster™ is positioned between the HME and the patient. A metal part is covered with a membrane that allows to heat external water. The membrane made of Gore-Tex™ allows the production of water vapor. This system can be used with any HME in order to improve their performance [80]. Another system, the Humid-Heat™, is based on a similar principle, with a heated humidifier piece surrounding a specific HME, also with a supply of extra water [81]. A third "active" HME has been described, the "performer," running on the same principle [82]. The latter was evaluated with the psychrometric method in the study conducted by Chiumello et al., which allows a comparison with our results. The system delivered inspiratory gases with a water content from 3 to 5 mgH_2O/L above HME with good performance [69, 82]. The active HME tested had higher humidification performances in comparison with effective HMEs: a gain of approximately 3 mgH_2O/L with Booster™ and about 5 mgH_2O/L with the Humid-Heat™ under standard conditions of use. However, the clinical benefit to increase humidity from 30 to 35 mgH_2O/L is not clear in the literature. In comparison with best-performing HMEs, the potential benefits of a few extra mgH_2O/L versus added complexity and cost without removing dead space make the use of active ECH questionable.

10.3 Mechanical Proprieties of Humidification Systems (Resistances and Dead Space)

In addition to the humidification properties, mechanical aspects of HME and HH (especially resistance and dead space) must be taken into consideration in specific clinical situations. There is significant heterogeneity of the dead space and resistance among humidification devices [9, 47, 83–85]. The dead space more than the resistance between HME and HH should be considered. Indeed, humidification systems' resistances are fairly similar [86]. The HH circuit's resistance is not negligible, especially if the heated wire is in the circuit. Resistance is probably less if the heated wire is integrated into the wall. Several studies showed that during assisted ventilation, HME increased the work of breathing and the minute ventilation and decreased alveolar ventilation in comparison with HH [87–92]. During controlled ventilation, HMEs decrease the alveolar ventilation in comparison with HH [92–98]. In patients with ARDS, it is possible to obtain the same alveolar ventilation with lower tidal volumes when using heated humidifiers due to the reduction of the instrumental dead space. In Moran study, when replacing the HME by a heated humidifier, with the same alveolar ventilation target, it was possible to reduce the tidal volume from 521 ± 106 to 440 ± 118 ml ($p < 0.001$) without significant changes in $PaCO_2$, and plateau airway pressure decreased from 25 ± 6 to 21 ± 6 cmH_2O ($p < 0.001$) [94]. Similar data were shown in Pitoni study in ARDS patients with brain injury [98].

The use of a heated humidifier in order to reduce dead space has a real impact mainly in patients in whom a ventilator strategy including "permissive hypercapnia" is required (especially in cases of ARDS or severe asthma). This is especially true during ARDS, as the high respiratory rate increases the dead space effect [12, 99, 100]. During a spontaneous breathing trial, performed with minimal pressure support levels, the interpretation of the breathing pattern should take into account the humidification system used [87, 101]. To compensate for the HME's dead space, the minimum level of pressure support should be increased by about 5 to 8 cmH$_2$O in comparison with a spontaneous breathing trial conducted in pressure support with a heated humidifier [87, 89, 91].

10.4 Comparison of Humidification Devices' Cost

Several studies have compared the costs of different humidification systems [32, 35–37, 41, 46, 77, 102–104]. The comprehensive studies are difficult to perform and should take into account the following:

1. The costs of devices and circuits.
2. The human costs: time to set up heated humidifiers, time to change HMEs, and time to empty the water traps (when heated wires are not used).
3. The miscellaneous costs: cleaning, storage, and maintenance of humidifiers, water used in humidifiers, water traps, etc.

Not surprisingly, most evaluations have shown that the costs associated with heated humidifiers are much larger compared with the HME. Branson et al. compared HME with heated humidifiers with and without heated wire [104]. In this study, the use of heated humidification without heated circuit caused a heavy workload in relation to water trap emptying (on average nine times per 24 h), a procedure whose duration was estimated to 5 min. Therefore, 45 min per day was spent to empty water traps with this system. The cost of using heated humidifiers (with or without heated wire) was much larger than the HMEs in this study (Table 10.3). Moreover, during this study, HMEs were changed every 24 h. With less frequent changes (every 2 to 3 days and up to 7 days), the daily costs of these devices are even lower [43, 77, 78, 102, 103].

The duration of ventilator circuit use was 24 h in the study of Craven who challenged this practice [56]. Other studies followed and showed that the spacing change and even the lack of change for the same patient resulted in a reduction of costs and especially the rate of ventilator-acquired pneumonia [105–109], which went against the generally accepted idea. The question of duration of use of HMEs follows the same path, but there is still a fear of prolonged use of these devices based on the

Table 10.3 Daily cost for different humidification devices (in US dollars (from reference 104))

Humidification device	Day 1	Day 2	Day 3	Day 4	Day 5
HME	5.2	4.6	4.5	4.4	4.7
HH with heated wire	30.2	16.1	12.6	9.9	9.0
HH without heated wire	27.8	21.7	19.6	18.6	18.0

HH heated humidifiers, *HME* heat and moisture exchangers

risks of poorer humidification performance and of increased resistance of the HMEs. Most manufacturers recommend changing these devices every 24 h. Yet many studies have argued for lifetimes greater than 24 h [40, 43, 46, 68, 77, 78, 102, 103, 110, 111] and up to 7 days [43, 46, 77]. With prolonged use, humidification performances do not change a lot with the most efficient HMEs, with the exception of the results in Ricard et al. study that showed in 3 COPD patients over 10 included, a reduction over time of HME's effectiveness with absolute humidity below 27 mgH$_2$O/L (with a minimum of 24.9 mgH$_2$O/L in a patient on day 5) after several days of use [77]. However, among 23 other patients without COPD included and the majority of COPD patients, the values of absolute humidity measured daily remained stable during the 7 days of use. Similarly, no endotracheal tube occlusion has occurred with this practice. In this same study, the resistances of the devices were not significantly changed after use [77].

In addition to the maximum duration of a single HME, the issue of the maximum duration of use of this humidification system in patients with prolonged ventilation has been raised. Branson et al. have proposed an algorithm which limited the use of HME to a maximum of 5 days [41, 112], replacing them with a heated humidifier after this period. There is no clear data now to limit the duration of HME use. Numerous studies have demonstrated that prolonged use of HME did not result in any particular risk for patients [36, 38, 113]. Especially in the study conducted by Lacherade et al., who compared HME and HH on the rate of ventilator-acquired pneumonia, the duration of use was 2 weeks on average in the HME group ($n = 185$) without specific problems being noted [38]. The rate of ventilator-acquired pneumonia (28.8% vs. 25.4%, $P = 0.48$), the duration of mechanical ventilation (14.9 ± 15.1 vs. 13.5 ± 16.3, $P = 0.36$), and the mortality (34.2% vs. 32.8%, NS) were similar. A trend for more endotracheal tube occlusion was noted in the heated humidifier group in comparison with HME group (6 vs. 1, $P = 0.12$).

10.5 Conclusion (Table 10.4 and Fig. 10.5)

Humidification of the gases delivered to the patients while upper airways are bypassed is mandatory *at all times* in intubated patients to avoid severe complications related to under-humidification, from mucus thickening to deadly endotracheal tube occlusions.

Table 10.4 Advantage and drawbacks for different humidification devices

Humidification device	Humidification performances	Circuit condensation (I/E)	Dead space	Resistance	Cost
Passive HME	− to ++	0/0	+ to +++	+	−
Active HME	++	0/0	++	+	+
Heated humidifier	− to +++	0 to ++/0 to +	0	0[a] to +	+
This system still does not exist	+++	0/0	0	0	−

[a] If heated wire are within the circuit wall
HME heat and moisture exchangers

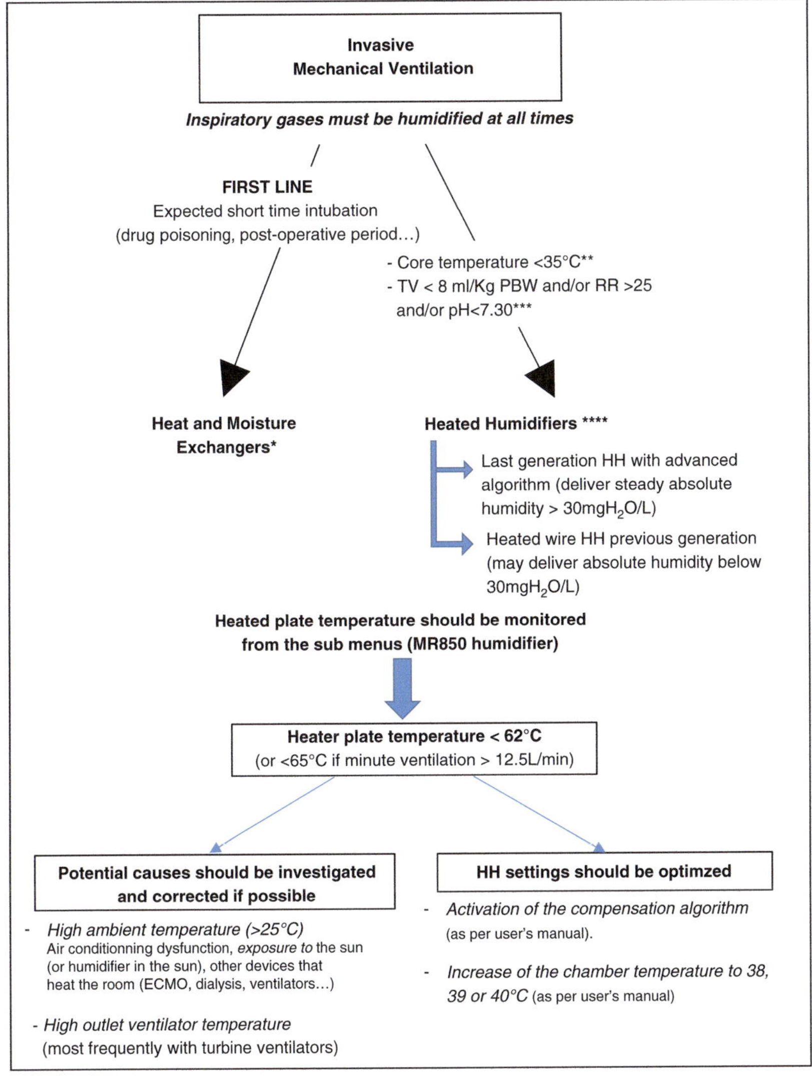

Fig. 10.5 Recommendations for humidification management during invasive mechanical ventilation. *Using a HME delivering at least 28 mgH₂O/L based on independent evaluation [9]. **The other contraindications of HME are the presence of bronchopleural fistula, hemoptysis/bloody secretions, or intoxication with substances with respiratory elimination. ***In the event of threatening hypercapnic or mixed acidosis with pH < 7.30 and when there is a risk of auto-PEEP limiting the increase in respiratory rate. When the minute ventilation before intubation was high (measured or estimated). ****Situations at risk of malfunction with heated humidifiers with heating wire should be avoided (using them in high ambient temperatures, humidifiers being directly exposed to the sun, utilization of turbine ventilators with high outlet temperature). Monitoring where possible of the HH heater plate's temperature (if heater plate temperature > 62 °C for the MR 850, the absolute humidity is probably adequate). Heater Plate Monitoring Video: (126) Monitoring of MR 850 humidification performances with heater plate temperature - YouTube. **Optimization of HH settings video:** (126) How to increase outlet chamber temperature on MR850 to improve humidity delivery - YouTube. *HH* Heated Humidifier, *TV* Tidal Volume, *RR* Respiratory Rate, *PBW* Predicted Body Weight

The choice of a humidification system during mechanical ventilation should take into account the humidification performance, of course, but also the mechanical properties and finally the cost of the device. For the majority of the patients, a good-performing HME can be used when mechanical ventilation is initiated. Clinicians should be aware of the wide heterogeneity in humidification performance among available devices and the inability to detect underperforming HMEs with current ISO standards. For specific situations, when instrumental dead space reduction is considered, especially when lung-protective ventilation is implemented with low tidal volumes and high respiratory rates [12], utilization of heated humidifiers is a better choice. Clinicians have to be aware of the impact of external conditions and especially ambient or outlet ventilator temperature (heated humidifiers) or patient core temperature (heat and moisture exchangers) on the humidification device performances.

Heated humidifiers with heated wire have very reduced performance if the inlet temperature of the humidification chamber is high, which can happen when the ambient temperature is high (absence of air conditioning or humidifier "in the sun") or when the outlet temperature of ventilator is high (using turbine ventilators). This issue is partially improved with compensation algorithm and with specific technologies (counter-flow humidifiers), but these systems are not available in all countries. The monitoring of the heater plate temperature with MR 850 may help clinicians to ensure adequate humidity is delivered to patients [60]. With last generation of heated humidifiers, humidity delivered seems steady around 35–40 mgH_2O/L or slightly above, and the question of the over-humidification is raised, and clinicians must be aware of this potential risk, which did not exist with previous systems [114].

The performances of *humidifiers without heated wire* are influenced by the settings as expected but are much less influenced by external conditions. Recommended settings with those humidifiers (Y-piece temperature around 30 to 32 °C) deliver gas around 30 mgH_2O/L or slightly above.

Heat and moisture exchangers have very heterogeneous humidification performances, and only a few reach 30 mgH_2O/L. Systems with similar external appearance can have very different humidification performances, which may be responsible for potentially serious confusion. The HME performance is mainly influenced by the expiratory humidity which is mainly related to patient's core temperature. In hypothermic patient whose water content of the expiratory gas is lower than the normothermic patients, HMEs have poor performance. However, there is a lack of clinical data for short-term periods of hypothermia (as for therapeutic hypothermia after cardiac arrest that is usually used for 24 h). The additional instrumental dead space with HME causes a reduction in alveolar ventilation. This may have an impact particularly in patients with protective ventilatory strategy (low tidal volume and high respiratory rate). In these cases, heated humidifiers should be used instead of HMEs. Also, HME can increase the work of breathing during assisted ventilation, which may be an issue for severe COPD patients, and the minimal level of pressure support used for spontaneous breathing trials should be 10 to 12 rather than 5 to 7 cmH_2O if a HME is used.

There is not much argument for using an active HME when effective HMEs exist, and the added complexity of these devices may not be worth it.

Independent data on humidification systems' performance should be known by the users [9, 50]. In addition, the other characteristics that differentiate HMEs and heated humidifiers (mainly resistance, dead space, and costs) must be known by the clinician to choose the optimal humidification system for the patients on mechanical ventilation.

References

1. Lassen HC. A preliminary report on the 1952 epidemic of poliomyelitis in Copenhagen with special reference to the treatment of acute respiratory insufficiency. Lancet. 1953;1:37–41.
2. Burton JDK. Effect of dry anaesthetic gases on the respiratory mucus membrane. Lancet. 1962;1:235.
3. Williams R, Rankin N, Smith T, Galler D, Seakins P. Relationship between the humidity and temperature of inspired gas and the function of the airway mucosa. Crit Care Med. 1996;24:1920–9.
4. British Standards Institution. Specifications for humidifiers for use with breathing machines. London: BS 4494; 1970.
5. American National Standards Institute. Standard for humidifiers and nebulizers for medical use. ASI. 1979;Z79(9):8.
6. International Organization of Standards. Humidifiers for medical use. ISO 8185 1988;60:14.
7. AARC clinical practice guideline. Humidification during mechanical ventilation. American Association for Respiratory Care. Respir Care. 1992;37:887–90.
8. American Association for Respiratory C, Restrepo RD, Walsh BK. Humidification during invasive and noninvasive mechanical ventilation: 2012. Respir Care. 2012;57:782–8.
9. Lellouche F, Taille S, Lefrancois F, et al. Humidification performance of 48 passive airway humidifiers: comparison with manufacturer data. Chest. 2009;135:276–86.
10. Ryan SN, Rankin N, Meyer E, Williams R. Energy balance in the intubated human airway is an indicator of optimal gas conditioning. Crit Care Med. 2002;30:355–61.
11. Lellouche L, Taillé S, Maggiore SM, et al. Influence of ambient air and ventilator output temperature on performances of heated-wire humidifiers. Am J Respir Crit Care Med. 2004;170:1073–9.
12. Lellouche F, Delorme M, Brochard L. Impact of respiratory rate and dead space in the current era of lung protective mechanical ventilation. Chest. 2020;158(1):45–7.
13. Lavoie-Berard CA, Lefebvre JC, Bouchard PA, Simon M, Lellouche F. Impact of airway humidification strategy in the mechanically ventilated COVID-19 patients. Respir Care. 2021;67(2):157–66.
14. Chamney AR. Humidification requirements and techniques. Including a review of the performance of equipment in current use. Anaesthesia. 1969;24:602–17.
15. Chatburn RL, Primiano FP Jr. A rational basis for humidity therapy. Respir Care. 1987;32:249–54.
16. International Organization of Standards. Humidifiers for medical use. General requirements for humidification systems. ISO 8185 1997.
17. Villafane MC, Cinnella G, Lofaso F, et al. Gradual reduction of endotracheal tube diameter during mechanical ventilation via different humidification devices. Anesthesiology. 1996;85:1341–9.
18. Mietto C, Pinciroli R, Piriyapatsom A, et al. Tracheal tube obstruction in mechanically ventilated patients assessed by high-resolution computed tomography. Anesthesiology. 2014;121:1226–35.

19. Moran I, Cabello B, Manero E, Mancebo J. Comparison of the effects of two humidifier systems on endotracheal tube resistance. Intensive Care Med. 2011;37:1773–9.
20. Kapadia FN. Factors associated with blocked tracheal tubes. Intensive Care Med. 2001;27:1679–81.
21. Kapadia FN, Bajan KB, Singh S, Mathew B, Nath A, Wadkar S. Changing patterns of airway accidents in intubated ICU patients. Intensive Care Med. 2001;27:296–300.
22. Perez Acosta G, Santana-Cabrera L. Necrotizing tracheobronchitis with endotracheal tube obstruction in COVID-19 patients. Rev Clin Esp. 2020;220:531–3.
23. Lavoie-Bérard CA, Lefebvre JC, Bouchard PA, Simon M, Lellouche F. Impact of the airway humidification strategy in mechanically ventilated COVID-19 patient. Retrospective analysis and literature review. Respir Care. 2022;67(2):157–66. https://doi.org/10.4187/respcare.09314.
24. Wiles S, Mireles-Cabodevila E, Neuhofs S, Mukhopadhyay S, Reynolds JP, Hatipoglu U. Endotracheal tube obstruction among patients mechanically ventilated for ARDS due to COVID-19: a case series. J Intensive Care Med. 2021;36(5):604–11.
25. Rubano JA, Jasinski PT, Rutigliano DN, et al. Tracheobronchial Slough, a potential pathology in endotracheal tube obstruction in patients with coronavirus disease 2019 (COVID-19) in the intensive care setting. Ann Surg. 2020;272:e63–e5.
26. Zaidi G, Narasimhan M. Lessons learned in critical care at a 23 hospital health system in New York during the coronavirus disease 2019 pandemic. Chest. 2020;158:1831–2.
27. Bottiroli M, Calini A, Pinciroli R, et al. The repurposed use of anesthesia machines to ventilate critically ill patients with coronavirus disease 2019 (COVID-19). BMC Anesthesiol. 2021;21:155.
28. Lellouche F, Lavoie-Bérard CA, Rousseau E, et al. How to avoid an epidemic of endotracheal tube occlusion. Lancet Respir Med. 2021;9:1215–6.
29. Al Dorzi HM, Ghanem AG, Hegazy MM, et al. Humidification during mechanical ventilation to prevent endotracheal tube occlusion in critically ill patients: a case control study. Ann Thorac Med. 2022;17:37–43.
30. Cohen IL, Weinberg PF, Fein IA, Rowinski GS. Endotracheal tube occlusion associated with the use of heat and moisture exchangers in the intensive care unit. Crit Care Med. 1988;16:277–9.
31. Martin C, Perrin G, Gevaudan MJ, Saux P, Gouin F. Heat and moisture exchangers and vaporizing humidifiers in the intensive care unit. Chest. 1990;97:144–9.
32. Misset B, Escudier B, Rivara D, Leclercq B, Nitenberg G. Heat and moisture exchanger vs heated humidifier during long-term mechanical ventilation. A prospective randomized study. Chest. 1991;100:160–3.
33. Roustan JP, Kienlen J, Aubas P, Aubas S, du Cailar J. Comparison of hydrophobic heat and moisture exchanger with heated humidifier during prolonged mechanical ventilation. Intensive Care Med. 1992;18:97–100.
34. Boots RJ, George N, Faoagali JL, Druery J, Dean K, Heller RF. Double-heater-wire circuits and heat-and-moisture exchangers and the risk of ventilator-associated pneumonia. Crit Care Med. 2006;34:687–93.
35. Boots RJ, Howe S, George N, Harris FM, Faoagali J. Clinical utility of hygroscopic heat and moisture exchangers in intensive care patients. Crit Care Med. 1997;25:1707–12.
36. Dreyfuss D, Djedaini K, Gros I, et al. Mechanical ventilation with heated humidifiers or heat and moisture exchangers: effects on patient colonization and incidence of nosocomial pneumonia. Am J Respir Crit Care Med. 1995;151:986–92.
37. Hurni JM, Feihl F, Lazor R, Leuenberger P, Perret C. Safety of combined heat and moisture exchanger filters in long-term mechanical ventilation. Chest. 1997;111:686–91.
38. Lacherade JC, Auburtin M, Cerf C, et al. Impact of humidification systems on ventilator-associated pneumonia: a randomized multicenter trial. Am J Respir Crit Care Med. 2005;172:1276–82.
39. Kirton OC, DeHaven B, Morgan J, Morejon O, Civetta J. A prospective, randomized comparison of an in-line heat moisture exchange filter and heated wire humidifiers: rates of

ventilator-associated early-onset (community-acquired) or late-onset (hospital-acquired) pneumonia and incidence of endotracheal tube occlusion. Chest. 1997;112:1055–9.

40. Thomachot L, Vialet R, Viguier JM, Sidier B, Roulier P, Martin C. Efficacy of heat and moisture exchangers after changing every 48 hours rather than 24 hours. Crit Care Med. 1998;26:477–81.

41. Branson RD, Davis K Jr, Campbell RS, Johnson DJ, Porembka DT. Humidification in the intensive care unit. Prospective study of a new protocol utilizing heated humidification and a hygroscopic condenser humidifier. Chest. 1993;104:1800–5.

42. Jaber S, Pigeot J, Fodil R, et al. Long-term effects of different humidification systems on endotracheal tube patency: evaluation by the acoustic reflection method. Anesthesiology. 2004;100:782–8.

43. Thomachot L, Leone M, Razzouk K, Antonini F, Vialet R, Martin C. Randomized clinical trial of extended use of a hydrophobic condenser humidifier: 1 vs. 7 days. Crit Care Med. 2002;30:232–7.

44. Thomachot L, Vialet R, Arnaud S, Barberon B, Michel-Nguyen A, Martin C. Do the components of heat and moisture exchanger filters affect their humidifying efficacy and the incidence of nosocomial pneumonia? Crit Care Med. 1999;27:923–8.

45. Thomachot L, Viviand X, Arnaud S, Boisson C, Martin CD. Comparing two heat and moisture exchangers, one hydrophobic and one hygroscopic, on humidifying efficacy and the rate of nosocomial pneumonia. Chest. 1998;114:1383–9.

46. Kollef MH, Shapiro SD, Boyd V, et al. A randomized clinical trial comparing an extended-use hygroscopic condenser humidifier with heated-water humidification in mechanically ventilated patients. Chest. 1998;113:759–67.

47. Branson R, Davis J. Evaluation of 21 passive humidifiers according to the ISO 9360 standard: moisture output, dead space, and flow resistance. Respir Care. 1996;41:736–43.

48. Lellouche F, Taille S, Maggiore SM, et al. Influence of ambient and ventilator output temperatures on performance of heated-wire humidifiers. Am J Respir Crit Care Med. 2004;170:1073–9.

49. Rathgeber J, Kazmaier S, Penack O, Zuchner K. Evaluation of heated humidifiers for use on intubated patients: a comparative study of humidifying efficiency, flow resistance, and alarm functions using a lung model. Intensive Care Med. 2002;28:731–9.

50. Thiery G, Boyer A, Pigne E, et al. Heat and moisture exchangers in mechanically ventilated intensive care unit patients: a plea for an independent assessment of their performance. Crit Care Med. 2003;31:699–704.

51. Lellouche F, Qader S, Taille S, Brochard L. Influence of ambient air temperature on performances of different generations of heated humidifiers. Intensive Care Med. 2003;

52. Lellouche F, Lyazidi A, Brochard L. Improvement of humidification performances with new heated humidifiers. Am J Respir Crit Care Med. 2007;175

53. Schumann S, Stahl CA, Moller K, Priebe HJ, Guttmann J. Moisturizing and mechanical characteristics of a new counter-flow type heated humidifier. Br J Anaesth. 2007;98:531–8.

54. Lellouche F, Rousseau E, Bouchard PA. Evaluation of the new heated wire heated humidifier F&P 950 under varying ambient temperature conditions. Intensive Care Med Exp. 2021;9:001220.

55. Bouchard PA, Rousseau E, Lellouche F. Evaluation of the performances of new generation of heated wire humidifiers. Intensive Care Med Exp. 2022;10:000606.

56. Craven DE, Connolly MG Jr, Lichtenberg DA, Primeau PJ, McCabe WR. Contamination of mechanical ventilators with tubing changes every 24 or 48 hours. N Engl J Med. 1982;306:1505–9.

57. Ricard JD, Hidri N, Blivet A, Kalinowski H, Joly-Guillou ML, Dreyfuss D. New heated breathing circuits do not prevent condensation and contamination of ventilator circuits with heated humidifiers. Am J Respir Crit Care Med. 2003;167:A861.

58. Lellouche L, Qader S, L'Her E, et al. Advantages and drawbacks of a heated humidifier with compensation of under-humidification. Am J Respir Crit Care Med. 2003;167:A909.

59. Qader S, Taillé S, Lellouche F, et al. Influence de la température et de l'humidité du gaz sur la mesure du volume courant expiré. Réanimation. 2002;11:141s.

60. Lellouche F, Simard S, Bouchard PA. Monitoring of heated wire humidifier MR850 hygrometric performances with heater plate temperature. Respir Care. 2022;67(9):1147–53.

61. Lellouche F, Simard S, Bouchard PA. Monitoring of heated wire humidifier hygrometric performances with heater plate temperature. Respir Care. 2022;67:1147–53.

62. Ricard JD, Cook D, Griffith L, Brochard L, Dreyfuss D. Physicians' attitude to use heat and moisture exchangers or heated humidifiers: a Franco-Canadian survey. Intensive Care Med. 2002;28:719–25.

63. Burns KE, Lellouche F, Loisel F, et al. Weaning critically ill adults from invasive mechanical ventilation: a national survey. Can J Anaesth. 2009;56:567–76.

64. Mapleson WW, Morgan JG, Hillard EK. Assessment of condenser-humidifiers with special reference to a multiple-gauze model. Br Med J. 1963;1:300–5.

65. Walley RV. Humidifier for use with tracheotomy and positive-pressure respiration. Lancet. 1956;270:781–2.

66. Hingorani BK. The resistance to airflow of tracheostomy tubes, connections, and heat and moisture exchangers. Br J Anaesth. 1965;37:454–63.

67. Steward DJ. A disposable condenser humidifier for use during anaesthesia. Can Anaesth Soc J. 1976;23:191–5.

68. Boisson C, Viviand X, Arnaud S, Thomachot L, Miliani Y, Martin C. Changing a hydrophobic heat and moisture exchanger after 48 hours rather than 24 hours: a clinical and microbiological evaluation. Intensive Care Med. 1999;25:1237–43.

69. Lellouche F, Qader S, Taillé S, Brochard L. Impact of ambient air temperature on a new active HME and on standard HMES: bench evaluation. Intensive Care Med. 2003;29:S169.

70. Croci M, Elena A, Solca M. Performance of a hydrophobic heat and moisture exchanger at different ambient temperatures. Intensive Care Med. 1993;19:351–2.

71. Lellouche F, Qader S, Taille S, Lyazidi A, Brochard L. Under-humidification and over-humidification during moderate induced hypothermia with usual devices. Intensive Care Med. 2006;32:1014–21.

72. Dery R. The evolution of heat and moisture in the respiratory tract during anesthesia with a nonrebreathing system. Can Anaesth Soc J. 1973;20:296–309.

73. Martin C, Papazian L, Perrin G, Bantz P, Gouin F. Performance evaluation of three vaporizing humidifiers and two heat and moisture exchangers in patients with minute ventilation >10 L/min. Chest. 1992;102:1347–50.

74. Martin C, Thomachot L, Quinio B, Viviand X, Albanese J. Comparing two heat and moisture exchangers with one vaporizing humidifier in patients with minute ventilation greater than 10 L/min. Chest. 1995;107:1411–5.

75. Nakagawa NK, Macchione M, Petrolino HM, et al. Effects of a heat and moisture exchanger and a heated humidifier on respiratory mucus in patients undergoing mechanical ventilation. Crit Care Med. 2000;28:312–7.

76. Lellouche F, Qader S, Taillé S, Brochard L. Under-humidification of inspired gas with HME during induced hypothermia. Intensive Care Med. 2004;30:S 201.

77. Ricard JD, Le Miere E, Markowicz P, et al. Efficiency and safety of mechanical ventilation with a heat and moisture exchanger changed only once a week. Am J Respir Crit Care Med. 2000;161:104–9.

78. Davis K Jr, Evans SL, Campbell RS, et al. Prolonged use of heat and moisture exchangers does not affect device efficiency or frequency rate of nosocomial pneumonia. Crit Care Med. 2000;28:1412–8.

79. Kapadia F, Shelly MP, Anthony JM, Park GR. An active heat and moisture exchanger. Br J Anaesth. 1992;69:640–2.

80. Thomachot L, Viviand X, Boyadjiev I, Vialet R, Martin C. The combination of a heat and moisture exchanger and a booster: a clinical and bacteriological evaluation over 96 h. Intensive Care Med. 2002;28:147–53.

81. Larsson A, Gustafsson A, Svanborg L. A new device for 100 per cent humidification of inspired air. Crit Care. 2000;4:54–60.
82. Chiumello D, Pelosi P, Park G, et al. In vitro and in vivo evaluation of a new active heat moisture exchanger. Crit Care. 2004;8:R281–8.
83. Ploysongsang Y, Branson R, Rashkin MC, Hurst JM. Pressure flow characteristics of commonly used heat-moisture exchangers. Am Rev Respir Dis. 1988;138:675–8.
84. Manthous CA, Schmidt GA. Resistive pressure of a condenser humidifier in mechanically ventilated patients. Crit Care Med. 1994;22:1792–5.
85. Lucato JJ, Tucci MR, Schettino GP, et al. Evaluation of resistance in 8 different heat-and-moisture exchangers: effects of saturation and flow rate/profile. Respir Care. 2005;50:636–43.
86. Lellouche F, Maggiore SM, Deye N, et al. Effect of the humidification device on the work of breathing during noninvasive ventilation. Intensive Care Med. 2002;28:1582–9.
87. Girault C, Breton L, Richard JC, et al. Mechanical effects of airway humidification devices in difficult to wean patients. Crit Care Med. 2003;31:1306–11.
88. Iotti GA, Olivei MC, Braschi A. Mechanical effects of heat-moisture exchangers in ventilated patients. Crit Care. 1999;3:R77–82.
89. Iotti GA, Olivei MC, Palo A, et al. Unfavorable mechanical effects of heat and moisture exchangers in ventilated patients. Intensive Care Med. 1997;23:399–405.
90. Le Bourdelles G, Mier L, Fiquet B, et al. Comparison of the effects of heat and moisture exchangers and heated humidifiers on ventilation and gas exchange during weaning trial from mechanical ventilation. Chest. 1996;110:1294–8.
91. Pelosi P, Solca M, Ravagnan I, Tubiolo D, Ferrario L, Gattinioni L. Effects of heat and moisture exchangers on minute ventilation, ventilatory drive, and work of breathing during pressure-support ventilation in acute respiratory failure. Crit Care Med. 1996;24:1184–8.
92. Campbell RS, Davis K Jr, Johannigman JA, Branson RD. The effects of passive humidifier dead space on respiratory variables in paralyzed and spontaneously breathing patients. Respir Care. 2000;45:306–12.
93. Hinkson CR, Benson MS, Stephens LM, Deem S. The effects of apparatus dead space on P(aCO2) in patients receiving lung-protective ventilation. Respir Care. 2006;51:1140–4.
94. Moran I, Bellapart J, Vari A, Mancebo J. Heat and moisture exchangers and heated humidifiers in acute lung injury/acute respiratory distress syndrome patients. Effects on respiratory mechanics and gas exchange. Intensive Care Med. 2006;32:524–31.
95. Prat G, Renault A, Tonnelier JM, et al. Influence of the humidification device during acute respiratory distress syndrome. Intensive Care Med. 2003;29:2211–5.
96. Prin S, Chergui K, Augarde R, Page B, Jardin F, Veillard-Baron A. Ability and safety of a heated humidifier to control hypercapnic acidosis in severe ARDS. Intensive Care Med. 2002;28:1756–60.
97. Richecoeur J, Lu Q, Vieira SR, et al. Expiratory washout versus optimization of mechanical ventilation during permissive hypercapnia in patients with severe acute respiratory distress syndrome. Am J Respir Crit Care Med. 1999;160:77–85.
98. Pitoni S, D'Arrigo S, Grieco DL, et al. Tidal volume lowering by instrumental dead space reduction in brain-injured ARDS patients: effects on Respiratory mechanics, gas exchange, and cerebral hemodynamics. Neurocrit Care. 2020;34(1):21–30.
99. Lellouche F. Decrease dead space prior to calling the ECMO! Chest. 2021;159:1682–3.
100. Lellouche F, Grieco DL, Maggiore SM, Antonelli M. Instrumental dead space in ventilator management. Lancet Respir Med. 2021;9(3):e22.
101. Hilbert G. Difficult to wean chronic obstructive pulmonary disease patients: avoid heat and moisture exchangers? Crit Care Med. 2003;31:1580–1.
102. Djedaini K, Billiard M, Mier L, et al. Changing heat and moisture exchangers every 48 hours rather than 24 hours does not affect their efficacy and the incidence of nosocomial pneumonia. Am J Respir Crit Care Med. 1995;152:1562–9.
103. Markowicz P, Ricard JD, Dreyfuss D, et al. Safety, efficacy, and cost-effectiveness of mechanical ventilation with humidifying filters changed every 48 hours: a prospective, randomized study. Crit Care Med. 2000;28:665–71.

104. Branson R, Davis J, Brown R. Comparison of three humidification techniques during mechanical ventilation: patient selection, cost, and infection considerations. Respir Care. 1996;41:809–16.
105. Dreyfuss D, Djedaini K, Weber P, et al. Prospective study of nosocomial pneumonia and of patient and circuit colonization during mechanical ventilation with circuit changes every 48 hours versus no change. Am Rev Respir Dis. 1991;143:738–43.
106. Fink JB, Krause SA, Barrett L, Schaaff D, Alex CG. Extending ventilator circuit change interval beyond 2 days reduces the likelihood of ventilator-associated pneumonia. Chest. 1998;113:405–11.
107. Hess D, Burns E, Romagnoli D, Kacmarek RM. Weekly ventilator circuit changes. A strategy to reduce costs without affecting pneumonia rates. Anesthesiology. 1995;82:903–11.
108. Kollef MH, Shapiro SD, Fraser VJ, et al. Mechanical ventilation with or without 7-day circuit changes. A randomized controlled trial. Ann Intern Med. 1995;123:168–74.
109. Long MN, Wickstrom G, Grimes A, Benton CF, Belcher B, Stamm AM. Prospective, randomized study of ventilator-associated pneumonia in patients with one versus three ventilator circuit changes per week. Infect Control Hosp Epidemiol. 1996;17:14–9.
110. Daumal F, Colpart E, Manoury B, Mariani M, Daumal M. Changing heat and moisture exchangers every 48 hours does not increase the incidence of nosocomial pneumonia. Infect Control Hosp Epidemiol. 1999;20:347–9.
111. Boyer A, Thiery G, Lasry S, et al. Long-term mechanical ventilation with hygroscopic heat and moisture exchangers used for 48 hours: a prospective clinical, hygrometric, and bacteriologic study. Crit Care Med. 2003;31:823–9.
112. Branson R. Humidification for patients with artificial airways. Respir Care. 1999;44:630–41.
113. Memish Z, Oni G, Djazmati W, Cunningham G, Mah M. A randomized clinical trial to compare the effects of a heat and moisture exchanger with a heated humidifying system on the occurrence rate of ventilator-associated pneumonia. Am J Infect Control. 2001;29:301–5.
114. Williams RB. The effects of excessive humidity. Respir Care Clin N Am. 1998;4:215–28.
115. Panchamia RK, Piracha MM, Samuels JD. Desperate times: repurposing anesthesia machines for mechanical ventilation in COVID-19. J Clin Anesth. 2020;66:109967.
116. Sugimoto R, Kenzaka T, Fujikawa M, Kawasaki S, Nishisaki H. Humidifier use and prone positioning in a patient with severe COVID-19 pneumonia and endotracheal tube impaction due to highly viscous sputum. Cureus. 2020;12:e8626.
117. van Boven EA, van Duin S, Ponssen HH. Endotracheal tube obstruction in patients diagnosed with COVID-19. Netherland J Crit Care. 2021;29:102–3.
118. Lellouche F, Taillé S, Maggiore SM, et al. Influence of ambient and ventilator output temperatures on performance of new heated humidifiers. Am J Respir Crit Care Med. 2002;165:A788.

Postoperative Mechanical Ventilation-Humidification

11

Gül Erdal Dönmez ⓘ and Zuhal Karakurt ⓘ

11.1 Introduction

After major surgery, such as cardiothoracic or abdominal surgery, or any emergency operation requiring general anesthesia, patients with chronic obstructive pulmonary disease (COPD) or neurologic comorbidities or who are active smokers require invasive mechanical ventilation (IMV). Following surgery, IMV-related complications such as atelectasis, acute lung damage, and pneumothorax may occur [1]. The requirement for a longer duration of IMV increased the risk of complication [1, 2].

The most often encountered complication in patients following surgery is atelectasis caused by insufficient inspiration. All these can cause airway obstruction and atelectasis [3]. The latest clinical practice guideline recommends that all patients receiving IMV should have their airways humidified to grade 1A [4]. The previous review by Lorente in 2012 is updated in this chapter [5].

G. E. Dönmez (✉) · Z. Karakurt
University of Health Sciences Hamidiye School of Medicine, Sureyyapasa Chest Diseases and Thoracic Surgery Teaching and Research Hospital, Respiratory Intensive Care Unit, Istanbul, Turkey

A. M. Esquinas (ed.), *Humidification in the Intensive Care Unit*,
https://doi.org/10.1007/978-3-031-23953-3_11

11.2   The Need for Humidification

The total needed moisture input of the airways to the alveoli is 44 mg/L, of which the upper airways supply 75%. Due to the bypass of the upper airway during IMV, the highest moisture support is lost. Mechanical ventilators provide postoperative patients with a blend of dry-cold medical gases that are not moistened. Patients who are intubated should require humidification due to the loss of 75% neutral upper airway moisture support [6, 7]. The loss of air moisture results in the evaporation of water from mucus and periciliary fluids, increasing mucus viscosity and causing the periciliary fluid layer to disappear. All of these factors contribute to decreased mucociliary clearance, and thick mucus cannot be easily cleared by cilia. The mobility and rate of cilia are reduced, and mucociliary transport is impaired. During IMV, the altered mucociliary physiology can result in decreased respiratory function and atelectasis. Humidification is required to maintain normal airway physiology during IMV [8]. External humidification during IMV can help prevent hypothermia, disturbance of the airway epithelium, bronchospasm, obstruction of the airway, and atelectasis [9, 10].

11.3   Humidification at an Optimal Level

The humidity in the trachea can fluctuate between 36 and 40 mg/L during normal respiration, and the optimal needed moisture below the carina is 44 mg/L (100% relative humidity [RH] at 37 °C). If patients are intubated, the moisture level needed should be as much as 75% of the airway moisture level. As the total needed moisture input of the airways to the alveoli is 44 mg/L, of which the upper airways supply 75 percent. The mathematical calculation is revealed that 33 mg/L (total amounth of reguire humudity multiple by a lost rate of upper airway moisture [44 mg/L × 75% = 33 mg/L) [4, 6, 8]. One study revealed that exposure to humidity levels less than 25 mgH$_2$O/L for 1 h or 30 mgH$_2$O/L for 24 h or more has been linked to airway mucosal dysfunction [7].

The currently used humidifiers are heat and moisture exchanger (HME) and heated humidifiers (HH). The HME is a passive humidifier device, also called artificial nose, which traps the heat and humidity from patient's exhaled gas and returns some of them to the patient on the subsequent inhalation. HH is an active humidifier, and the inspired gas passes across or over a heated water bath and turn the patients inspirium circuit. There were two old studies that showed patients on mechanical ventilation should be given with humidification devices that deliver at least 28 mgH$_2$O/L and have a reliable humidity monitoring method and measurements that are obtained independently from the manufacturer [9, 11]. The last guidelines published by the American Association for Respiratory Care (AARC) recommend a temperature of 33 °C (standard deviation 2) with relative humidity of 100% and a water vapor level of 44 mg/L [4]. The assurance of humidification level can be possible with active humidifiers. Almost every HME or filter used in endotracheal tube occlusion cases during the COVID-19 pandemic met the ISO standard [12]. The literatures addressed that by using a psychrometric method to determine the degree of humidity given by HME devices, using the identical bench previously described [9, 11], they showed an unacceptably low humidity output (mean 25.8 mgH$_2$O/L [SD 09]), despite manufacturers' claims of a comfortable humidity [13]. The authors pointed out that the validity of standards should be reevaluated and how these measurements are controlled to know which HMEs are efficient and which HMEs are not in patients receiving IMV [13]. Very recently, at the beginning of the COVID-19 pandemic, the mean absolute humidity of inspiratory gases was 7.8 mgH$_2$O/L when the heated humidifiers were turned off, and that is an extremely low level of humidity [14]. The recommended minimum inspiratory humidity level for HME is 30 mgH$_2$O/L (International Organization for Standardization [ISO] 9360), and for heated humidifiers, it is 33 mgH$_2$O/L [11].

11.4 Type of Humidifiers, Advantages, and Disadvantages for Postoperative Invasive Mechanical Ventilation

For postoperative period, the need for IMV increases the morbidity and mortality. It is accepted that humidification is necessary for all invasive mechanical ventilation. In previous review of Lorente in 2012, it was mentioned that ventilator-associated pneumonia (VAP) was a controversial by influencing humidifier devices [5]. In 2014, the Centers for Disease Control and Prevention (CDC) recommended to not choose the humidification device based on infection control (CDC 2014).

11.5 The Latest Type of Humidifiers (See Detail in Sect. 11.2)

1. Active humidifiers (heated humidifiers).
2. Passive humidifiers.

Table 11.1 summarizes the type of humidifiers and their advantages-disadvantages.

Table 11.1 Type of humidifiers and their advantages and disadvantages in invasive mechanical ventilation[a]

	Active humidifiers (heated humidifiers)	Passive humidifiers [16]
Device classification (based on their mechanism)	1. Bubble humidifiers 2. Pass-over humidifiers	1. Heat and moisture exchangers (HMEs) 2. Hygroscopic condenser humidifiers (HCHs) or hygroscopic heat and moisture exchangers (HHMEs) 3. Heat and moisture exchangers with filter 4. Combined heat and moisture exchangers
Implementation and monitoring	Observe that the tubing drains the water Downward and not toward the artificial airway or the ventilator Water level, temperature level; check the presence of condensation	It should always be placed before the "Y" part of the circuit The recommended limit of 30 mg/L had a dead space of approximately 60 mL; therefore, the volume should be taken into account when selecting an HME
Advantages	1. They do not have contraindications 2. As they are placed in the inspiratory branch, they do not add instrumental dead space 3. If used correctly, they do not increase the resistance 4. They have alarm systems 5. They are more efficient and can deliver accurate temperatures	1. Their use is simple 2. They do not have risks related to the treatment equipment 3. They are light in weight 4. They are cheaper 5. They are easily available in the intensive care unit
Disadvantages	1. Possibility of electrocution of the patient and the operator 2. They expose the airway lesion to excessive temperature 3. The presence of water in the circuit can limit the airflow 4. Condensation generates changes in the airway pressure and can lead to asynchronies 5. Colonization of the circuit 6. They require more monitoring to ensure correct performance	1. They are contraindicated in some pathologies or clinical conditions 2. Because they are placed before the "Y" in the circuit, they increase the instrumental dead space 3. They increase the resistance (negligible in most cases) 4. They have lower performance or efficiency compared with an active humidifier 5. They should be retired to be able to apply aerosol therapy (except Gibeck humid-Flo HME®)
Clinical condition in postoperative patients		
Lung-protective strategies	Implement the use of active humidifiers	

Table 11.1 (continued)

	Active humidifiers (heated humidifiers)	Passive humidifiers [16]
Comorbid diseases: COPD	It does not increase the instrumental dead space or the ventilatory demand, without the risk of generating auto-PEEP	Not first choice; when used, change every 48 h
Burn [17]	Especially in patients with large body surfaces affected and inhalatory lesions due to its stable performance	
Bronchopleural fistula	Patient with an exhaled volume below 70 percent of the inhaled volume	
Hypothermia [18]	For patients under a hypothermia strategy since they have demonstrated a better performance than HMEs and active HMEs	
ARDS	It maintains its performance despite the ventilatory strategy used. It allows the optimization of the effective alveolar ventilation and decreases the VT and the instrumental dead space	–
Weaning process [19]	In patients with a problem in PaCO2 due to their pathology or who present significant muscle weakness, the use of an active humidifier is recommended	
VAP	No any humidification device selection to prevent VAP	No any humidification device selection to prevent VAP

[a]Table is adapted from Plotnikow GA and coworkers [15]

11.6 Recommendations About the Type of Humidification in International Guideline Based on Invasive Mechanical Ventilation

As the latest international guideline of the American Association for Respiratory Care, Clinical Practice Guideline for Humidification During Invasive and Noninvasive Mechanical Ventilation 2012 [4]:

- *"Humidification is recommended on every patient receiving invasive mechanical ventilation"* (1A).
- *When providing* **active humidification** *to patients who are invasively ventilated, it is suggested that the device provide a humidity level between* **33 mgH$_2$O/L** *and* **44 mgH$_2$O/L** *and gas temperature between* **34 °C** *and* **41 °C** *at the circuit Y-piece, with an RH of 100 percent (2B).*

- *When providing humidification to **patients with low tidal volumes,** such as when lung-protective ventilation strategies are used, **HMEs are not recommended** because they contribute additional dead space, which can increase the ventilation requirement and PaCO$_2$ (2B).*
- *It is suggested that **HMEs are not used** as **a prevention strategy** for **ventilator-associated pneumonia** (2B).*

11.7 Conclusions

Every patient undergoing IMV should have their airways humidified. The postoperative airway mucosa should be moisturized to protect it from the drying effect of the gas-dry air mixture and to prevent mucosal fragility, bleeding, and atelectasis. Airway humidification can be accomplished with either a heat and moisture exchanger (HME) (cost-effective) or a heated humidifier (HH) (expensive). All types of humidification devices are not recommended for preventing VAP. Although HME and HH have comparable airway protective efficacy, when thick secretion, atelectasis, burn, or hypothermia is present in patients with postoperative IMV, HH should be suggested.

References

1. Ferguson MK. Preoperative assessment of pulmonary risk. Chest. 1999;115(5 Suppl):58S–63S.
2. Zochios V, Chandan JS, Schultz MJ, Morris AC, Parhar KK, Giménez-Milà M, Gerrard C, Vuylsteke A, Klein AA. The effects of escalation of respiratory support and prolonged invasive ventilation on outcomes of cardiac surgical patients: a retrospective cohort study. J Cardiothorac Vasc Anesth. 2019;34(5):1226S–34S.
3. Tenling A, Hachenberg T, Tydén H, Wegenius G, Hedenstierna G. Atelectasis and gas exchange after cardiac surgery. Anesthesiology. 1998;89(2):371S–8S.
4. American Association for Respiratory Care, Restrepo RD, Walsh BK. Humidification during invasive and noninvasive mechanical ventilation. Respir Care. 2012;57(5):782S–8S.
5. Lorente L. Postoperative mechanical ventilation-humidification. In: Esquinas A, editor. Humidification in the intensive care unit. Berlin, Heidelberg: Springer; 2012. p. 157S–62S.
6. Zuchner K. Humidification: measurement and requirements. Respir Care Clin N Am. 2006;12(2):149S–63S.
7. Williams R, Rankin N, Smith T, Galler D, Seakins P. Relationship between the humidity and temperature of inspired gas and the function of the airway mucosa. Crit Care Med. 1996;24(11):1920S–9S.
8. Kilgour E, Rankin N, Ryan S, Pack R. Mucociliary function deteriorates in the clinical range of inspired air temperature and humidity. Intensive Care Med. 2004;30(7):1491S–4S.
9. Lellouche F, Taillé S, Lefrançois F, Deye N, Maggiore SM, Jouvet P, Ricard JD, Fumagalli B, Brochard L, Groupe de travail sur les Respirateurs de l'AP-HP. Humidification performance of 48 passive airway humidifiers: comparison with manufacturer data. Chest. 2009;2009(135):276S–86S.
10. Al Dorzi HM, Ghanem AG, Hegazy MM, AlMatrood A, Alchin J, Mutairi M, Aqeil A, Arabi YM. Humidification during mechanical ventilation to prevent endotracheal tube occlusion in critically ill patients: a case control study. Ann Thorac Med. 2022;17:37S–43S.

11. Branson R, Davis J. Evaluation of 21 passive humidifiers according to the ISO 9360 standard: moisture output, dead space, and flow resistance. Respir Care. 1996;41:736S–43S.

12. Standardization of humidifiers for mechanical use: general requirements for humidification systems. International Organization for Standardization ISO 2007;8185(Third edition):2007.

13. Lellouche F, Lavoie-Bérard CA, Rousseau E, Bouchard PA, Lefebvre JC, Branson R, Brochard L. How to avoid an epidemic of endotracheal tube occlusion. Lancet Respir Med. 2021;9(11):1215S–6S.

14. Zaidi G, Narasimhan M. Lessons learned in critical care at a 23 hospital health system in New York during the coronavirus disease 2019 pandemic. Chest. 2020;158:1831S–2S.

15. Plotnikow GA, Accoce M, Navarro E, Tiribelli N. Humidification and heating of inhaled gas in patients with artificial airway. A narrative review. Rev Bras Ter Intensiva. 2018;30(1):86S–97S.

16. Siempos II, Vardakas KZ, Kopterides P, Falagas ME. Impact of passive humidification on clinical outcomes of mechanically ventilated patients: a meta-analysis of randomized controlled trials. Crit Care Med. 2007;35(12):2843S–51S.

17. McCall JE, Cahill TJ. Respiratory care of the burn patient. J Burn Care Rehabil. 2005;26(3):200S–6S.

18. Lellouche F, Qader S, Taille S, Lyazidi A, Brochard L. Under-humidification and over-humidification during moderate induced hypothermia with usual devices. Intensive Care Med. 2006;32(7):1014S–21S.

19. Girault C, Breton L, Richard JC, Tamion F, Vandelet P, Aboab J, Leroy J, Bonmarchand G. Mechanical effects of airway humidification devices in difficult to wean patients. Crit Care Med. 2003;31(5):1306S–11S.

Humidification in Laparoscopy

12

Guniz Meyanci Koksal and Ulgen Zengin

12.1 Brief Discussion

1. Today, laparoscopic procedures are widely preferred with an increasing rate for they are more cosmetic and surgical stress is lower when compared with conventional techniques.
2. The cold (-21 °C) and dry (0%) CO_2 used in laparoscopic surgery causes an increase in the postoperative pain and need for analgesics and a decrease both in preoperative and postoperative patient comfort accompanied by morphological and metabolic changes in the peritoneum.
3. Cold and dry CO_2 causes the patient to be hypothermic, and external heating is insufficient in preventing hypothermia.
4. Warming and humidification of CO_2 is the order of the day although some studies suggest that warming and humidification does not prevent the effect of cold and dry gas.
5. The side effects of cold and dry CO_2 must be prevented. New prospective, blind clinical studies must be carried on with different techniques of warming-humidification and different temperatures and humidification concentrations using constant wide patient groups by skilled surgical and anesthesia teams.

Laparoscopic interventions were firstly described in 1987 as minimally invasive techniques which were widely used especially in abdominal surgery. Laparoscopy

G. M. Koksal (✉)
Department of Anesthesiology and Reanimation, Cerrahpasa Medical School, Istanbul Cerrahpasa University, İstanbul, Turkey

U. Zengin
Department of Anaesthesiology and Reanimation, Marmara University Medical Faculty, İstanbul, Turkey

A. M. Esquinas (ed.), *Humidification in the Intensive Care Unit*,
https://doi.org/10.1007/978-3-031-23953-3_12

is used not only for the abdomen but also for invasive procedures to be performed in cavities such as the thorax and pelvis [1].

In abdominal surgery, pneumoperitoneum is created by insufflation of gas into the abdominal cavity through the peritoneum. The insufflated gas is frequently carbon dioxide (CO_2) gas. Pneumoperitoneum causes an increase in intra-abdominal pressure. The increase in pressure impairs the perfusion of the intra-abdominal organs, especially the mesenteric region and kidneys. Moreover, the cardiac output decreases, which pushes the diaphragm up, causing atelectasis in the basal parts of the lungs, and the ventilation perfusion ratio is also impaired. Also, moderate hypoxia and hypercarbia are observed, and urine output is decreased (<0.5 mL/kg) [2].

However, since it is a minimally invasive procedure, the incision size and pain are less, and early mobilization is possible. The patient's fluid loss and infection rates are also reduced.

The CO_2 gas used during peritoneal insufflation is a dry and cold gas. For every 50 L of gas insufflation, the body temperature drops by 0.3 °C. CO_2 gas is stored as liquid in cylinders at an average of −90 °C, its temperature is between −19 °C and, −21 °C, and its relative humidity is 0. The temperature of the peritoneal cavity is 36 °C, and the relative humidity is virtually 100%. The constant presence of CO_2 gas in the peritoneal cavity in the peritoneal mesothelium causes morphological and biochemical damage. In fact, using heated and humidified gas will prevent hypoxemia, reduce pain, and decrease the amount of analgesic used in the postoperative period. Even just warming the patient will have a positive effect and results in the prevention of hypothermia. Even insufflation of heated-non-humidified CO_2 gas has been demonstrated to reduce humoral inflammation in the peritoneum [3, 4].

Hypothermia causes significant perioperative morbidity, and it is important to the anesthesiologists. We have noted in our daily practice that prolonged abdominal laparoscopy is responsible for a significant drop in core body temperature. This results from the combination of specific heat losses, particularly via convection and evaporation, leading to less energy loss from the body due to the insufflated gas, and nonspecific heat losses caused by the imbalance of thermoregulatory mechanisms during general anesthesia [5]. The warm abdomen and the organs therein make a large internal surface area for heat exchange, and because gas is constantly circulating and being renewed, there is a significant energy transfer from the patient to the intraperitoneal gas as the gas is warmed [6]. The focus of many studies was to evaluate in a prospective, randomized, controlled study the postoperative outcomes of pain and narcotic use with patient having different kinds of procedures comparing conventional dry-cold, dry-warmed, and humidified-warmed gas [6].

Pneumoperitoneum damages the mesothelial cells of the peritoneum. Mesothelial cells contain an average of 230 microvilli per 10 μm^2. These microvilli allow the exchange of molecules by providing tissue mobility between the peritoneum and organs. CO_2 gas causes bulging, delaminization, and loss of villi and death in mesothelial cells. The effect of CO_2 gas also increases in the organism where inflammatory markers increase with a rise in peritoneal pressure. Especially in patients who will be scheduled for laparoscopic cancer surgery, mesothelial tissue defect and inflammatory process should be minimal in order to prevent the spread of cancerous cells [7].

In laparoscopic surgery, low peritoneal pressure (>12 mmHg), normothermia, and heating and humidification of CO_2 gas will reduce many of the mentioned processes, although these cannot be completely prevented. The vavless or CO_2 recirculating systems specifically used in robotic surgery, effective methods for reducing systemic and localized inflammation. Temperature control is also important in terms of reducing surgical infections [8].

Devices such as HumiGard and AirSeal (iFS, USA) are used to humidify and heat the CO_2 gas used during insufflation. The tube system of these devices is disposable and expensive. Fisher & Paykel's systems can be preferred, which heat the CO_2 gas up to 37 °C and humidify 98%. The use of these systems, especially in elderly patients, will result in a more stable hemodynamics and decrease in lactic acid level and shorten the recovery [9].

Savel et al. [10] performed a randomized double-blind, prospective, controlled clinical trial of 30 patients undergoing laparoscopic Roux-en-Y gastric bypass. Patients received postoperative analgesia from morphine, delivered via a patient-controlled analgesia pump, and pain scores and amount of morphine were measured postoperatively. Their trial was unable to provide evidence of any significant reduction in postoperative pain as measured by either morphine requirements or pain scores with the use of warmed-humidified CO_2. They were able to demonstrate a statistically significant increase in end-of-case temperature with the use of this device, but this result is not clinically significant.

Mouton et al. [11] advocated that the use of humidified insufflation gas reduces postoperative pain following laparoscopic cholecystectomy, but the heat-preserving effect of humidified gas insufflation is not significant.

Peng et al. [12] suggest that heated (37 °C)-humidified (95% relative humidity) insufflation results in significantly less hypothermia, less peritoneal damage, and decreased adhesion formation as compared with cold-dry CO_2 insufflation.

12.2 Conclusion

It has been proved that the use of cold and dry CO_2 in laparoscopic surgery causes an increase in the postoperative pain, hypothermia, acidosis in the peritoneum, and a decrease both in preoperative and postoperative patient comfort. The loss of heat during perioperative period causing hypothermia is an important concern for the anesthesiologists and intensivists. Hypothermia not only causes some metabolic changes but also prolongs the recovery from the anesthesia, resulting in the increased use of supplies and drugs that might lead to a need to ICU. All of these will result in increased hospital stay, morbidity, and cost. To avoid this, we try to keep the patients' temperature between physiological limits by warming out patients perioperatively. In laparoscopic surgery, it is not possible to keep the patients' temperature in normal values with external heating for the surgeons prefer to use cold-dry CO_2. Although many studies were made in the past decade on the warming and humidification of CO_2, there are still two different opinions, one supporting the warming and humidification and the other against it. The most important factor on these two different opinions is the discrepancy between the protocols of the studies. The warming temperature and the rate of humidification, the patient groups, and the type and the duration of the operations differ in study groups. It is more appropriate to standardize the patient groups and warming and humidification rate of the gas, in prospective, blind clinical trials. In these studies, different warming levels and different concentrations of humidification that are suitable for human physiology must be used. As commonly accepted, the results of the animal trials are not thoroughly concordant with the human studies. Especially in studies where pain and the amount of analgesic used are evaluated, using animal model may not be correct. This discordance is more evident in small animals like rats. It is also an issue who the surgeon doing the laparoscopic surgery is. The use of laparoscopic surgery has increased dramatically in the last decade because of cosmetic concerns and its lower surgical stress. It is essential that the surgical team must be experienced in the procedure and must give a proper position to the patient and the gas must be thoroughly emptied. All of these factors affect the postoperative waking from the anesthesia, pain, amount of analgesic used, and the hemodynamics of the patient. Hence, the study protocols dealing with the warming and humidification of CO_2 in humans must be accomplished by skilled teams.

In the future studies, the techniques of warming and humidification must also be evaluated. Different techniques will surely affect the results of the studies. Nowadays, different techniques such as HME Booster, modified Aeroneb, and Pall system are worked on, and still no distinction has been shown on any technique.

Wang et al. [9] introduced in a pig model that the acidosis created on the peritoneum by the CO_2 gas in laparoscopy increases the implantation of tumor cells and the warming and humidification of CO_2 or buffering with bicarbonate does not decrease this impact. Therefore, a detailed study is needed on the consequences of CO_2 insufflations in laparoscopic surgery in oncologic patients.

As a result, although there are negatory concerns on the warming and humidification of CO_2 used – to raise the abdominal wall – during the laparoscopic surgery, wide series of human studies in different physiological temperatures and humidification concentrations are needed to eliminate the side effects of cold and dry gas.

References

1. Liu L, Lv N, Hou C. Effects of a multifaceted individualized pneumoperitoneum strategy in elderly patients undergoing laparoscopic colorectal surgery A retrospective study. Medicine. 2019;98:14(e15112). https://doi.org/10.1097/MD.0000000000015112.
2. Wong YT, Shah PC, Birkett DH, D. M. Brams carbon dioxide pneumoperitoneum causes severe peritoneal acidosis, unaltered by heating, humidification, or bicarbonate in a porcine model. Surg Endosc. 2004;18:1498–503. https://doi.org/10.1007/s00464-003-9290-7.
3. Erikoglu M, Yol S, Avunduk MC, Erdemli E, Can A. Electron-microscopic alterations of the peritoneum after both cold and heated carbon dioxide pneumoperitoneum. J Surg Res. 2005;125:73–7.
4. Hamza MA, Schneider BE, White PF, et al. Heated and humidified insufflation during laparoscopic gastric bypass surgery: effect on temperature, postoperation pain, and recovery outcomes. J Laparoendosc Adv Surg Tech A. 2005;15:6.

5. Schlotterbeck H, Greib N, Dow AW, Schaeffer R, Geny B, Diemunsch P. Changes in core temperature during peritoneal insufflation: comparison of two CO_2 humidification devices in pigs. J Surg Res. 2010;1–6 https://doi.org/10.1016/j.jss.2010.04.003.

6. Schlotterbeck H, Schaeffer R, Dow AW, Diemunsch P. Cold nebulization used to prevent heat loss during laparoscopic surgery: an experimental study in pigs. Surg Endosc. 2008;22:2626–0.

7. Sampurno S, Chittleborough TJ, Carpinteri S, Hiller J, Heriot A, Lynch AC, Ramsay RG. Modes of carbon dioxide delivery during laparoscopy generate distinct differences in peritoneal damage and hypoxia in a porcine model. Surg Endosc. 2020;34:4395–402.

8. Sammour T, Kahokehr A, Hayes J, Hulme-Moir M, Hill AG. Warming and humidification of insufflation carbon dioxide in laparoscopic colonic surgery a double-blinded randomized controlled trial. Ann Surg. 2010;251:1024–33. https://doi.org/10.1097/SLA.0b013e3181d77a25.

9. Sammour T, Kahokehr A, Andrew G. Hill independent testing of the Fisher & Paykel Healthcare MR860. Minim Invasive Ther Allied Technol. 2010;19:219–23.

10. Savel RH, Balasubramanya S, Lazheer S, Gaprindashuili T, Arabou E, Fazylou RM, Lazzaro RS, Macura JM. Beneficial effects of humidified, warmed carbon dioxide insufflation during laparoscopic bariatric surgery: a randomized clinical trial. Obes Surg. 2005;15:64–9.

11. Mauton WG, Bessell JR, Millard SH, Baxter PS, Maddein GJ. A randomized controlled trial assessing the benefits of humidified insufflation gas during laparoscopic surgery. Surg Endosc. 1999;13:106–8.

12. Peng Y, Zheng M, Ye Q, Chen X, Yu B, Liu B. Heated and humidified CO_2 prevents hypothermia peritoneal injury, and intra-abdominal adhesions during prolonged laparoscopic insufflations. J Surg Res. 2009;151:40–7.

Humidification in Intensive Care Medicine: Humidification and Complications in Invasive Mechanical Ventilation

13

Dara D. Regn

13.1 Introduction

When the tracheal mucosa is bypassed via endotracheal tube (ETT) intubation or from a surgically placed tracheostomy, humidification is essential to preserve tracheobronchial mucosal integrity and is an accepted standard of care in the intensive care unit [1]. Without humidification, the tracheal mucosa will lose ciliary function and develop inspissated secretions, and the underlying connective tissue will undergo structural changes [2–5]. Williams et al. performed a meta-analysis evaluating the relationship between the humidity and temperature of inspired gas and airway mucosal function [6]. They developed a model suggesting above or below optimal temperature, and humidity conditions can lead to impaired airway mucosal dysfunction, or, vice versa, that adequate mucociliary function is an indicator of ideal humidification. Oostdam et al. showed animals that inspired dried air demonstrated a significant reduction of extravascular water of the loose connective tissue of the airways and an increase in airway resistance to histamine resulting in reduced bronchospasm threshold [2]. ETT occlusion secondary to thickened or dried secretions is also strongly linked to suboptimal humidification [5, 7]. The most common way to avoid these and other potential complications (Box 13.1) is accomplished by applying humidification from non-heated wire humidifiers, heated wire humidifiers (HWHs), or a heat and moisture exchangers (HMEs) [4, 8]. The goal of each of these humidification devices is to provide tracheal humidification consisting of heat and moisture to the inspired gas with a minimum of 30 mgH$_2$O/L or 100% relative

D. D. Regn (✉)
Pulmonary/Critical Care/Sleep Medicine, Aeromedical Consultation Service,
United States Air Force School of Aerospace Medicine, Wright Patterson AFB, OH, USA

© The Author(s), under exclusive license to Springer Nature
Switzerland AG 2023
A. M. Esquinas (ed.), *Humidification in the Intensive Care Unit*,
https://doi.org/10.1007/978-3-031-23953-3_13

> **Box 13.1 Complications of Mechanical Ventilation with Suboptimal Humidification**
>
> **Cyto-morphologic airway modifications**
>
> Decrease in sol phase depth.
> Hyperviscosity of airway secretions.
> Tracheal inflammation.
> Deciliation, epithelial ulceration, and then necrosis.
>
> **Functional airway modifications**
>
> Decrease in the humidification capabilities.
> Downward shift of the isothermic saturation boundary (ISB) further down the respiratory tract.
> Decrease in the mucus transport velocity, secretion retention.
> Decrease in the bronchospasm threshold.
> Alteration of the ciliary function, ciliary paralysis.
> Airway obstruction and increase in airflow resistance.
>
> **Pulmonary, mechanical, and functional alterations**
>
> Atelectasis.
> Decrease in functional reserve capacity and compliance.
> V/Q mismatching, increase in intrapulmonary shunt, hypoxemia.
> Pulmonary infection.
> *Source*: ref. [5]

humidity with a delivered gas at 30 °C [4, 5]. The level of humidification delivered to the patient is also dependent upon room temperature, variance in minute ventilation, and ventilator gas temperature [8].

13.2 Humidification Device Selection Considerations

Selection of a humidifier should be based upon clinical context. The American Association for Respiratory Care (AARC) guidelines recommend a temperature of 33 ± 2 °C with relative humidity (RH) of 100% and a water vapor level of 44 mg/L [4]. Heated humidifiers should provide an AH level between 33 and 44 mgH_2O/L, whereas HMEs should provide a minimum of 30 mgH_2O/L. In general, HMEs probably improved baseline variables of humidification and temperature, but whether they perform according to specification is arduous to actually measure [3].

Multiple independent studies have raised concerns about validity of manufacturer data. An independent assessment of humidification capacity of 32 HMEs was performed by Lellouche et al. and found 36% of the tested HMEs had an absolute humidity (AH) of 4 mgH$_2$O/L lower than what was listed by the manufacturer, with some AHs varying by as much as 8 mgH$_2$O/L [17]. Lemmens et al. reviewed three different HMEs, and their main findings showed that following manufacturers' expectations did not reliably predict performance during routine anesthesia procedures; only one HME performed according to expectations [16]. The other two performed at less than the values specified by the manufacturers, but did provide humidification.

Solomita evaluated non-heated wire humidification, heated wire humidification, and HMEs to determine the effects of humidification on the volume of airway secretions in mechanically ventilated patients [8]. Their results revealed that measurement of temperature alone was inadequate to predict humidification and non-heated wire humidification was associated with greater secretion volume. In practice, humidity is measured by a combination of temperature and arbitrary clinical observation of secretion characteristics and accumulation, visual observation of condensate in the tubing system, and requirement for saline instillation because formal measurement of humidity with such devices as a hygrometer-thermometer system is limited by technology and cost [3, 5].

Non-heated wire humidifiers are becoming increasingly less popular because of the concerns over respiratory condensation [8]. In patients requiring long-term mechanical ventilation >96 h, the HWHs are the device of choice [4, 8]. Other indications for heated humidifiers (HHs) include contraindications for HMEs as listed in Box 13.2 [4]. Heated humidification devices are capable of delivering gases with 100% relative humidity near 37 °C body temperature. However, HHs are more expensive than HMEs and have been associated with a potential for electrical shock, hyperthermia, thermal injury, and nosocomial infections [4, 9, 10]. Inappropriate settings of temperature or humidification can also lead to increased resistive work of breathing due to mucous plugging and/or life-threatening occlusions of endotracheal or tracheostomy tubes [8, 11].

Box 13.2 HME Contraindications According to AARC Clinical Practice Guidelines 2012

Thick, copious, or bloody secretions.
When there is loss in expired tidal volume (e.g., expired tidal volume less than 70% of the delivered volume, those with large bronchopleurocutaneous fistulas or incompetent or absent endotracheal tube cuffs).
In patients managed with low tidal volumes like those with ARDS.
In difficult to wean patients and those with limited respiratory reserve.
Hypothermic patients with body temperature less than 32 °C.
In patient with high minute volumes (>10 L/min).
When the patient is receiving aerosol treatments when the nebulizer is placed in the patient circuit.
Source: ref. [4].

HMEs are disposable devices that function by passively storing heat and moisture from the patients' exhaled gas and releasing it to the inhaled gas acting as an "artificial nose" because it mimics nasal cavity humidification [4, 9]. Their regulation of humidity is slightly lower than that of HHs, but their clinical efficacy is similar [12]. HMEs are hydrophobic, hygroscopic, or a combination of both. Hydrophobic HMEs have the best antimicrobial properties and lower humidity retention but cause more narrowing in ETT diameter [9]. Hygroscopic HMEs have less antimicrobial filtration but better humidity qualities, and all HMEs are able to absorb moisture in the expired air. HME humidity and temperature settings are predetermined by the manufacturer based on in vivo studies. The International Organization for Standardization (ISO) states the appropriate HME should have at least 70% efficiency, providing at least 30 mg/L of water vapor. Lellouche suggests an absolute humidity (AH) <30 mgH$_2$O/L is associated with a risk of ETT occlusion (Fig. 13.1) [13]. The airway resistance has been shown to be less in hygroscopic models compared to hydrophobic or combination HMEs [14]. Certain new models of HMEs can be converted from a passive to active device with an addition of an active heated water source which may increase AH by 2–3 mg/L [18].

HMEs are more attractive than heated humidifiers for patients requiring mechanical ventilation of short duration because they are less costly and easier to use [9–11]. They are recommended for shorter durations <96 h or during patient transport and have been used safely for up to 7 days [4, 10]. Multiple studies have advocated for the use of HMEs for >48 h; however, less frequent HME changes increase the risk of airway occlusion [10]. HMEs appeared to lose the ability to maintain humidity for more than 48 h in patients with COPD. They do not require electricity, and there is no risk of thermal injury or concerns about excessive condensation. Like HHs, they possess a unique set of complications, i.e., hypothermia, hypoventilation due to increased dead space, impaction of secretions in extreme circumstances resulting in complete occlusion of airway, and increased airway resistance and work of breathing. HMEs also have contraindications (Box 13.2) [4].

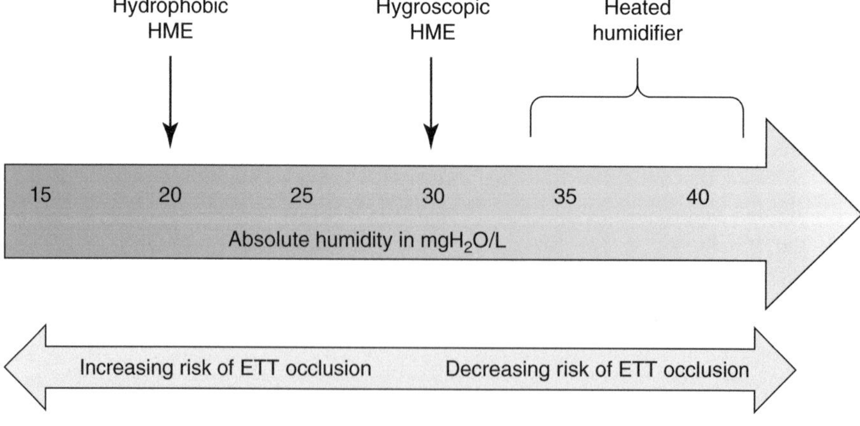

Fig. 13.1 Recommendation of Lellouche et al. [26]

Heated humidifiers are generally used for long-term ventilation and patients with thick secretions. However, a Cochrane systematic review revealed no difference in outcomes between HMEs and HHs; however, $PaCO_2$ and minute ventilation were found to be higher in HMEs [19]. HMEs that possess a large dead space present another problem that clinicians need to be aware of, particularly when using low tidal volume for lung-protective strategies in patients with limited respiratory reserve [3]. Resultant hypercarbia and/or increased minute ventilation may ensue. Acute respiratory distress syndrome is now considered a contraindication for use of HMEs, and HHs are recommended.

13.3   Risk of Infection with Each Device

Relative risk of ventilator-associated pneumonia (VAP) or nosocomial infections with humidifiers has been the subject of numerous meta-analyses [15]. Other etiologies with stronger relationships to VAP include microaspirations from around the endotracheal tube cuff, re-intubation or prolonged mechanical ventilation, prolonged sedation and paralysis, and previous antibiotic exposure [23–25]. Nevertheless, the humidifier can be a real threat if not managed correctly. Routine inspection of the humidification device for secretions and/or condensate in the patient circuit should be scheduled [14]. Cook et al. found lower rates of VAP with the use of HMEs; however, since then, various HMEs and HHs were analyzed in recent meta-analyses, and no differences were found in the rates of VAP [20–22]. A recent Cochrane review also found no difference in pneumonia prevalence when HME was used; however, it was suggested that the use of hydrophobic HME without hygroscopic properties may reduce the risk of pneumonia compared to an HH [19].

13.4   Conclusion

Adequate humidification is essential in patients who are mechanically ventilated or undergo tracheostomy as tracheal mucosa and ciliary function can be severely impaired without it [1]. Selection of appropriate humidification based upon clinical parameters is essential in order to avoid potential complications such as endotracheal occlusions, damaging mucosa, or increased work of breathing [2, 5]. The goal of humidification is to maintain minimal physiologic conditions of 32–34 °C and 100% relative humidity [4, 5]. Objective assessment of humidity is difficult to make, so routine clinical monitoring of the quantity of secretions and condensate in the tubing system is recommended [4]. HMEs are generally preferred if there are no contraindications in patients who require mechanical intubations for short duration [4, 10]. If mechanical ventilation is prolonged, optimal humidification is required to ensure tracheal mucosal function. Ultimately, the humidification devices and target settings will change as more studies emerge, but the indications will remain the same.

References

1. Forbes AR. Humidification and mucous flow in the intubated trachea. Br J Anaesth. 1973;45:874–8.
2. Oostdam JC, Walker DC, Knudson K, et al. Effect of breathing dry air on structure and function of airways. J Apply Physiol. 1986;61(1):312–7.
3. Branson R. Conditioning inspired gases: the search for relevant physiologic end points. Respir Care. 2009;54(4):450–2.
4. AARC Clinical Practice Guideline. Humidification during invasive and non-invasive mechanical ventilation: 2012. Respir Care. 2012;57(5):782–8.
5. Sottiaux T. Consequences of under- and over-humidification. Respir Care Clin. 2006;12(2):233–52.
6. Williams R, Rankin N, Smith T, Galler D, Seakins P. Relationship between the humidity and temperature of inspired gas and the function of the airway mucosa. Crit Care Med. 1196;24(11):1920–9.
7. Branson RD. The effects of inadequate humidity. Respir Care Clin N Am. 1998;4(2):199–214.
8. Solomita M, et al. Humidification and secretion volume in mechanically ventilated patients. Respir Care. 2009;54(10):1329–35.
9. Ricard JD, Miere EL, Markowicz P, et al. Efficiency and safety of mechanical ventilation with a heat and moisture exchanger changed only once a week. Am J Respir Crit Care Med. 2000;161:104–9.
10. Kollef M, et al. A randomized trial comparing an extended-use hygroscopic condenser humidifier with heated-water humidification in mechanically ventilated patients. Chest. 1998;113:759–67.
11. Jaber S, et al. Long-term effects of different humidification systems on endotracheal tube patency. Anesthesiology. 2004;100:783–8.
12. Misset B, et al. Heat and moisture exchanger vs. heated humidifier during long-term mechanical ventilation. Chest. 1991;100:160–3.
13. Lellouch F, Taille S, Qader S, et al. Humdification des voies aeriennes: difficile mais vital. In: Programs and abstracts of the 12eme journee d' assistance ventilatoire en ventilation artificielle. France: Cretieil; 2004. p. 23–40.
14. Lucatao JJ, et al. Evaluation of resistance in 8 different heat-and-moisture exchangers: effects of saturation and flow rate/profile. Respir Care. 2005;50(5):636–43.
15. Shaw MJ. The ventilator circuit and ventilator associated pneumonia. Respir Care. 2005;50(6):774–85.
16. Lemmens HJ, Brock-Utne JG. Heat and moisture exchange devices: are they doing what are supposed to do? Anesth Analg. 2004;98:382–5.
17. Lellouch F, Taile S, Lefrancois F, et al. Humidification performance of 48 passive airway humidifiers: comparison with manufacturer data. Chest. 2009;135(2):276–86.
18. Chiumello D, Pelos P, Park G, et al. In vitro and in vivo evaluation of new active heat moisture exchanger. Crit Care. 2004;8(5):R281–8.
19. Gillies D, Todd A, Foster JP. Heat and moisture exchangers versus heated humidifiers for mechanically ventilated adults and children (review). Cochrane Database Syst Rev. 2017;9:CD004711.
20. Kirton OC, DeHaven B, Morgan J, Morejon O, Civetta J. A prospective, randomized comparison of an in-line heat and moisture exchange filter and heated wire humidifiers: rates of ventilator-associated early-onset (community-acquired) or late-onset (hospital-acquired) pneumonia and incidence of endotracheal tube occlusion. Chest. 1997;112(4):1055–9.
21. Hess DR, Kallstrom TJ, Mottram CD, Myers TR, Sorenson HM, Vines DL. Care of the ventilator circuit and its relation to ventilator-associated pneumonia. Respir Care. 2003;48(9):89–879.
22. Siempos II, Vardakas KZ, Kopterides P, Falagas ME. Impact of passive humidification on clinical outcomes of mechanically ventilated patients: a meta-analysis of randomized controlled trials. Crit Care Med. 2007;35(12):2843–51.

23. Ranjan N, Chaudhary U, Chaudhary D, Ranjan KP. Ventilator associated pneumonia in a tertiary care intensive care unit: analysis of incidence, risk factors and mortality. Indian J Crit Care Med. 2014;18(4):200–4.
24. Charles MP, Kali A, Easow JM, et al. Ventilator associated pneumonia. Australas Med J. 2014;7(8):334–44.
25. Walaszek M, Kosiarka A, Gniadek A, et al. The risk factors for hospital-acquired pneumonia in the intensive care unit. Przegl Epdiemiol. 2016;70:15.
26. Lellouche F, Taille S, Qader S, et al. Humidification des voies aeriennes: diffi cle mais vital. In: Programs and abstracts of the 12eme journee d' assistance ventilatoire en ventilation artifi cielle. France: Creteil; 2004. p. 23–40.

Humidification in Postextubation Respiratory Failure

14

Kishore Kumar, Sulochana Kumari, Antonio Esquinos, and Meenakshi Narasimhan

14.1 Introduction

The inspired gas is heated and moistened significantly by the human airway [1]. During normal breathing, inspiratory gases are warmed and humidified in the nasal passage and pharynx of the upper airways [2]. Humidification is especially necessary in the care of mechanically ventilated and postextubated patients; however, dry and cold gas causes mucosal dryness of the upper respiratory system [3]. The physiology of gas transfer and the protective mechanism of airways such as filtering and warming of inspired air are altered after endotracheal intubation and extubation [4]. Postextubation respiratory failure is common in intensive care unit (ICU) which leads to reintubation in up to 24% of patients and increasing cost, length of stay and mortality [5]. Postextubated respiratory failure patients require meticulous clinical assessment, and the underlying medical condition of the patient's respiratory failure should resolve significantly with adequate oxygenation with humidification, good weaning criteria and rapid shallow breathing index of less than 105 breaths/min/L

K. Kumar (✉)
Department of Respiratory Medicine, Chettinad Hospital and Research Institute (CHRI), Chettinad Academy and Research and Education (CARE), Chennai, India

S. Kumari
Department of Respiratory Medicine, Chettinad Hospital and Research Institute (CHRI), Chettinad Academy and Research and Education (CARE), Chennai, India

Dr. D. Y Patil Hospital and Research Centre, Pune, India

A. Esquinos
Intensive Care Unit, Hospital Morales Meseguer, Murcia, Spain

M. Narasimhan
Department of Respiratory Medicine, Chettinad Hospital and Research Institute (CHRI), Chennai, India
e-mail: respiratorymedicine@care.edu.in

143

[6]. The management of postextubation incorporates oxygenation with facemask, and numerous therapeutic contexts have employed administration of high-flow nasal oxygen (HFNO) and non-invasive ventilation (NIV) with adequate humidification that augment patients with respiratory failure [7, 8]. The routine use of humidification in postextubation respiratory failure is controversial, and there are no widely accepted discourse practices, indications, equipments, etc. In terms of enhancing patient comfort and a few clinical indicators, the literature offers some evidence. However, in order to give convincing data to encourage the use of humidification in postextubation, further clinical investigations are required.

14.2 Need for Humidification During Postextubation Respiratory Failure

Humidity is the amount of water vapour in gaseous environment that varies with the temperature and can be expressed as absolute and relative humidity [4]. Unlike gas exchange, heat and moist exchange is the respiratory system's important function. The connective tissue of the nose is distinguished by a dense vascular system with numerous thin-walled veins. This system is in charge of warming the inspired air to increase its humidity capacity. Isothermic saturation boundary (ISB) is as the air travels down to the respiratory tract reaches the body temperature of 37 °C and 100% relative humidity [9]. Tracheal reintubation is generally used to treat extubation failure, which has been defined as 'the inability to tolerate removal of the endotracheal tube'. [10] It is essential to focus on removal of the artificial airway and oxygenated humidification rather than the mechanical support to prevent the extubation respiratory failure. Postextubation respiratory failure includes all the causes but is not limited to glottis oedema, laryngospasm, inspissated respiratory secretion and tracheal collapse [11]. The mucosa of the respiratory system is lined with goblet cells and pseudo-stratified columnar ciliated epithelial cells which preserve the mucous layer from the foreign barriers and act as a point of humidity exchange [12]. After endotracheal intubation, the upper airway loses its capacity to heat and moisture inhaled gas due to artificial airway bypassing the respiratory tract; hence, partial delivery of dry and cold medical gases damages the respiratory epithelium which may be one of the causes of respiratory failure after extubation which leads to increased work of breathing, atelectasis, thick secretions and bronchospasm [13].

14.3 Indication of Humidification in Postextubation

The goal of the humidification is to continue the normal physiologic function of the smaller airways. Dry gas administration at a flow rate greater than 4 L/min leads to rapid heat and water loss in the upper airways causing further damage to the epithelial structure. Overcoming humidity deficit and humidifying the dry air to oxygenation are the primary indication for humidification [14]. Secondary indications to humidification are bronchospasm, thick secretions and high minute volume of

>10 L/min which leads to respiratory failure after extubation. Cool humidified gas is used to treat upper airway inflammation caused by croup, epiglottitis and postextubation oedema. Physical principles such as temperature, surface area, contact time and heating affect the humidifier's performances [15].

14.4 High-Flow Nasal Cannula Therapy as a Prevention of Postextubation Hypoxemic Respiratory Failure

Unlike conventional oxygen therapy (COT), HFNC allows warmed and humidified gas to the airways. Mucociliary function can be impaired by cold and dry oxygen which causes increased airway resistance and secretion clearance [16]. After extubation, patients with acute respiratory failure demand inspiratory flow rate of 30–120 L/min which cannot be achieved by COT resulting in low oxygen concentration at the alveolar level. The other benefit of HFNC is that it reduces dead space by washing out air from the patient's upper airway and it also proved some amount of positive end-expiratory pressure (PEEP) to the patients. HFNC with good humidification has been used as a frontline respiratory adjunct for acute respiratory failure after extubation in immunocompetent and immunocompromised patients [17, 18]. HFNC is often used as a standard treatment for recent extubation failure underlying respiratory failure; in supporting this, two randomized cross-over trials compared the short-term interventions in patients with extubated failure after passing spontaneous breathing trial (SBT). Both investigations showed better outcome in HFNC with good humidification and no significant changes in gas exchange [19, 20]. Maggiore and colleagues conducted a randomized study with 105 unselected postextubation patients receiving either conventional oxygen therapy (COT) with a Venturi mask or HFNC over a period of 48 hours. The included patients had PaO_2/FiO_2 ratio less than 300 at extubation, and HFNC leads to better oxygenation [21].

Fernandez and colleagues conducted a multicentre study comparing HFNC vs. COT for 24-h postextubation in high-risk extubation failure patients, but the study was stopped due to poor recruitment and failed to provide definitive findings with postextubation failure [22].

14.5 High-Flow Nasal Cannula Therapy as a Prevention of Postextubation Hypercapnic Respiratory Failure

There is a lack of literature that justifies the use of HFNC to minimize extubation failure in hypercapnic respiratory failure due to the well-established role of NIV in the clinical settings. Patients with $PaCO_2 > 45$ mm Hg are included in the RCT by Maggiore et al., who need NIV after extubation [21]. Hypercapnic respiratory failure was a criterion for exclusion in both RCTs conducted by the Spanish group on patients with low or high risk of extubation failure. It is not appropriate to employ preventive HFNC postextubation in hypercapnic respiratory failure in the absence of high-quality evidence supporting its usage [22].

14.6 Conclusion

In many therapeutic settings for adults, infants, children and preterm neonates, devices that give high-flow heated and humidified oxygen through nasal cannulae (HFNC) have become the standard care of postextubation respiratory failure. Optimizing patient outcomes requires preventing extubation failure and reintubation and maintaining a patent airway. Additional randomized controlled studies on a variety of patient population are required to confirm the clinical benefits of humidification in postextubation hypoxemic and hypercapnic respiratory failures.

Key Determinants

1. Postextubation respiratory failure is common in intensive care unit (ICU) which leads to reintubation in up to 24% of patients.
2. Postextubated respiratory failure patients require meticulous clinical assessment.
3. Tracheal reintubation is defined as the inability to tolerate removal of the endotracheal tube.
4. The goal of the humidification is to continue the normal physiologic function of the smaller airways.
5. Cool humidified gas is used to treat upper airway inflammation caused by croup, epiglottitis and postextubation oedema.

References

1. Shelly MP. The humidification and filtration functions of the airways. Respir Care Clin N Am. 2006;12(2):139–48.
2. Chikata Y, Oto J, Onodera M, Nishimura M. Humidification performance of humidifying devices for tracheostomized patients with spontaneous breathing: a bench study. Respir Care. 2013;58(9):1442–8.
3. Oto J, Nakataki E, Okuda N, Onodera M, Imanaka H, Nishimura M. Hygrometric properties of inspired gas and oral dryness in patients with acute respiratory failure during noninvasive ventilation. Respir Care. 2014;59(1):39–45.
4. Cerpa F, Cáceres D, Romero-Dapueto C, Giugliano-Jaramillo C, Pérez R, Budini H, Hidalgo V, Gutiérrez T, Molina J, Keymer J. Suppl 2: M5: humidification on ventilated patients: heated Humidifications or heat and moisture exchangers? Open Respir Med J. 2015;9:104.
5. Demling RH, Read TR, Lind LJ, Flanagan HL. Incidence and morbidity of extubation failure in surgical intensive care patients. Crit Care Med. 1988;16(6):573–7.
6. Nugent K. Postextubation management of patients at high risk for reintubation. J Thorac Dis. 2016;8(12):E1679.
7. Frat JP, Brugiere B, Ragot S, Chatellier D, Veinstein A, Goudet V, Coudroy R, Petitpas F, Robert R, Thille AW, Girault C. Sequential application of oxygen therapy via high-flow nasal cannula and noninvasive ventilation in acute respiratory failure: an observational pilot study. Respir Care. 2015;60(2):170–8.
8. Sotello D, Rivas M, Mulkey Z, Nugent K. High-flow nasal cannula oxygen in adult patients: a narrative review. Am J Med Sci. 2015;349(2):179–85.

9. Kacmarek RM, Stoller JK, Heuer A. Egan's fundamentals of respiratory care e-book. Elsevier Health Sciences; 2019.
10. Epstein S. Decision to extubate. Intensive Care Med. 2002;28(5):535–46.
11. Hartley M, Vaughan RS. Problems associated with tracheal extubation. Br J Anaesth. 1993;71(4):561–8.
12. Anderson SD, Holzer K. Exercise-induced asthma: is it the right diagnosis in elite athletes. J Allergy Clin Immunol. 2000;106(3):419–28.
13. Al Ashry HS, Modrykamien AM. Humidification during mechanical ventilation in the adult patient. Biomed Res Int. 2014;25:2014.
14. Restrepo RD, Walsh BK. Humidification during invasive and noninvasive mechanical ventilation: 2012. Respir Care. 2012;57(5):782–8.
15. Ari A, Fink J. Humidity and aerosol therapy. Mosby's Respiratory Care Equipment-E-Book. 2017;24:156.
16. Chanques G, Constantin JM, Sauter M, Jung B, Sebbane M, Verzilli D, Lefrant JY, Jaber S. Discomfort associated with underhumidified high-flow oxygen therapy in critically ill patients. Intensive Care Med. 2009;35(6):996–1003.
17. Frat JP, Thille AW, Mercat A, Girault C, Ragot S, Perbet S, Prat G, Boulain T, Morawiec E, Cottereau A, Devaquet J. High-flow oxygen through nasal cannula in acute hypoxemic respiratory failure. N Engl J Med. 2015;372(23):2185–96.
18. Coudroy R, Jamet A, Petua P, Robert R, Frat JP, Thille AW. High-flow nasal cannula oxygen therapy versus noninvasive ventilation in immunocompromised patients with acute respiratory failure: an observational cohort study. Ann Intensive Care. 2016;6(1):1–1.
19. Tiruvoipati R, Lewis D, Haji K, Botha J. High-flow nasal oxygen vs. high-flow face mask: a randomized crossover trial in extubated patients. J Crit Care. 2010;25(3):463–8.
20. Rittayamai N, Tscheikuna J, Rujiwit P. High-flow nasal cannula versus conventional oxygen therapy after endotracheal extubation: a randomized crossover physiologic study. Respir Care. 2014;59(4):485–90.
21. Maggiore SM, Idone FA, Vaschetto R, Festa R, Cataldo A, Antonicelli F, Montini L, De Gaetano A, Navalesi P, Antonelli M. Nasal high-flow versus venturi mask oxygen therapy after extubation. Effects on oxygenation, comfort, and clinical outcome. Am J Respir Crit Care Med. 2014;190(3):282–8.
22. Fernandez R, Subira C, Frutos-Vivar F, Rialp G, Laborda C, Masclans JR, Lesmes A, Panadero L, Hernandez G. High-flow nasal cannula to prevent postextubation respiratory failure in high-risk non-hypercapnic patients: a randomized multicenter trial. Ann Intensive Care. 2017;7(1):1–7.

Part V

Humidification and Ventilator Associated Pneumonia

Humidification During Invasive Mechanical Ventilation: Selection of Device and Replacement

Jean-Damien Ricard

15.1 Which Device for which Patients

As stated earlier on, adding heat and moisture to the inspired gas during invasive mechanical ventilation is mandatory. This can be adequately achieved both by HMEs and heated humidifiers [1]. There are very few and rare contraindications to the use of HMEs. Because they act passively, the amount of heat and moisture they deliver to the inspired gases depends on the amount of heat and moisture they retain during expiration. Therefore, patients with profound hypothermia or important broncho-pleural fistula should preferably be ventilated with a heated humidifier. In addition, a heated humidifier may be preferable in patients ventilated for acute asthma or acute respiratory distress syndrome, in whom a drastic tidal volume reduction induces extreme respiratory acidosis (to avoid increased dead space with HMEs) [2] until improvement in the patient's respiratory condition enables the use of an HME. Apart from these specific situations, HMEs should be considered first to heat and humidify inspired gases of all mechanically ventilated patients. As mentioned earlier, they are as effective clinically as heated humidifiers, and they are much cheaper and much easier to use. Importantly, medical as well as surgical patients can benefit from them. Indeed, despite former algorithms that tended to restrict their use to patients without a history of respiratory disease and for the first 5 days of mechanical ventilation only, several studies have clearly shown that they can be used in any patient requiring mechanical ventilation, even in patients with COPD and for any length of mechanical ventilation. Because patients with COPD represent the most important subgroup of mechanically ventilated ICU patients in the United States and because their

J.-D. Ricard (✉)
INSERM U1137, UFR de Médecine, Université Paris Cité, Paris, France

AP-HP, Hôpital Louis Mourier, DMU ESPRIT, Service de Médecine Intensive Réanimation, Colombes, France
e-mail: jean-damien.ricard@lmr.aphp.fr

151

A. M. Esquinas (ed.), *Humidification in the Intensive Care Unit*,
https://doi.org/10.1007/978-3-031-23953-3_15

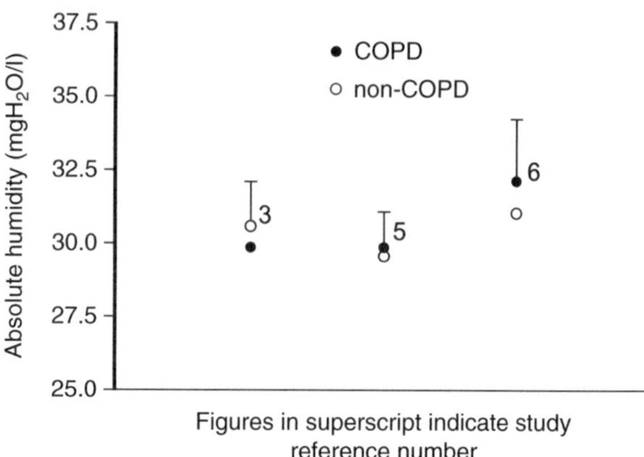

Fig. 15.1 Comparison of levels of absolute humidity delivered by HMEs in COPD and non-COPD patients in three different studies. Very similar levels are obtained, indicating that HMEs can be used in COPD patients

duration of ventilation is longer than that of other patients, adequate humidification is probably more critical in such patients than in those ventilated for shorter periods of time. Numerous studies have shown that long-term mechanical ventilation can be safely conducted in such patients with HMEs [3–6]. Three studies have specifically compared the humidity output of HMEs in COPD and non-COPD patients and consistently found that values for absolute humidity measured in COPD and non-COPD patients were very similar (Fig. 15.1) [3, 5, 6].

15.2 Humidification During Invasive Mechanical Ventilation

15.2.1 Frequency of HME Replacement

There is now considerable evidence that HMEs can be used for longer than the 24 h recommended by the manufacturers (reviewed in [7]). These compelling results stem either from rigorous clinical evaluation [8, 9] or extensive bedside measurement of humidity delivery [3–6, 10]. Figure 15.2 shows that humidity delivery of a combined HME (Hygrobac®, DAR, Mirandola, Italy) used for 7 days without change was remarkably stable during this period of time. Progressive clogging of the device with tracheal secretions (that seriously increase its resistance to airflow) could have been a potential drawback to the prolonged use of the HME. Repeated measurements of the resistance of the HME over 7 days indicate that this phenomenon did not occur [3] (Fig. 15.2). Maintaining the HME vertically above the tracheal tube (Fig. 15.3), as well as having nurses and doctors repeatedly check the position of the HME, prevents secretions from refluxing from the tracheal tube and obstructing the HME [3, 5]. Use of HMEs can be extended in both medical patients

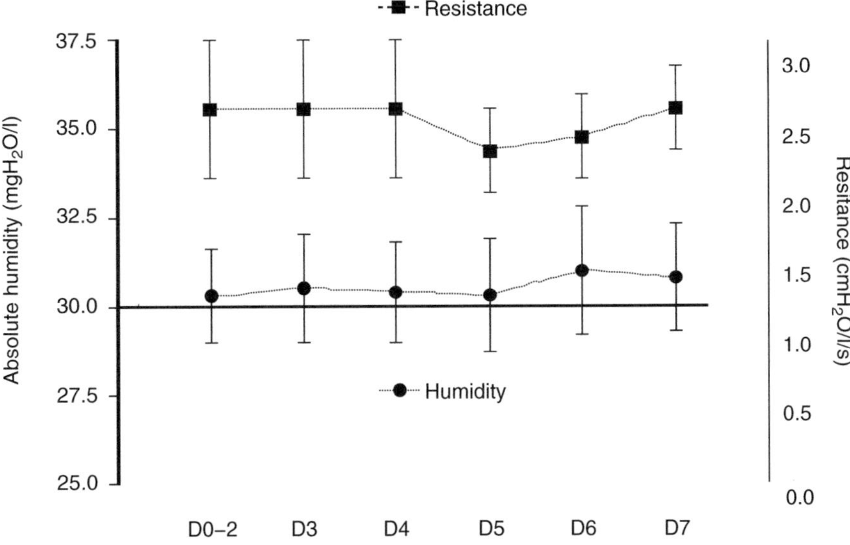

Fig. 15.2 Levels of absolute humidity (*left Y axis*) and resistance (*right Y axis*) measured with HMEs kept during 7 days in mechanically ventilated patients. Both parameters remained remarkably stable during the 7 days of use (reproduced from Ricard JD [3])

(including those with COPD [3–6]) and surgical patients [10–12]. This practice is now widely accepted, and recommendations have been made to change HMEs only once a week [13]. In our own published [3, 6] and unpublished experience, we have been changing HMEs only once a week since 1997 and haven't encountered endotracheal tube occlusions.

15.2.2 Bedside Adjustment

Assessing adequate humidification at the bedside is desirable if not essential for at least two reasons: (1) a potentially life-threatening tracheal tube occlusion [14] may occur without any precursory clinical signs of insufficient humidification and (2) devices may not deliver, in some instances, the heat and humidity that is expected from them, either because they are malfunctioning or because performances measured in the clinical setting do not attain those publicized by the manufacturer [6].

There are two aspects to this assessment: (1) Is the device delivering enough heat and humidity (according to the standards)? (2) Is the amount of heat and moisture delivered appropriate for a given patient?

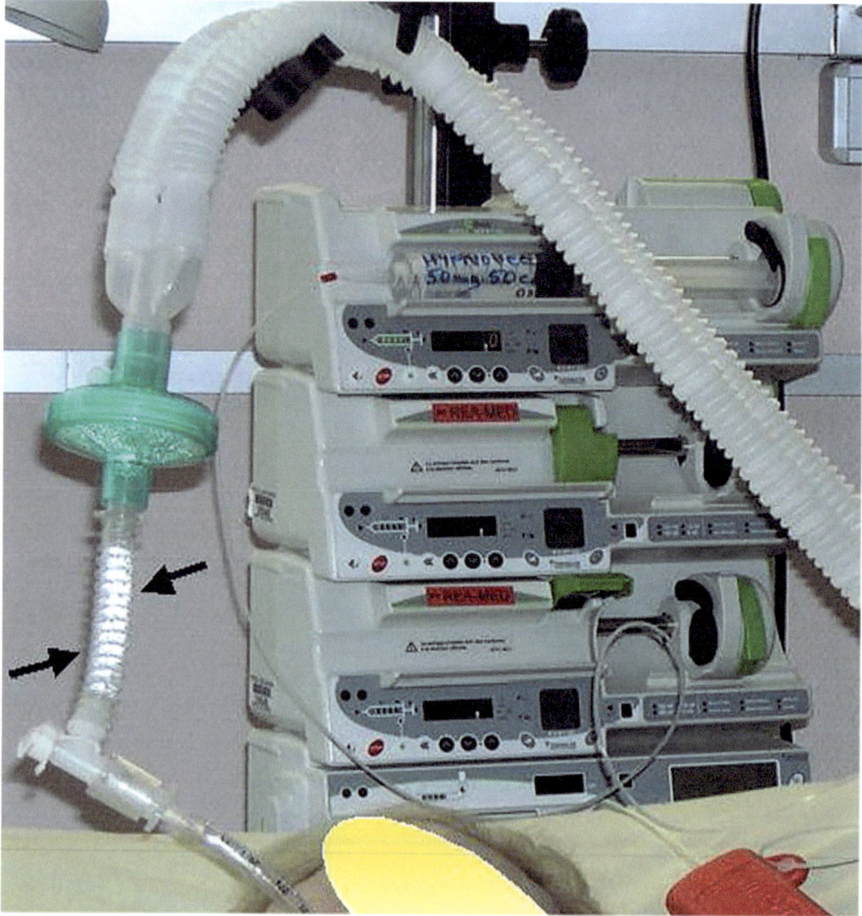

Fig. 15.3 Photograph of an HME and its flex tube in a mechanically ventilated patients. Black arrows show the presence of abundant condensation in the flex tube. The flex tube and the HME are positioned vertically above the endotracheal tube, so as to limit secretions reaching the HME

15.3   Assessing HMEs and Heated Humidifiers at the Bedside

A simple means of evaluating the humidity delivered by a given device is to rate the amount of condensation seen in the flex tube that connects either the Y piece (when using a heated humidifier) or the HME to the endotracheal tube [15]. Indeed, a positive correlation has been found between the amount of condensation seen in the flex tube (black arrows, Fig. 15.3) and the absolute humidity measured at the bedside [15]. When, with a given device, the flex tube is constantly dry over time or if only very few droplets of water are seen, then the absolute humidity delivered by this device is probably below 25 mgH$_2$O/L and the patient at risk of endotracheal tube occlusion. On the other hand, when numerous droplets are seen in the flex tube or when it is dripping wet, then the device is more likely to deliver an absolute humidity sufficient to avoid endotracheal tube occlusion [15].

15.4   Assessing Adequacy of Inspired Gas Conditioning

Though it is conceivable that some patients have special humidification needs, the prevailing literature indicates that heated humidifiers and HMEs equally meet the humidification requirements of the vast majority of mechanically ventilated patients. Therefore, monitoring the aspect of the secretions (thick and tenacious or on the contrary watery and abundant) in order to detect insufficient or excessive humidification may be of limited value, since changes in the mucus aspect may be entirely due to the patient's condition (respiratory status, fluid balance, etc.) and not the consequence of the humidifying device. As a matter of fact, it has been shown that air humidification with either an HME or a heated humidifier had similar effects on mucosal rheological properties, contact angle, and transportability by cilia in patients undergoing mechanical ventilation. Finally, results from a recent meta-analysis indicate that both HMEs and heated humidifiers should be considered the gold standard of humidification since no difference in outcome was found between patients ventilated with an HME and those with heated humidifiers [1, 16]. For obvious practical and economic reasons, HMEs should be systematically used in the first place.

References

1. Ricard JD. Gold standard for humidification: heat and moisture exchangers, heated humidifiers, or both? Crit Care Med. 2007;35:2875–6.
2. Prin S, Chergui K, Augarde R, Page B, Jardin F, Vieillard-Baron A. Ability and safety of a heated humidifier to control hypercapnic acidosis in severe ARDS. Intens Care Med. 2002;28:1756–60.
3. Ricard JD, Le Mière E, Markowicz P, Lasry S, Saumon G, Djedaïni K, Coste F, Dreyfuss D. Efficiency and safety of mechanical ventilation with a heat and moisture exchanger changed only once a week. Am J Respir Crit Care Med. 2000;161:104–9.
4. Markowicz P, Ricard JD, Dreyfuss D, Mier L, Brun P, Coste F, Boussougant Y, Djedaïni K. Safety, efficacy and cost effectiveness of mechanical ventilation with humidifying filters changed every 48 hours: a prospective, randomized study. Crit Care Med. 2000;28:665–71.
5. Boyer A, Thiery G, Lasry S, Pigné E, Salah A, de Lassence A, Dreyfuss D, Ricard JD. Long-term mechanical ventilation with hygroscopic heat and moisture exchangers used for 48 hours: a prospective, clinical, hygrometric and bacteriologic study. Crit Care Med. 2003;31:823–9.
6. Thiéry G, Boyer A, Pigné E, Salah A, de Lassence A, Dreyfuss D, Ricard JD. Heat and moisture exchangers in mechanically ventilated intensive care unit patients: a plea for an independent assessment of their performance. Crit Care Med. 2003;31:699–704.
7. Ricard JD. Humidification. In: Tobin M, editor. Principles and practice of mechanical ventilation. New York: McGraw-Hill; 2006. p. 1109–20.
8. Djedaïni K, Billiard M, Mier L, Le Bourdellès G, Brun P, Markowicz P, Estagnasie P, Coste F, Boussougant Y, Dreyfuss D. Changing heat and moisture exchangers every 48 hour rather than

every 24 hour does not affect their efficacy and the incidence of nosocomial pneumonia. Am J Respir Crit Care Med. 1995;152:1562–9.

9. Kollef M, Shapiro S, Boyd V, Silver P, Von Hartz B, Trovillion E, Prentice D. A randomized clinical trial comparing an extended-use hygroscopic condenser humidifier with heated-water humidification in mechanically ventilated patients. Chest. 1998;113:759–67.

10. Davis K Jr, Evans SL, Campbell RS, Johannigman JA, Luchette FA, Porembka DT, Branson RD. Prolonged use of heat and moisture exchangers does not affect device efficiency or frequency rate of nosocomial pneumonia. Crit Care Med. 2000;28:1412–8.

11. Thomachot L, Vialet R, Viguier JM, Sidier B, Roulier P, Martin C. Efficacy of heat and moisture exchangers after changing every 48 hours rather than 24 hours. Crit Care Med. 1998;26:477–81.

12. Thomachot L, Boisson C, Arnaud S, Michelet P, Cambon S, Martin C. Changing heat and moisture exchangers after 96 hours rather than after 24 hours: a clinical and microbiological evaluation. Crit Care Med. 2000;28:714–20.

13. Dodek P, Keenan S, Cook D, Heyland D, Jacka M, Hand L, Muscedere J, Foster D, Mehta N, Hall R, Brun-Buisson C. Evidence-based clinical practice guideline for the prevention of ventilator-associated pneumonia. Ann Intern Med. 2004;141:305–13.

14. Martin C, Perrin G, Gevaudan MJ, Saux P, Gouin F. Heat and moisture exchangers and vaporizing humidifiers in the intensive care unit. Chest. 1990;97:144–9.

15. Ricard JD, Markowicz P, Djedaïni K, Mier L, Coste F, Dreyfuss D. Bedside evaluation of efficient airway humidification during mechanical ventilation of the critically ill. Chest. 1999;137(115):1646–52.

16. Siempos I, Vardakas K, Kopterides P, Falagas M. Impact of passive humidification on clinical outcomes of mechanically ventilated patients: a meta-analysis of randomized controlled trials. Crit Care Med. 2007;35(12):2843–51.

Part VI

Humidification Tracheostomized

Giuseppe Fiorentino, Maurizia Lanza, Anna Annunziata,
and Antonio M. Esquinas

Abbreviations

HME	Passive heat and moisture exchangers
HH	Active humidifiers
ICU	Intensive care unit
VAP	Ventilator-associated pneumonia
TV	Tidal volume

16.1 Introduction

The inhaled air, during the passage through the upper airways, undergoes alterations of some of its characteristics up to having at the alveolar-capillary interface body temperature (37 °C), relative humidity of 100% and absolute humidity of 44 mg/L [1]. These conditions are reached at the level of the fourth or fifth bronchial generation, known as the isothermal saturation limit. This limit is of fundamental importance to keep the ciliary epithelium intact, essential for eliminating dust and inhaled particles through the clearance of ciliary mucus and bypassing damage to the muscle [2]. As a result, the upper airways are known to play an essential role in the physical defence of the lung by filtering, humidifying and heating inhaled gases before they reach the trachea, controlling secretions from dehydrating and

G. Fiorentino (✉)
Monaldi Hospital, Naples, Italy

M. Lanza · A. Annunziata
AO dei Colli PO Monaldi Hospital, Naples, Italy

A. M. Esquinas
Intensive Care Unit, Hospital General Universitario Morales Meseguer, Murcia, Spain

159

A. M. Esquinas (ed.), *Humidification in the Intensive Care Unit*,
https://doi.org/10.1007/978-3-031-23953-3_16

preserving the clearance system respiratory mucosa intact [3]. Placement of the tracheostomy results in upper airway bypass, and as a result, these patients have deficient humidification and heating of the inspired gases. The most typical pathological changes in these patients are thickening and increased viscosity of secretions, injury to the ciliated tracheal mucosa, which will be inflamed and ulcerated, frequent formation of mucus plugs in the airways and crusts, the latter persistent in the postoperative period after tracheostomy, resulting in a higher incidence of airway infections, obstruction or atelectasis due to retained secretions [4]. These alterations involve cleaning operations with repeated aspirations through the tracheostomy, which cause discomfort to the patient and, in turn, increase the likelihood of airway obstruction and the risk of infections. Therefore, humidification achieved by devices is necessary for all mechanically ventilated patients and tracheostomized patients, although the optimal humidity value of these patients remains unclear.

16.2 Humidification for Tracheostomy

Mechanical ventilation uses dry gas to ventilate the lungs by bypassing the body's average warming and humidifying mechanisms. Thus, this causes damage to the respiratory epithelium of patients by making secretions stickier and activating the mechanisms described in the introductory chapter. Different types of humidifiers have been produced for clinical use to prevent this from happening, and each has its advantages and disadvantages [5]. Humidifiers are devices that add water molecules to the gas. These devices are classified as active or passive based on external sources of heat and water or the use of patients' temperature and hydration to achieve humidification.

Regardless of the device chosen, it should meet the minimum requirements to replace upper airway functions, which according to the American Association for Respiratory Care, are:

- 30 mg/l of absolute humidity, 34 °C and 100% relative humidity for HME.
- Between 33 and 44 mg/l of absolute humidity; between 34 °C and 41 °C; 100% relative humidity for active humidifiers.

In addition, the risk of infection of each device must be considered [6].

16.3 Passive Heat and Moisture Exchangers (HME)

The operating principle of passive humidifiers is based on the ability to retain heat and humidity during the expiratory cycle and deliver 70% of the gas inhaled during inspiration. They use the individual's temperature and hydration to achieve humidification.

Passive heat and moisture exchangers (HME) are those filters that are placed between the respiratory circuit and the patient (between mount or tracheostomy and ventilation lines). They are also known as artificial noses and feature a cellulose fibre surface with a hygroscopic coating that absorbs water in the exhaled air. They represent a simple, practical and effective way to humidify and heat the air, and mechanical ventilation is widely used. Made of materials with high conduction and thermal resistance, they have the task of retaining heat and condensing the humidity of the exhaled air, then returning them to the patient in the form of heated vapour. With inhalation, the air passes over the hygroscopic surface and humidifies and heats the air that passes into the airways during the next inhalation.

The HME can be attached directly to the tracheostomy tube for an person who respires spontaneously with a tracheostomy [7].

They are divided into:

- hygroscopic; they have a large condensation surface with a hygroscopic coating that allows them to chemically absorb most of the humidity and heat exhaled by the patient;
- hydrophobic; characterized by a weak electrical conductivity, they are less efficient in terms of gas conditioning but have a high bacterial filtration capacity;
- mixed; hydrophobic and hygroscopic, they combine thermal conditioning and humidification performance with an adequate quality of microbiological filtration.

Despite the theoretical advantages of hygroscopic HMEs over hydrophobic devices, no differences were shown in the number of tracheal aspirates, mucus viscosity, atelectasis, tracheal tube occlusion, bacterial colonization, and colonization ventilator-associated pneumonia (VAP) [8].

Under optimal conditions, this can provide an absolute humidity more significant than 30–32 mg H_2O/l at a temperature of 27–30 °C. However, overall their performance depends on many variables such as the flow rate of the inspiratory/expiratory flow, the ambient temperature, the quantity of water vapour in the average flow and their size.

They have some drawbacks:

- they increase the dead space by about 90/100 ml;
- they can become clogged with condensation and secretions and cause them to accumulate in the respiratory circuit (with consequent resistance to the airflow, risk of infections and malfunction of machinery);
- the ambient temperature can affect their performance;
- they are not recommended in certain clinical conditions, such as in patients who have a low tidal volume (TV) (a condition where the dead space of the HME can represent an essential volume of air), and inappropriate elimination of CO_2 or abundant tracheobronchial secretions.

HME filter manufacturers provide general specifications for the care and management of specific issues. These filters require regular checking to ensure they are not blocked by secretions or condensation. Good management of HME filters is of paramount importance to avoid flow obstructions, leading to increased resistance during lung ventilation. An artificial nose positioned at the end of the tracheostomy, the end of the airway in some patients also increases dead space [9]. In patients undergoing mechanical ventilation, the HME filter must be positioned before the "Y" of the circuit in order to come into contact with both inhaled and exhaled air. Here too, the position before the "Y" increases the dead space and adversely affects ventilation parameters.

Several authors have observed the adverse effects of additional dead space on respiratory mechanics. This typically becomes relevant when the disease requires lung protection strategies (low TV). Prat Hinkson's studies explain this, demonstrating significant changes in the partial pressure of arterial carbon dioxide ($PaCO_2$) (and pH) under these circumstances [10].

We know that the respiratory rate, the TV, or both must increase; otherwise, arterial carbon dioxide will increase. This consequence is most prominent in spontaneously breathing patients and is a role of the association between TV and dead space [11].

The presence of HME makes it more challenging to administer drugs through small volume nebulizers. Therefore, these filters are not recommended in patients who require frequent administration. A metered-dose inhaler can be used with an HME if its adapter is placed between the HME and the endotracheal tube or tracheostomy tube. It should be noted that to increase the amount of humidity produced, HMEs use calcium chloride or lithium chloride as hygroscopic additives. At the same time, other manufacturers also use chlorhexidine for bacteriostatic effects. In 2009, the European Respiratory Society (ERS), the European Society of Clinical Microbiology and Infectious Diseases (ESCMID) and the European Society of Intensive Care Medicine (ESICM) published a statement choosing HMEs over HHs for the prevention of VAP. In the same year, the VAP Guidelines Committee and the Canadian Critical Care Trials Group declared that there was no difference in the incidence of VAP between HME and HH. The inclination of the European guidelines towards HMES coincides with the trend of clinical practice. The piece of lithium contained in these filters, which could be released into the trachea and then absorbed, was also examined and found that the small amount of lithium in these devices seems to make this concern unwarranted [12].

However, as a general recommendation, the HME should be changed:

- Due to excessive condensation, which increases its resistance.
- Due to the visible impact with secretions or blood.
- Every 48 h in patients with chronic obstructive pulmonary disease.
- Every 96 h and up to 1 week in the remaining patients

16.4 Active Humidifiers (HH)

Active humidifiers (HH) can deliver gas at approximately 37 °C at an absolute humidity of 44 mg H_2O/l and are traditionally considered the gold standard of inspired gas humidification. Active humidifiers consist of heating plates that heat by increasing the temperature of sterile water contained in a humidification chamber and thus generating steam. The air intended for the patient passes through this chamber contained in a humidification chamber, saturates with water vapour and reaches the set temperature [13].

The management of active humidification devices includes:

- the correct positioning of the humidifier, which must be interposed on the inspiratory line of the circuit at least 20–30 cm lower than the patient and the ventilator, in order to avoid the danger of condensation entering the machine, causing damage or being directed towards the patient's airways (infectious risk);
- an adequate environment. Active humidifiers must be set to deliver an inspiratory gas temperature (usually monitored by a sensor located in the Y-piece of the circuit) between 34 °C and 41 °C and a humidity between 33 mg/l and 44 mg/l of water vapour;
- careful monitoring. Active humidifiers can be equipped with displays to view temperatures, alarms to ensure greater safety and servo-controlled thermostats to avoid excessive humidification.

The regulation of humidification is crucial [14] as insufficient humidification, and insufficient heating can cause damage such as tracheal inflammation and ulceration of the tracheobronchial mucosa, loss of body water and heat, retention of secretions that become thick viscous, thus inhibiting ciliary activity. This can cause an increase in respiratory work and obstructive phenomena affecting the airways and related frequent bronchopulmonary infections and more or less extensive atelectasis.

On the other hand, excessive humidification can sometimes be counterproductive. It reduces the viscosity of secretions, increases mucociliary clearance, and determines a dilution of the surfactant by recalling neutrophils in the bronchioles and lungs. This could also lead to retention of secretions with consequent atelectasis, worsening lung compliance. All these changes increase local susceptibility to bacterial infections, with the risk of bronchopneumonia.

Also, the heating of the inspired gases must be obtained with the right measure as an excess can damage the bronchial mucosa causing a weakening of the cycling clearance. The ISO (International Organization of Standardization) has established that the gas supply at temperatures above 41 °C represents a risk of damage to the patient's bronchial epithelium [14]. While active plate humidifiers are more accurate than HMEs in providing heat and humidification, they are less practical. Furthermore, they have a higher cost, and they have the problems of electrical equipment such as overheating, and the humidification chambers can be the site of colonization. Although data demonstrate that the risk of infection of active humidifiers does not significantly exceed that of passive ones, demonstrating the mismatch between the filter used and the incidence of ventilator-associated pneumonia [15].

Active humidifiers are classified into: (1) bubble; (2) passover; (3) counter-flow; and (4) inline vaporizer. All use an external device to provide both heat and humidification and consist of an electric heater on which is positioned a plastic container with a metal base in which there is sterile water. When this base is heated, the temperature of the water increases by convection. They have different designs and techniques for humidification. When used with mechanical ventilation, as previously mentioned, they are positioned in line with the inspiratory branch of the respirator. The circuit leaving the inhalation valve is connected to the inlet hole of the plastic casing, which must always be filled with water to the level indicated by the manufacturer. Subsequently, a second section of the circuit (of standard length) is connected to the outlet hole of the casing and to the "Y" of the circuit responsible for supplying gas to the patient. With this type of humidification device, it is mandatory to use water wells, i.e. tanks with one-way circulation systems that allow the deposition of excess condensate without air leaks. Excessive water accumulation in the circuit can lead to self-priming, incorrect reading of the ventilator monitor, or even the drainage of infected material into the patient's airways.

Some types of active humidifiers are regulated by a heating wire that maintains the temperature of the gas in the passage and by two sensors connected to another wire connected to the output of the heater (distal) and a part of the circuit (near the patient), which has the objective of maintaining the temperature of the system.

The heated wire breathing circuit keeps the temperature stable along its entire path and decreases condensation [16].

16.5 Bubble Humidifier

The bubble humidifiers are no longer used. Their mechanism for acquiring heat and humidity was constituted by a tube immersed in a water tank where the gas was directed. The gas that comes out from the other side of the pipe, heated by diffusers or grilles, enters the fan circuit, having acquired both humidity and heat during its passage towards the surface. The moisture content of the gas depends on various factors, first of all on the amount of water present in the container and on the flow rate; therefore, if the water column in the container is higher, the gas-water interface will increase. On the other hand, as the circulating flow increases, the device's performance decreases [17].

16.6 Passover

In this type of humidifier, the gas passes over the surface of a water tank which constitutes the humidifier chamber, which is heated and transports water vapor to the patient, exiting in the ventilator circuit. It is presented in the wick or membrane variant. Passover devices have a lower resistance than bubble humidifiers and have replaced most of these and are commonly used in invasive and non-invasive mechanical ventilation. They are very simple and the reservoir is powered through a closed system [18].

16.7 Counterflow

In the counterflow humidifier, the water is heated outside the vaporizer and is subsequently pumped into the upper portion of the humidifier through pores. These pores are tiny in diameter, and therefore, water comes into contact with a large surface. The gas flows in the opposite direction. The air is hydrated and heated to body temperature as it passes through the humidifier chamber. Schumann et al. compared the counter-current humidifier with a Passover and a heat and humidity exchanger (HME) in an artificial lung model. The authors highlighted that the counter-current device needed less breathing work than the others. Additionally, the humidification performance of the counter-current model was separated of flow and respiratory rate, in contrast to the heated Passover humidifier, where humidification performance decreased as fan speed increased. This technology is promising, but more studies are needed before it becomes widely adopted [19].

16.8 Inline Vaporizer

The new inline vaporizer was designed for high-frequency percussion ventilation [20]. Use a small plastic capsule where water vapour enters the gas at the inspiratory end of the ventilator circuit near the patient. A peristaltic pump supplies the water, and its quantity is set by the doctor based on some parameters of the ventilator and, in particular, the minute volume. In addition to water vapour, the gas heating is supplemented by a small disc heater in the capsule. Temperature and humidity are entirely adjustable and can be constantly displayed.

16.9 High Flow Humidifiers

High flow humidifiers consist of a heating structure, water tank and a temperature and alarm probe. Most of these types of humidifiers fall into pass-over humidifiers, wick humidifiers or bubble humidifiers. All are, however, capable of providing a wide range of temperatures and humidity [21].

These devices are heated and prevent the patient from losing body heat. This is of fundamental importance, especially in neonatal realities.

When using heated humidifiers, the patient's airway temperature must be monitored continuously with a thermometer or thermistor. This is to avoid damage to the mucosa caused by heat.

It may also be desirable to monitor the relative humidity of the proximal airways, although this is not commonly done. With high flow humidifiers, the water level in the tank can be maintained manually by adding water from a bag through a fill set connected to the humidifier or from a floating feed system to keep the water level constant. Manual methods tend to increase the risk of tank contamination and carry the additional risk of spillage and overfilling, so float fill and feed systems are preferred [22].

Most humidifiers are servo-controlled; the operator selects the preferred gas temperature on the thermistor. The system maintains control of the gas temperature regardless of gas flow or tank level changes. These systems are equipped with audiovisual alarms to signal high-temperature conditions. It is essential to recognize that the thermistors in these systems have a relatively slow response and reflect only the average temperature of the inspired gas. Actual temperatures can fluctuate above and below the average temperature with cyclic gas flow, as can happen in a mechanical ventilation circuit.

It has become popular to heat the tube that carries the gas from the humidifier to the patient in recent years. These circuits contain electrical wires that heat the gas passing through the heated fan wire circuit. Heated wire rings provide a more accurate gas temperature supplied to the patient and prevent water condensation in the tube. The wire temperature can be controlled by the humidifier temperature control or separately. If the temperature of the heating cables is controlled separately from the humidifier, this can affect the umidity furnished to the patient if the tube temperature is higher than the temperature of the gas leaving the humidifier, the relative humidity of the gas decreases, which can cause drying of secretions and obstruction of the endotracheal tube. If, on the other hand, the temperature of the tube is lower than the temperature of the gas leaving the humidifier, condensation will occur in the tube [23].

Precautions and monitoring

- Observe that the hose drains water downwards and not towards the artificial airways or the ventilator.
- Correctly position the water separators to receive the drained water
- Frequently monitor the active humidifier device (water level, temperature level, check for condensation)
- Never fill above the recommended level
- Do not drain the condensate towards the humidifier chamber

16.10 Advantages and Disadvantages of Passive and Active Humidifiers

There are some data for acceptance of HMEs over active humidifiers especially concerning the prevention of ventilation-associated pneumonia.

But generally, considering the humidification capacity and the advantages and disadvantages, both passive and active humidifiers are suitable for conditioning inhaled gas. Device selection should not be based solely on infection control.

Active plate humidifiers, compared to HMEs, are more efficient in terms of precision in providing humidification and heat to the inspired gases. But they are less practical and have higher costs and risks such as overheating, all the usual problems relating to electrical equipment and the colonization of the liquid present in the humidification chamber [24]. Regarding the latter eventuality and, in general, the risk of infection, it should be specified that the active humidification systems do not seem to be more or less at risk than the passive ones: various scientific studies show no correspondence between the humidification method [25, 26]. Used and the incidence of pneumonia associated with mechanical ventilation. When deciding which humidification system to use, several clinical scenarios need to be considered as each device has particular properties that can affect the patient's clinical situation. Below are the advantages and disadvantages of both devices to consider (Tables 16.1 and 16.2).

Table 16.1 Advantage and disadvantage of HH

	Advantages	Disadvantages
Active	Universal application	Cost
	Reliability	Using water
	Alarms	Condensation
	Wide ranges of temperature and humidity	Risk of contamination
	Temperature monitoring	Low possibility of electrical shock and burns
	Reaches the maximum absolute humidity	No filter

Table 16.2 Advantage and disadvantage of HME

	Advantages	Disadvantages
Passive	Cost	Does not apply all patients
	Passive operation	Increase dead space
	User friendly	Increase resistance
	Removal of condensation	Potential occlusion
	Portable	Misting problems

16.11 Aerosol Therapy Humidifiers

The Gibeck Humid-Flo HME for Aerosol Therapy is an HME that does not need to be removed but can remain on the line while aerosol is applied in mechanical ventilation.

This consequently avoids the opening of the circuit and reduces the potential contamination of the pipes and the exposure of the medical personnel to contaminated gases. This humidifier is equipped with two modes: "HME and AEROSOL".

They can be selected by rotating the device's central axis. With HME mode, the device serves as a conventional passive humidifier. In AEROSOL mode, the humidifier part is skipped; then the aerosol goes directly to the patient without coming into contact with the material of the filter humidifier. However, there are some critical issues. The absolute humidity provided with this device would appear low as it provides 30.4 mg/L, but with a TV of 1000 ml.

However, various studies, albeit only in laboratory, attest that the presence of modified HME for aerosol therapy does not interfere with drug deposition [27]. Recently, in a bench study, Ari et al. evaluated the performance of different HMEs to be used in combination with aerosol therapy. Those authors found no significant differences in drug deposition (albuterol) in the artificial lung without HME (control) compared to HME, using a hydrated circuit (simulating a patient's actual gas exhalation) [28].

16.12 Conclusion

Humidification of the inspired gas is necessary and mandatory for all mechanically ventilated patients and even more so in tracheostomized patients [29]. It is necessary to prevent retention with increased viscosity of the secretion, any blockages or obstructions of the tracheal tube or tracheostomy tube and alterations in the epithelium of the respiratory tract. Patients requiring long-term tracheostomy or tracheostoma can benefit from artificial noses and especially patients with upper airway disease. The device not only helps maintain moisture, but also acts as a filter to prevent inhalation of large particles of dust and other airborne detritus. Various authors have emphasised how the use of an HME in patients with tracheostomy reduces the sputum production and the number of coughing episodes per day. These results can be very important to the patient's quality of life and often also allow for improved sleep habits and greater safety when traveling away from home [30]. HMEs exhibit a wide variation in performance and are the cheapest systems to use. Jet nebulizers can be efficient at delivering aerosolized solutions to the lungs and trachea in mechanically ventilated patients, but in spontaneously breathing patients, a heated humidifier and HMEs have better humidification and thermal capabilities. Nebulizers are also said to be potentially harmful. Heated humidification has shown a potential advantage over cold air nebulization in newly tracheostomized patients with respect to physiological and clinically relevant parameters [31]. Patients who require tracheostomy and prolonged mechanical ventilation in subacute hospitals and long-term care facilities can use the artificial nose for much longer periods. Inadequate humidifier settings or the selection of inappropriate devices can adversely affect clinical outcomes by damaging the airway mucosa, prolonging mechanical ventilation, or increasing work of breathing. Humidifier devices can work passively or actively, depending on the source of heat and humidity. Depending on the clinical scenario, the humidifier selection may change over time. The choice is commonly one of the doctor's preferences and costs. There is no one humidification method suitable for all patients and clinicians must adapt the method used to the patient's needs [32].

References

1. http://www.cdc.gov/hicpac/pdf/guidelines/HApneu2003guidelines.pdf.
2. Sahin-Yilmaz A, Naclerio RM. Anatomy and physiology of the upper airway. Proc Am Thorac Soc. 2011;8(1):31–9.
3. Keck T, Leiacker R, Heinrich A, Kühnemann S, Rettinger G. Humidity and temperature profile in the nasal cavity. Rhinology. 2000;38(4):167–71.
4. Stannard W, O'Callaghan C. Ciliary function and the role of cilia in clearance. J Aerosol Med. 2006;19(1):110–5.
5. Restrepo RD, Walsh BK, American Association for Respiratory Care. Humidification during invasive and noninvasive mechanical ventilation: 2012. Respir Care. 2012;57(5):782–8.
6. Davis K Jr, Evans SL, Campbell RS, et al. Prolonged use of heat and moisture exchangers does not affect device efficiency or frequency rate of nosocomial pneumonia. Crit Care Med. 2000;28(5):1412–8.
7. Chikata Y, Oto J, Onodera M, Nishimura M. Humidification performance of humidifying devices for tracheostomized patients with spontaneous breathing: a bench study. Respir Care. 2013;58(9):1442–8.
8. Kola A, Eckmanns T, Gastmeier P. Efficacy of heat and moisture exchangers in preventing ventilator-associated pneumonia: meta-analysis of randomized controlled trials. Intensive Care Med. 2005;31(1):5–11.
9. Campbell RS, Davis K Jr, Johannigman JA, Branson RD. The effects of passive humidifier dead space on respiratory variables in paralyzed and spontaneously breathing patients. Respir Care. 2000;45(3):306–12.
10. Hinkson CR, Benson MS, Stephens LM, Deem S. The effects of apparatus dead space on P(aCO2) in patients receiving lung-protective ventilation. Respir Care. 2006;51(10):1140–4.
11. Prat G, Renault A, Tonnelier JM, Goetghebeur D, Oger E, Boles JM, et al. Influence of the humidification device during acute respiratory distress syndrome. Intensive Care Med. 2003;29(12):2211–5.
12. Birk R, Händel A, Wenzel A, et al. Heated air humidification versus cold air nebulization in newly tracheostomized patients. Head Neck. 2017;39:2481–7.
13. Roux NG, Plotnikow GA, Villalba DS, Gogniat E, Feld V, RiberoVairo N, et al. Evaluation of an active humidification system for inspired gas. Clin Exp Otorhinolaryngol. 2015;8(1):69–75.
14. Sottiaux TM. Consequences of under- and over-humidification. Respir Care Clin N Am. 2006;12(2):233–52.
15. Kelly, Gillies D, Todd DA, Lockwood C. Heated humidification versus heat and moisture exchangers for ventilated adults and children. Cochrane Database Syst Rev. 2010;4:CD004711.
16. Schena E, Saccomandi P, Cappelli S, Silvestri S. Mechanical ventilation with heated humidifiers: measurements of condensed water mass within the breathing circuit according to ventilatory settings. Physiol Meas. 2013;34(7):813.

17. Thomachot L, Leone M, Razzouk K, Antonini F, Vialet R, Martin C. Randomized clinical trial of extended use of a hydrophobic condenser humidifier: 1 vs. 7 days. Crit Care Med. 2002;30(1):232–7.
18. Roux NG, Feld V, Gogniat E, Villalba D, Plotnikow G, Ribero Vairo N, et al. El frasco humidificador como sistema de humidificación del gas inspirado no cumple con las recomendaciones. Evaluación y comparación de tres sistemas de humidificación. Estudio de laboratorio. Med Intensiva. 2010;27(3):257.
19. Schumann S, Stahl CA, Moller K, Priebe H-J, Guttmann J. Moisturizing and mechanical characteristics of a new counter-flow type heated humidifier. Br J Anaesth. 2007;98(4):531–8.
20. Jones SW, Short KA, Joseph M, Sommer C, Cairns BA. Use of a new novel humidification system with high frequency percussive ventilation in a patient with inhalation injury. J Burn Care Res. 2010;31(3):499–502.
21. Chikata Y, Izawa M, Okuda N, Itagaki T, Nakataki E, Onodera M, et al. Humidification performance of two high-flow nasal cannula devices: a bench study. Respir Care. 2014;59(8):1186–90.
22. Eaton Turner E, Jenks M. Cost-effectiveness analysis of the use of high-flow oxygen through nasal cannula in intensive care units in NHS England. Expert Rev Pharmacoecon Outcomes Res. 2018;18(3):331–7.
23. Lellouche F, Qader S, Taille S, Lyazidi A, Brochard L. Influence of ambient temperature and minute ventilation on passive and active heat and moisture exchangers. Respir Care. 2014;59(5):637–43.
24. Cuquemelle E, Lellouche F. Assessment of humidification performance: still no easy method! Respir Care. 2013;58(9):1559–61.
25. Siempos II, Vardakas KZ, Kopterides P, Falagas ME. Impact of passive humidification on clinical outcomes of mechanically ventilated patients: a meta-analysis of randomized controlled trials. Crit Care Med. 2007;35(12):2843–51.
26. Klompas M, Branson R, Eichenwald EC, Greene LR, Howell MD, Lee G, et al. Strategies to prevent ventilator-associated pneumonia in acute care hospitals: 2014 update. Infect Control Hosp Epidemiol. 2014;35(Suppl 2):133–54.
27. Diot P, Morra L, Smaldone GC. Albuterol delivery in a model of mechanical ventilation: comparison of metered-dose inhaler and nebulizer efficiency. Am J Respir Crit Care Med. 1995;152(4):1391–4.
28. Ari A, Alwadeai KS, Fink JB. Effects of heat and moisture exchangers and exhaled humidity on aerosol deposition in a simulated ventilator-dependent adult lung model. Respir Care. 2017;62(5):538–43.
29. Yu M. Tracheostomy patients on the ward: multiple benefits from a multidisciplinary team? Crit Care. 2010;14(1):109.
30. Solomita M, Palmer LB, Daroowalla F, et al. Humidification and secretion volume in mechanically ventilated patients. Respir Care. 2009;54(10):1329–35.
31. Lewarski JS. Long-term care of the patient with a tracheostomy. Respir Care. 2005;50(4):534–7.
32. De Leyn P, Bedert L, Delcroix M, et al. Tracheotomy: clinical review and guidelines. Eur J Cardiothorac Surg. 2007;32(3):412–42.

Ineffective Complications in Tracheostomized Patients

17

Jose Luis Sandoval Gutierrez

Over 100,000 tracheostomies are performed annually in the USA. More than 12,000 tracheostomies are inserted annually in the UK, and up to 20% of patients in Intensive Care Unit (ICU) are managed with a tracheostomy [1, 2].

A tracheostomy is a surgical procedure during which a prosthesis is placed through a conduit created between the skin and the trachea [3, 4].

Is performed to bypass airway obstruction, aid in the management of secretions, to a reduction of anatomic dead space, and to aid in weaning from mechanical ventilation in patients with respiratory failure [5, 6].

Tracheostomy can be one of the easiest or most difficult, dangerous, and frustrating of surgical procedures. Securing the airway is fundamental to the success of carrying out a tracheostomy and preventing complications.

Indications for tracheostomy placement include upper respiratory tract obstruction, prolonged ventilation, copious secretions, severe obstructive sleep apnea and head/neck surgery [7, 8].

Is necessary a equipment for tracheostomy humidification (Table 17.1).

Complications of tracheostomy can be life threatening. Patients requiring tracheostomy placement may have multiple comorbidities that can contribute to the risk of complication.

Tracheostomy tube placement can be performed surgically via open surgical tracheostomy (OST) o percutaneously via percutaneous dilational tracheostomy (PDT). The preprocedure use of ultrasound and bronchoscopy appears to reduce periprocedural complications.

The potential complications of tracheostomy range from minor bleeding to life-threatening airway obstructions.

J. L. S. Gutierrez (✉)
Pneumology Department, Instituto Nacional de Enfermedades Respiratorias
"Ismael cosió Villegas", Mexico City, Mexico

171

A. M. Esquinas (ed.), *Humidification in the Intensive Care Unit*,
https://doi.org/10.1007/978-3-031-23953-3_17

Table 17.1 Equipment for tracheostomy humidification

Air compressor
Nebulizer bottle
Aerosol tubing
Trach mask
Sterile water
Saline ampules
Heat moisture exchanger

Table 17.2 Tracheostomy early complications

Bleeding
Infection
Membrane injury
Obstruction
Extubation

Table 17.3 Short term complications

Blockage
Displacement
Pneumothorax
Emphysema
Infections
Tracheal necrosis

Early complications of tracheostomy are those occurring withing the first week following placement (Table 17.2).

Short term complications (Table 17.3).

Prolonged tracheostomy tube placement in critically ill patients with multiple comorbities can lead to a number of late complications (Table 17.4).

Assessing the prevalence of late complications of tracheostomy may be particularly challenging. Late complications can occur in up to 65% of patients.

The onset of the COVID-19 pandemic has resulted in an increase in patients with severe acute respiratory distress síndrome (ARDS) in intensive ICU worldwide. Tracheostomy is often performed to facilitate the process of weaning form mechanical ventilation, reducing sedation in patients in need of prolonged mechanical ventilation.

The are practical tips to minimizing complications of tracheostomy (Table 17.5).

Tracheostomy tubes are devices that are increasingly being used in patients with chronic airway diseases. The placement of tracheostomy tubes facilities liberation from mechanical ventilation, increases the ability to mobilize patients with chronic respiratory failure, and reduces the dosage of sedation. Although these devices may be essential in facilitating recovery in chronic airway disease, they are not without risk for complication. Understanding the possible early and late complications of tracheostomy placement and identifying symptoms of such complications allow physicians to provide the optimal care for patients following tracheostomy.

Table 17.4 Tracheostomy late complications

Stenosis
Fracture
Tracheomalacia
Granulation tissue
Fistula
Aspiration
Nosocomial pneumonia
Reduce phonation
Dysphagia
Device related complications
Mortality

Table 17.5 Practical tips to minimizing complications of tracheostomy

Transverse incision
Dissection in the midline
The isthmus of the thyroid gland can usually be retracted superiorly to expose trachea
The insertion of the tracheostomy tube must be done under direct visión
Subcutaneous emphysema can be avoided
Prior to the end of the procedure, silk traction sutures should be placed above and below the cut tracheal rings
The use of a high volume low pressure cuff has greatly decreased the incidence of tracheal stenosis

References

1. Sancho J, Ferrer S, Lahosa C, Posadas T, Bures E, Bañuls P, Fernandez-Presa L, Royo P, Blasco ML, Signes CJ. Tracheostomy in patients with COVID19: predictors and clinical features. Eur Arch Otorhinolaryngol. 2021;278:3911–9.
2. Yaghoobi S, Kayalha H, Ghafouri R, Yazdi Z, Beigom KM. Comparison of complications in percutaneous dilatational tracheostomy versus surgical tracheostomy. Global J Health Sci. 2014;6(4):221–5.
3. Kligerman MP, Saraswathula A, Sethi RK, Divi V. Tracheostomy complications in the emergency department: a national analysis of 38,271 cases. ORL. 2020;2020:1–7.
4. Fernandez Bussy S, Mahajan B, Folch E, Caviedes I, Guerrero J, Majid A. Tracheostomy tube placement early and late complications. J Bronchol Intervent Pulmonol. 2015;22:357–64.
5. Tracheostomy humidification. https://www.hopkinsmedicine.org/tracheostomy.
6. Pauli N, Olofsson ME, Bergquist H. Tracheotomy in COVID19 patients: a retrospective study on complications and timing. Laryngos Invest Otolaryngol. 2021;6:446–52.
7. Lewith H, Athanassoglou V. Update on management of tracheostomy. BJA Educ. 2019;19(11):370–6.
8. Cernea C, Dias FL, Fliss D, Lima RA, Myers EN, Wei WI. Pearls and pitfalls in head and neck surgery. Basel: Larger; 2012. p. 166–7.

Humidification Tracheostomized Patients

18

Uğur Özdemir and Antonio M. Esquinas

18.1 Introduction

As it is known, the upper airway is responsible for heating and humidifying the inspired air that will be delivered to the lung in the normal situation. In this way, lung damage is prevented and breathing can be continued regularly without any complications. Percutaneous tracheostomy or surgical tracheotomy is frequently performed in intensive care units, especially in patients who need prolonged invasive mechanical ventilation (IMV) requirement. Patients with a tracheostomy cannula may not need IMV support over time, but the tracheostomy cannula can still be used under the patient's spontaneous breathing in order to clear secretions of the lower respiratory tract and maintain airway patency. Therefore, respiratory support treatments in tracheostomized patients continue under IMV support or under spontaneous breathing without IMV support. In this cases, the airway humidification capacity and ability of the patients undergoes serious changes. If a cuffed tracheostomy tube is used in tracheostomy patients with or without IMV support, the humidifying capacity of the upper airway is bypassed as well. Sufficiently humidified air reaching the lungs is very important in terms of continuation of muco-ciliary activity, preservation of epithelial integrity, softening and facilitating removal of secretions in the lower airway, prevention of lower airway obstruction, and prevention of lower respiratory tract infections. Apart from these, adequate humidification of inspired air is essential for reduction in work of breathing, better oxygenation, better

U. Özdemir (✉)
Division of Critical Care Medicine, Department of Internal Medicine, Ankara Training and Research Hospital, Ankara, Turkey

A. M. Esquinas
Intensive Care Unit, Hospital General Universitario Morales Meseguer, Murcia, Spain

A. M. Esquinas (ed.), *Humidification in the Intensive Care Unit*,
https://doi.org/10.1007/978-3-031-23953-3_18

175

ventilation/perfusion ratio, and more effective respiratory support. If a cuffless tracheostomy cannula is used, some air may enter to the lower airways of the patient from the upper airway, but due to the higher airway resistance of the upper airway, most part of the breathing will still be through the tracheostomy cannula. Therefore, adequate humidification and heating of the air-oxygen mixture given to the patient's airway is required in tracheostomized patients.

Under a certain pressure and temperature, a liter of air can carry a certain weight of water vapor, and the water vapor above this amount condenses into visible water. For example, 1 l of air at 37° at sea level can contain up to 33.9 mg of water vapor. During physiological respiration, a humidity rate close to this value is obtained at the carina level. In the case of physiological respiration without any air supplementation, the moisture amount observed at the carina level is 36–40 mgH$_2$O/L [1]. The recommended minimum humidity level at the carina is 33 mgH$_2$O/L to maintain mucociliary activity and facilitate excretion of endobronchial secretions [1]. In order to achieve these the specified humidity levels, the air breathed in artificial respiratory support treatments must be humidified and applications without humidification should be avoided, even for a short time. Considering that the air applied during the respiratory support given to the patients is completely dry, the importance of humidification will be better understood. The humidification applied to the airways of the patients in the ICU can basically be provided passive or active route. Active humidifiers work independently from the patient and allow the distilled water in a water tank to be mixed with the inspiratory air by evaporation with temperature regulation. On the other hand, passive humidifiers act like an artificial nose. Moisture in the exhaled air is maintained in a artificial surface, and this retained moisture is similarly used to passively humidify the inspired dry air by transferring of the water to the air.

18.2 Active Humidifiers

This type of heaters are called "Heated Humidifiers (HHs)". These types of humidifiers are placed on the inspiratory air connection line. Thus, the oxygen-air mixture, which has reached the desired temperature and humidity percentage, is delivered to the patient. The temperature and humidity of the air mixture transmitted to the patient are continuously monitored by the microprocessor through sensors placed on the inspiratory line and the values set by the operator are tried to be achieved by the device. This sensor-controlled targeted temperature and humidity levels will prevent patients from being damaged by low temperature and humidity, as well as being damaged by excessive temperature (>41 °C) and humidity levels (>44 mg/L at 37 °C temperature). The level of humidification can be changed (0–100%), and in some devices, a fixed level of humidification is provided as a pre-set. Some active humidifiers prevent air condensation along the breathing circuit by better controlling the temperature of the air to be inhaled with a resistance wire extending along the inspiratory line.

Heated humidifiers can be configured in two different patterns as cascade (bubble) or passover [2]. Cascade type heated humidifier allows the air to pass through the water in the reservoir, producing air bubbles and humidifying the air in the meantime. This type of humidifier causes an increase in airway resistance. Passover type heated humidifiers provide humidification of the air during contact with the water surface. The performance of this type of humidifiers can be increased by a porous membrane, which has the ability to absorb water, has placed partly above the water surface, and partly in the water. In this case, the system is called "wick" humidifier. In Wick humidifier, more active humidification can be achieved due to increased the contact surface area between water and air flow. In active humidifiers, unwanted water condensation in the breathing circuit should be monitored. As a result of water condensation, ventilator monitoring may be impaired, patient-ventilator dyssynchrony may be occur or contaminated fluid in the breathing circuit may reach the lungs.

18.3 Passive Humidifiers

This type of heaters are called "Heat and moisture exchangers (HMEs)". HMEs have the ability to store heat and moisture in the exhaled air in the respiratuar loop. Conversely, stored heat and moisture are returned to the inhaled air during inspiration. There are 3 different types of HMEs, they are hydrophobic, hygroscopic (HHME), and a filtered HME [3]. In simple terms, hydrophobic HMEs produce from disposable foam or paper for the creating large hydrophobic surface area. Due to the hydrophobic feature of the created surface, the air passing through the membrane continues on its way by leaving some of the moisture it contains. In the hygroscopic HMEs, the fibers are coated with hygroscopic chemicals (calcium chloride or lithium chloride). In this way, the humidification of the air during each inspiration is optimized. At the same time, a reduction in liquid condensation occurs within the HME. Finally, filtered HMEs have an electrostatic filter in addition to the hydrophobic or hygroscopic surface described above. By this way, as a result of the interaction of water molecules with the electrostatic artificial surface, the water absorption and adsorption properties of the material are increased.

HMEs are placed before the Y-connector in the ventilator circuit. Therefore, they cause an increase in the dead space in proportion to their volume. In clinical practice, this situation does not have significant consequences in patients followed up with the IMV. However, they can become a significant problem in patients without IMV support. Passive humidifiers can cause an increase in airway resistance over time due to condensation of the water or accumulation of patient secretions. Therefore, HMEs need to be replaced at regular intervals. It is stated that HMEs do not lose their moisturizing properties for up to 4 days and can be used safely from a bacteriological point of view [4]. However, it would be an appropriate approach to change HMEs at least every 48 h, especially considering possible obstructive lung diseases in patients. Also, HMEs should be changed in the presence of visible secretions and blood in the their chamber.

18.4 Clinical Comparison of Active and Passive Humidifiers

Although there are no significant differences between HMEs and HHs in terms of infection rate, mortality and airway obstruction, both methods have some advantages and disadvantages compared to each other [5]. The fact that they are easily accessible, inexpensive, light in weight, and easy to apply highlights the use of HMEs. However, the use of HMEs is limited by the fact that they increase dead space and airway resistance, they have lower performance compared to HHs, and they are not suitable if the patient suffers from abundant amounts of sticky or bloody secretions. On the other hand, HHs may not be first choice for every patient because they increase the workload of ICU staffs, they are more expensive and need to more cost for maintenance. Therefore, the choice should be made considering the clinical characteristics of each patient. An algorithm that can be used clinically to select HME or HH is shown in Fig. 18.1. It is accepted that with proper use, HHs do not increase the risk of infection compared to HMEs. However, they can become a source of infection in inappropriate use. It is very important to monitor the HHs in terms of water condensation in the artificial airway and to position the breathing circuit in such a way as to prevent the water flow into the endotracheal tube during possible water condensation in the inspiratory line. For this purpose, the breathing circuit can be positioned lower than the endotracheal tube.

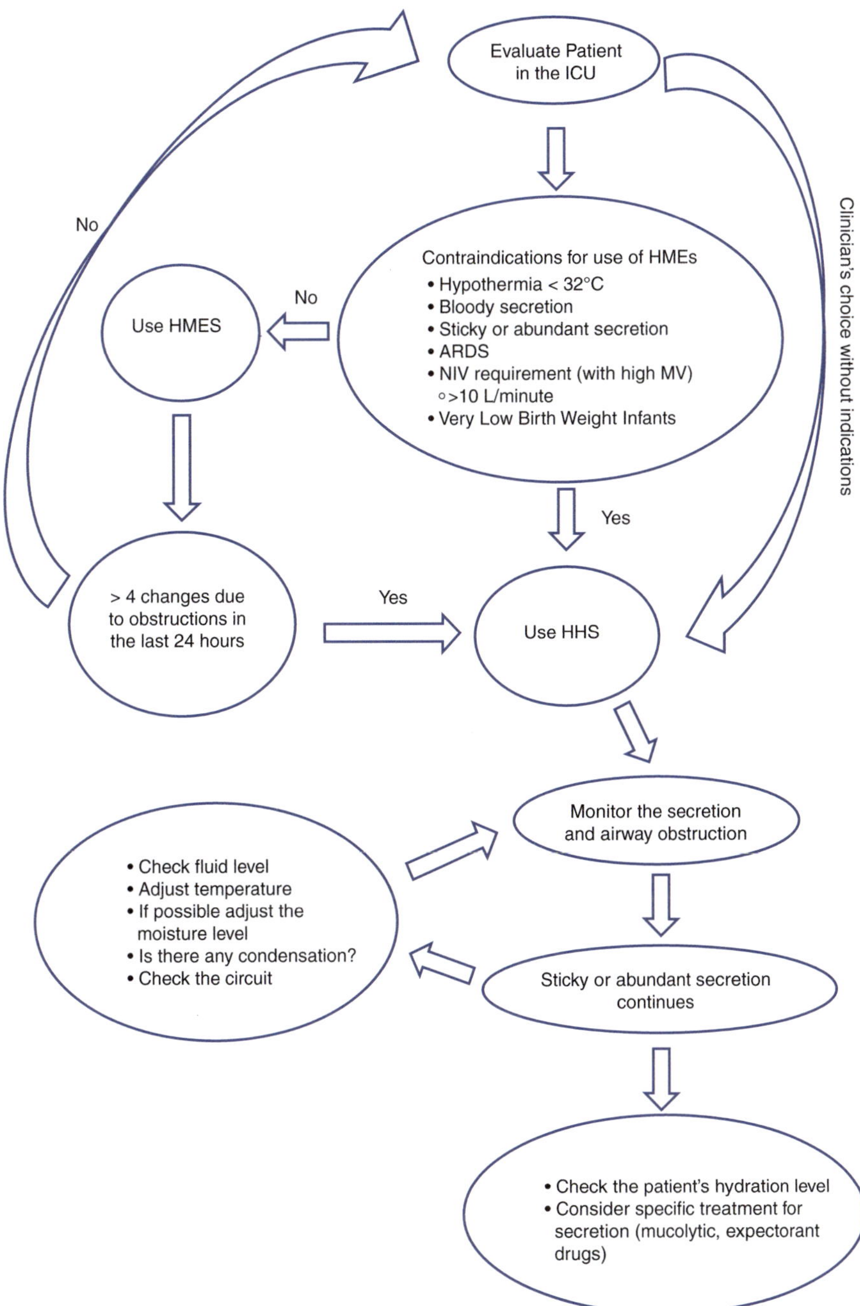

Fig. 18.1 Clinical selection algorithm for the humidifiers, adapted from Branson's algorithm [6]. *HHs* heated humidifiers, *HMEs* heat and moisture exchangers, *ARDS* acute respiratory distress syndrome

18.5   Combination of the Active and Passive Humidification

It may be beneficial to use active and passive humidifiers in the combination. For this purpose, the combination concept of an active heated humidifier and a hygroscopic HME was introduced by Shelley in 1991 [7]. With its introduction, this new device was named as the active hygroscopic heat and moisture exchanger (AHHME), the Humid-Heat (Gibeck AB, Sweden). The AHHME is placed between the Y-connector of the breathing circuit and the endotracheal tube like the HMEs. In this system, a membrane located in the airway direction inside the chamber of AHHME is fed from the outside with a closed circuit water connection and active humidification is provided by actively adjusting the temperature inside the chamber. This system also has a hygroscopic HME at the exit of the chamber. Therefore, even if active humidification is turned off, it can at least continue to be used as an HHME. The advantages of this system are low water consumption, elimination of water condensation, continued use passively when active humidification is stopped, temperature setting, alarm content. The disadvantages are that the dead space and the weight is more than the HMEs, the possibility of obstruction, the heat source is close to the patient, and the temperature range is narrow. With these systems, the temperature can be maintained in the range of 36–38° and a humidification as 90–95% can be achieved in the airway of the patients [8]. There is no difference between AHHME, HH and HH with Heated Wire Circuit in terms of the viscosity of the material aspirated from the lower respiratory tract, airway humidification level, airway temperature, and frequency of aspiration. Therefore, active airway humidification can be provided with this device, with lower water consumption and less water condensation, when more humidification capacity is required in patients whose dead space increase is not a problem.

Booster technology can be given as another example of the combination of active and passive humidification. This system is placed between the already used HMEs and the endotracheal tube or fasial masks. In this system, there is a ceramic electric heater and a Gore Tex membrane inside the chamber. Water is transferred into this membrane with a closed circuit connection and the ceramic heater evaporates the water from the membrane. In this way, the evaporated and heated air reaches the lower respiratory tract at each inspiration. In expiration, heat and humidity are retained by the HME being used. The additional humidification contribution of this system to the HME is 3–4 mg H_2O/L [8]. This contribution is quite small, but they can be preferred because they are simpler and easier to use.

18.6   Use of the Humidifier in the in Tracheostomized Patients

When mechanical ventilation is provided through an endotracheal tube, the inspired gas must be humidified and heated. HMEs are often preferred in patients who are ventilated invasively because they are inexpensive and easily accessible. The algorithm presented in Fig. 18.1 can be used for humidifier selection for invasively ventilated patients. Figure 18.1 also lists some contraindications for the use of HMEs.

Apart from these factors, obtaining an expiratory air volume less than 70% of the inspiratory air volume given to the patient is also a contraindication. In this situation, which can be observed as a result of bronchopleuralcutaneous fistula and endotracheal cuff air leakage, most of the exhaled air will come out without HMEs [9]. Therefore, the humidification features of HMEs will be disabled. Apart from this, the fact that the patient is receiving aerosol therapy is another contraindication for the use of HME. Also, active heated humidification can be considered in patients followed by IMV and humidified with HMEs, in patients whose lung function does not improve to the desired degree within the first 5 days, or in patients whose atelectasis findings continue on direct chest X-ray. HHs have no contraindications during IMV administration and can be used as first choice before HMEs. However, in order to see the beneficial effects expect than hazardous effect of HHs, ICU staff must have sufficient experience in the appropriate use of HHs. Because, undesirable conditions such as thermal damage, hyperthermia, electrical shock, nosocomial infection may occur with inappropriate use of HHs. For example, choosing a high temperature or ignoring the condensation on the inspiratory line can cause serious airway obstruction, on the contrary.

Humidification is a standard practice during the application of IMV in tracheostomized patients. Humidification during IMV in tracheostomized patients in the early period is similar to that in patients followed up with endotracheal intubation. While there may be a need for active humidification in the first period after surgical procedure, the use of HME may be sufficient in the following period. Also, most HMEs also have the ability to filter bacteria and viruses. This feature can be important feature in tracheostomized patients who need IMV for a long time. However, there may be serious airway obstruction during the use of HME in tracheostomized patients. To prevent this, the tracheostomy cannula can be observed for water condensation, HME can be selected in the appropriate patient group (Fig. 18.1), hygroscopic HME type can be selected [10].

HME is generally not used in spontaneously breathing patients without IMV support. If HME is to be used in this patient group, HMEs with small chamber volumes can be selected, but their humidifying capacity is considerably reduced. At the same time, it should be observed whether the increased dead space is tolerated or no by the patient who use HME in the clinical sense. For this purpose, it can be investigated whether there is an increase in partial carbon dioxide pressure in the blood gas analysis and whether there is an increase in the respiratory rate of the patient. In patients who do not proper for HME use, humidification is often provided by applying a heated or cool aerosol to the proximal trachea. However, these aerosol applications should be avoided in patients whose airways are reactive, since severe bronchospasm can be triggered by these treatments. Passover active humidification systems should be used in this patient group [10]. The air humidification capacity of patients who are followed up with tracheostomy for a long time may increase as a result of modification in the lower airway epithelium, so the need for additional external humidification may decrease. Therefore, HMEs with low chamber volume may be beneficial especially in the chronic period in patients who develop bronchospasm with aerosol therapy due to active airway.

In tracheostomized patients, humidification with aerosol therapy can be done by spray or evaporation ways. The tracheal spray is easy to use and has a ready-to-use hand spray module to deliver the NaCl (0.9%) solution into the proximal trachea. Humidification can be provided by this way, once every 6–8 h during the day. Apart from this, water molecules can be nebulized and given in a longer time. Both methods do not have an advantage over each other. As mentioned above, for both methods, it should be observed whether the patients are complicated with bronchospasm and whether there is clinically adequate humidification.

References

1. Restrepo RD, Walsh BK, American Association for Respiratory Care. Humidification during invasive and noninvasive mechanical ventilation: 2012. Respir Care. 2012;57(5):782–8. https://doi.org/10.4187/respcare.01766. PMID: 22546299.
2. Gupta V, Sharma SK. Heated humidifier. In: Esquinas A, editor. Humidification in the intensive care unit. Berlin: Springer; 2012. https://doi.org/10.1007/978-3-642-02974-5_3.
3. Plotnikow GA, Accoce M, Navarro E, Tiribelli N. Humidification and heating of inhaled gas in patients with artificial airway. A narrative review. Rev Bras Ter Intensiva. 2018;30(1):86–97. https://doi.org/10.5935/0103-507x.20180015.
4. Thomachot L, Boisson C, Arnaud S, Michelet P, Cambon S, Martin C. Changing heat and moisture exchangers after 96 hours rather than after 24 hours: a clinical and microbiological evaluation. Crit Care Med. 2000;28(3):714–20. https://doi.org/10.1097/00003246-200003000-00019.
5. Vargas M, Chiumello D, Sutherasan Y, Ball L, Esquinas AM, Pelosi P, Servillo G. Heat and moisture exchangers (HMEs) and heated humidifiers (HHs) in adult critically ill patients: a systematic review, meta-analysis and meta-regression of randomized controlled trials. Crit Care. 2017;21(1):123. https://doi.org/10.1186/s13054-017-1710-5.
6. Branson RD. Humidification of respired gases during mechanical ventilation: mechanical considerations. Respir Care Clin N Am. 2006;12(2):253–61. https://doi.org/10.1016/j.rcc.2006.03.011.
7. Branson RD, Campbell RS, Ottaway M, Johannigman JA. Comparison of conventional heated humidification to a new active heat and moisture exchanger in the ICU. Crit Care. 1999;3(Suppl 1):P017. https://doi.org/10.1186/cc392.
8. Branson RD, Durbin R, Reibel. Humidification for patients with artificial airways. Respir Care. 1999;44:630–42.
9. American Association for Respiratory Care. AARC clinical practice guideline. Humidification during mechanical ventilation. Respir Care. 1992;37(8):887–90. PMID: 10145779.
10. Heffner JE, Hess D. Tracheostomy management in the chronically ventilated patient. Clin Chest Med. 2001;22(1):55–69. https://doi.org/10.1016/s0272-5231(05)70025-3. PMID: 11315459.

Part VII

Humidification in Critically Ill Neonates

Humidification in Critically Ill Neonates

M. O'Reilly and Georg M. Schmölzer

Preterm birth interrupts normal lung maturation [1]. As a result, preterm infants are born before the lungs are sufficiently mature to sustain adequate gas exchange and they often require respiratory support in the delivery room and neonatal intensive care unit (NICU). Owing to their immaturity, the structurally underdeveloped lungs are highly susceptible to injury and altered development arising from the use of supplemental oxygen and other interventions aimed at maintaining adequate gas exchange [2, 3]. However, these life-saving clinical interventions can also perturb the normal process of lung development, contributing to the development of bronchopulmonary dysplasia (BPD)—a serious form of lung injury that carries irreversible damage and life-long respiratory consequences. Improvements in long-term respiratory outcomes can result from employment of clinical practice aimed at minimizing exposure to known injurious respiratory support interventions.

Humidity is the amount of water vapour in a gas, and is usually expressed as absolute humidity (mg H_2O/L) or relative humidity (%). The relationship between absolute humidity, relative humidity, and temperature is fixed; the relative humidity of a gas depends on its absolute water content and the temperature of the gas [4]. Warmer air has the ability to carry more water vapour and thus can have a higher absolute humidity when fully saturated (100% relative humidity). Under normal physiological conditions, gas entering the lungs is fully saturated and has a temperature of 37 °C; the resulting absolute humidity is 44 mg H_2O/L [5]. The average temperature of unconditioned inspired ambient air is approximately 23 °C and is closely associated with ambient room temperature; the average relative humidity is extremely low at 5.4% [6]. The nose and upper airways play a key role in conditioning the inspired ambient air. The inspired air gains heat and water vapour from the

M. O'Reilly · G. M. Schmölzer (✉)
Centre for the Studies of Asphyxia and Resuscitation, Neonatal Research Unit, Royal Alexandra Hospital, Edmonton, AB, Canada

Department of Pediatrics, University of Alberta, Edmonton, AB, Canada

© The Author(s), under exclusive license to Springer Nature Switzerland AG 2023

A. M. Esquinas (ed.), *Humidification in the Intensive Care Unit*,
https://doi.org/10.1007/978-3-031-23953-3_19

ciliated epithelial cells lining the upper airway, so that once it reaches the alveoli it is fully saturated with water vapour at core body temperature [4]. However, respiratory support in preterm infants can compromise the normal physiological process of gas warming and humidification. The humidity of the medical gas used in respiratory support devices is extremely low (absolute humidity <5 mg H_2O/L, relative humidity <20%), and when combined with the use of an endotracheal tube for invasive respiratory support (which bypasses the upper airways), essentially eliminates the ability for gas warming and humidification [5]. To overcome this, a humidifier placed in the ventilatory circuit will condition the gas before it reaches the patient, ideally in a manner that matches or closely resembles physiological conditions.

19.1 Unconditioned Gases and Pulmonary Damage

The inspiration of unconditioned gases (dry and cold) can have detrimental effects on the function and structure of the lungs and airways. Early animal studies have shown that inadequate conditioning of inspired gases can cause severe damage to the respiratory epithelium [7, 8]. Hirsch et al. ventilated dogs with dry compressed air (23 °C, <10% relative humidity) or heated humidified air (38 °C, 100% relative humidity). Dry air breathing significantly lowered tracheal mucous velocity, producing an almost complete cessation of the flow of tracheal mucous after 4 h of ventilation. Histological examination of the trachea revealed focal areas of sloughing of the ciliated epithelium and submucosal inflammation following ventilation with dry air. Breathing of heated humidified air produced no significant change in tracheal mucous velocity after the 4-hour ventilation period [8]. Marfatia et al. showed similar outcomes in rabbits ventilated with dry gases (23 °C, 18% relative humidity) compared to humidified gases (23 °C, 90% relative humidity) for 6 h. Histological damage to the respiratory epithelium was greater following ventilation with dry gases, and included destruction of cilia and mucous glands, disorganization and flattening of pseudostradified columnar or more distal cuboidal epithelium, disorganization of the basement membrane leading to loss of elasticity and ultimate collapse of the bronchioles, sloughing of cells into the airway lumen, ulcerations of the epithelium, and bronchial plugging [7]. More recently, Pillow et al. ventilated near-term lambs for 3 h using (1) heated humidified 21% oxygen, (2) cold dry 21% oxygen, (3) heated humidified 100% oxygen, or (4) cold dry 100% oxygen [9]. Exposure to hyperoxia (100% oxygen) was associated with poorer gas exchange and increased expression of inflammatory cytokines in lung tissue, with a trend towards higher IL-1β mRNA expression in the tracheal mucosa. In contrast, 3 h exposure to cold dry air had no effect on gas exchange or lung mechanics, and was associated only with a trend towards increased IL-1β mRNA expression in lung tissue [9]. Impaired cilial integrity (denuded and flattened cilia) in the tracheal tissue was marked in the group treated with cold dry 100% oxygen [9], demonstrating the sensitivity of the mucociliary transport system to inhalation of cold dry air. Pillow et al. observed a strong trend toward increased IL-1β in lung tissue after 3 h of ventilation with cold dry gas; however cold dry gas ventilation did not result in abnormal gas exchange or pulmonary mechanics [9]. These animal studies demonstrate the impact that aberrant inspired gas temperatures and humidity levels can have on pulmonary structure and inflammatory responses. This is particularly alarming for preterm infants who, owing to their structurally immature lungs and increased likelihood of being resuscitated with unconditioned gases in the delivery room, may be at significant risk of pulmonary trauma.

19.2 Resuscitation Gases in the Delivery Room

Humidification and warming of inspired gases during ventilatory support in the neonate may lessen or even prevent a pulmonary inflammatory response. Although ventilatory support in the NICU usually involves the delivery of heated and humidified gases, delivery room resuscitation is often undertaken without heating or humidification of the ventilatory gas, and this may be continued for some hours if transport to the NICU is required [9]. Dawson et al. measured the temperature and relative humidity of piped gases in the delivery room and showed that they are extremely dry, with a temperature similar to ambient temperature. The mean (SD) ambient temperature at test sites was 23.0 (0.95) °C, and the temperatures of piped oxygen and air were 23.3 (0.9) and 23.4 (0.9) °C, respectively [10]. The mean (SD) ambient relative humidity at test sites was 41.1 (2.2)%, and the relative humidity of piped oxygen and air were 2.1 (1.1) and 5.4 (0.7)%, respectively; the piped oxygen was significantly ($p < 0.001$) drier than piped air [10]. Humidification of ventilator gases is particularly important to newborn infants, due to their delicate lungs, and problems maintaining normal temperature and fluid balance [10]. The use of heated humidified gases in the delivery room could improve outcomes by reducing hypothermia, preserving mucosal function, and reducing respiratory complications [10].

19.3 Humidification and Thermoregulation

Thermoregulation is an essential component of neonatal care in the delivery room. A recent meta-analysis investigated the use of heated humidified gases for initial stabilization of preterm infants [11]. Heating and humidification of inspired gases immediately after birth and during transport to the NICU improved admission temperature in preterm infants; admission hypothermia was reduced by 36% (CI 17–50%), while admission normothermia was significantly increased [11]. The number of infants with more severe hypothermia (<35.5 °C) was significantly reduced (RR 0.32 CI 0.14–0.73) [11]. Furthermore, preterm infants <28 weeks' gestational age had significantly less admission hypothermia (RR 0.61 CI 0.42, 0.90) [11]. There was also a trend toward improved respiratory measures, however as the studies were not powered for these outcomes, they were not significantly different [11].

19.4 Over-humidification

Although inspiration of heated and humidified gas during respiratory support in the preterm infant is critical to prevent dehydration of respiratory mucosa and subsequent airway injury, excessive heating and over-humidification can also have adverse effects, including pulmonary edema, fluid overload, and impaired airway patency and lung mechanics [5]. During non-invasive respiratory support, the upper airways are still able to contribute to the humidification of the inspired gas; therefore, the ventilator humidifier should condition the gas to a lesser extent than during invasive respiratory support. However, in some circumstances the invasive humidification mode is used during non-invasive respiratory support, with the rationale that more humidification is superior. In a neonatal bench study, Flink et al. investigated the humidity delivered using invasive and non-invasive humidification modes during NCPAP and showed that the invasive humidification mode delivered gas with absolute humidity exceeding the recommended values for NCPAP [5]. This in turn could increase condensation and impair airway patency.

19.5 Summary

The inspiration of unconditioned gases (dry and cold) can have detrimental effects on the function and structure of the lungs and airways. Humidification is an important aspect of temperature management in premature infants.

References

1. Smith LJ, McKay KO, van Asperen PP, Selvadurai H, Fitzgerald DA. Normal development of the lung and premature birth. Paediatr Respir Rev. 2010;11:135–42. https://doi.org/10.1016/j.prrv.2009.12.006.
2. Keszler M. Novel ventilation strategies to reduce adverse pulmonary outcomes. Clin Perinatol. 2022;49:219–42. https://doi.org/10.1016/j.clp.2021.11.019.
3. O'Reilly M, Sozo F, Harding R. Impact of preterm birth and bronchopulmonary dysplasia on the developing lung: long-term consequences for respiratory health. Clin Exp Pharmacol. 2013;40:765–73. https://doi.org/10.1111/1440-1681.12068.
4. Schulze A. Respiratory gas conditioning and humidification. Clin Perinatol. 2007;34:19–33. https://doi.org/10.1016/j.clp.2006.12.009.
5. Flink RC, Kaam AH, Jongh FH. A humidifier in the invasive mode during noninvasive respiratory support could increase condensation and thereby impair airway patency. Acta Paediatr. 2018;107:1888–92. https://doi.org/10.1111/apa.14383.
6. Ralphe JL, Dail RB. Temperature and humidity associated with artificial ventilation in the premature infant. Adv Neonatal Care. 2018;18:366–77. https://doi.org/10.1097/anc.0000000000000519.
7. Marfatia S, Donahoe PK, Hendren WH. Effect of dry and humidified gases on the respiratory epithelium in rabbits. J Pediatr Surg. 1975;10:583–92. https://doi.org/10.1016/0022-3468(75)90360-7.
8. Hirsch JA, Tokayer JL, Robinson MJ, Sackner MA. Effects of dry air and subsequent humidification on tracheal mucous velocity in dogs. J Appl Physiol. 1975;39:242–6. https://doi.org/10.1152/jappl.1975.39.2.242.

9. Pillow JJ, Hillman NH, Polglase GR, Moss TJM, Kallapur SG, Cheah F-C, et al. Oxygen, temperature and humidity of inspired gases and their influences on airway and lung tissue in near-term lambs. Intensive Care Med. 2009;35:2157–63. https://doi.org/10.1007/s00134-009-1624-z.
10. Dawson JA, Owen LS, Middleburgh R, Davis PG. Quantifying temperature and relative humidity of medical gases used for newborn resuscitation. J Paediatr Child Health. 2014;50:24–6. https://doi.org/10.1111/jpc.12393.
11. Meyer MP, Owen L, Pas AB. Use of heated humidified gases for early stabilization of preterm infants: a meta-analysis. Front Pediatr. 2018;6:92–8. https://doi.org/10.3389/fped.2018.00319.

Humidification During Non-invasive Respiratory Support of the Newborn

20

M. O'Reilly and Georg M. Schmölzer

The lungs of preterm infants are structurally immature, deficient in surfactant, and not supported by a stiff chest wall, which makes them easily being damaged by invasive mechanical ventilation. As an alternative approach, non-invasive ventilation using either nasal continuous positive airway pressure (CPAP) or heated humidified high-flow nasal cannula (HHHFNC) has been advocated at the initiation of respiratory support.

20.1 Bubble Continuous Positive Airway Pressure (BCPAP)

Bahman-Bijari et al. compared the survival rates of preterm infants (body weight 1000–2000 grams) treated with BCPAP versus ventilator-derived CPAP (VCPAP) ($n = 50$) [1]. There was a significant greater success rate of BPCAP within the first 24 h compared with the VCPAP group (24/25 [96%] vs. 18/25 [77%]; $P = 0.02$). Treatment duration and length of hospital stay for infants treated with BCPAP compared to VCPAP was comparable between groups (treatment duration, mean (SD), 39.8 (38.04) h vs. 49.4 (33.7) h, $P = 0.3$; hospital stay, mean (SD), 8.9 (3.4) days vs. 10.6 (7.3) days, $P = 0.3$) [1].

Tagare et al. conducted a randomized controlled trial to compare the efficacy and safety of BCPAP with VCPAP in preterm infants <37 weeks' gestational age ($n = 114$) [2]. The proportion of infants with successful CPAP respiratory support was significantly higher in the BCPAP group compared to VCPAP (47/57 [82.5%] vs. 36/57 [63.2%]; $P = 0.03$).

M. O'Reilly · G. M. Schmölzer (✉)
Centre for the Studies of Asphyxia and Resuscitation, Neonatal Research Unit, Royal Alexandra Hospital, Edmonton, AB, Canada

Department of Pediatrics, University of Alberta, Edmonton, AB, Canada

A. M. Esquinas (ed.), *Humidification in the Intensive Care Unit*, https://doi.org/10.1007/978-3-031-23953-3_20

A randomized controlled trial conducted by Bhatti et al. compared the use of variable-flow Jet CPAP (JCPAP) with BCPAP in preterm infants <34 weeks' gestation ($n = 170$) with onset of respiratory distress within 6 h of life [3]. CPAP failure rates within 72 h were similar between study groups (JCPAP 29% vs. BCPAP 21%; RR 1.4 (0.8–2.3), $P = 0.25$). The time to CPAP failure was also comparable (mean (95% CI), JCPAP 59 (54–64) h vs. BCPAP 65 (62–68) h, log rank $P = 0.19$) [3].

A recent meta-analysis by Bharadwaj et al. indicated that BCPAP resulted in lower incidence of CPAP failure compared with VCPAP but not variable-flow CPAP. BCPAP did not favor improvement in mortality, BPD, or air leak. However, nasal injury was found to be higher with the use of BCPAP: twice the risk of nasal injury compared to other forms of CPAP [4].

20.2 Heated Humidified High-Flow Nasal Cannula (HHHFNC)

Heated humidified high-flow nasal cannula (HHHFNC) ventilatory support has recently been applied as an alternative non-invasive respiratory support technique in the NICU. The HHHFNC system is comprised of three components, (1) a fixed oxygen concentration system, (2) a humidification system, and (3) a high-flow system [5], which enables HHHFNC to constantly provide a prescribed FiO_2 while warming and humidifying the gas flow (37 °C, relative humidity 100%) that is delivered at a high-flow rate (usually 2–8 L/min) [5]. The heated and humidified gas is delivered through small binasal prongs, which are smaller than nasal CPAP (NCPAP) and are suggested to be more comfortable for the infant. Several studies have demonstrated that HHHFNC may be as effective as NCPAP and non-invasive intermittent positive pressure ventilation (NIPPV) [6–12].

Yoder et al. conducted a randomized controlled trial to evaluate the safety and efficacy of HHHFNC [6]. Infants ($n = 432$) ≥28 weeks' gestational age received either HHHFNC or NCPAP for non-invasive respiratory support in the NICU. There was no difference in early failure for HHHFNC (23/212 [10.8%]) compared to NCPAP (18/220 [8.2%]; $P = 0.344$), subsequent need for any intubation (32/212 [15.1%] vs. 25/220 [11.4%]; $P = 0.252$), or any of several adverse outcomes analyzed, including air leak [6]. Although the HHHFNC infants required a significantly longer duration of non-invasive respiratory support compared to NCPAP (median (25–75%): 4 (2–7) days vs. 2 (1–4) days, $P < 0.001$), there were no differences between HHHFNC and NCPAP infants for the days on supplemental oxygen (median (25–75%): 10 (5–27) days vs. 8 (5–24) days; $P = 0.357$). Furthermore, there were no differences between HHHFNC and NCPAP study groups for bronchopulmonary dysplasia (20% vs. 16%; $P = 0.575$) and discharge from hospital on supplemental oxygen (19% vs. 18%; $P = 0.698$) [6]. In addition, the absence of nasal trauma was significantly greater in HHHFNC infants compared to NCPAP (187/212 [91%] vs. 180/220 [84%]; $P = 0.047$) [6].

Manley et al. also investigated the efficacy of HHHFNC compared to NCPAP for non-invasive respiratory support following extubation in a randomized controlled trial in very preterm infants <32 weeks' gestational age ($n = 303$) [7]. The use of

HHHFNC was non-inferior to the use of NCPAP, with treatment failure occurring in 52/152 infants (34.2%) in the HHHFNC group and in 39/151 infants (25.8%) in the NCPAP group (risk difference, 8.4 percentage points; 95% confidence interval, −1.9 to 18.7). No significant differences were reported between HHHFNC and NCPAP in the number of days on respiratory support (median (IQR): 34 (7–55) days vs. 38 (11–57) days; $P = 0.44$) or the number of days on oxygen therapy (median (IQR): 38 (0–78) days vs. 49 (8–83) days; $P = 0.15$). Furthermore, there were no differences between HHHFNC and NCPAP study groups for oxygen supplementation at 36 weeks' gestational age (47/152 [30.9%] vs. 52/151 [34.4%]; $P = 0.51$) and discharge from hospital on supplemental oxygen (21/152 [13.8%] vs. 15/151 [9.9%]; $P = 0.30$). In addition, the occurrence of nasal trauma was significantly lower in HHHFNC infants compared to NCPAP (60/152 [39.5%] vs. 82/151 [54.3%]; $P = 0.01$).

Collins et al. also investigated the use of HHHFNC as an alternative method of non-invasive respiratory support post-extubation, compared to NCPAP, in a randomized controlled trial of very preterm infants <32 weeks' gestational age ($n = 132$) [9]. There was no difference in the rates of extubation failure between HHHFNC and NCPAP groups (15/67 [22%] vs. 22/65 [34%]; $P = 0.14$), subsequent need for any intubation (14/67 [21%] vs. 16/65 [25%]; $P = 0.61$), or bronchopulmonary dysplasia at 36 weeks' gestational age (24/67 [36%] vs. 28/65 [43%]; $P = 0.30$) [9]. Furthermore, the nasal trauma score in the first week of non-invasive respiratory support was significantly lower in HHHFNC infants compared to NCPAP (mean (SD): 3.1 (7.2) vs. 11.8 (10.7); $P < 0.01$) [9].

In another randomized controlled trial, Kugelman et al. compared the requirement for endotracheal ventilation in preterm infants <35 weeks' gestational age ($n = 76$) treated with HHHFNC with those treated with NIPPV [10]. There was no significant difference in the need for endotracheal ventilation between HHHFNC and NIPPV study groups (11/38 [28.9%] vs. 13/38 [34.2%]; $P = 0.80$) [10]. The rate of neonatal morbidities (pneumothorax, intraventricular hemorrhage, necrotizing enterocolitis, patent ductus arteriosus) was also comparable in both groups. Although the HHHFNC infants required a significantly longer duration of non-invasive respiratory support compared to NIPPV (median (range): 4.0 (1.0–15.0) days vs. 2.0 (0.3–6.5) days; $P < 0.006$), there were no differences between HHHFNC and NIPPV infants for the days on supplemental oxygen (median (range): 5.0 (0–69.0) days vs. 3.0 (0–90.0) days; $P = 0.18$) [10]. Furthermore, there were no differences between HHHFNC and NIPPV study groups for bronchopulmonary dysplasia (1/38 [2.6%] vs. 2/38 [5.2%]; $P = 1.00$) [10]. In addition, there were no reported cases of nasal trauma in both study groups [10].

More recently, a randomized controlled trial by Yengkhom et al. compared the safety and efficacy of HHHFNC with NCPAP following extubation in preterm infants ≥28 weeks' gestational age ($n = 128$) [11]. There was no significant difference in extubation failure within 72 h following extubation between the study groups (HHHFNC 22.2% vs. NCPAP 18.5%, risk difference 3.7%, 95% CI −10.3 to 17.6, $P = 0.604$). No significant differences were reported between HHHFNC and NCPAP in the duration on non-invasive respiratory support (mean (SD): 52.3 (46.1) h vs. 72.8 (96.6) h; $P = 0.787$) or the number of days on oxygen therapy (mean (SD): 12.9 (15.6) days vs. 10.5 (12.4) days; $P = 0.952$) [11]. Furthermore, there were no differences between HHHFNC and NCPAP study groups for incidence of bronchopulmonary dysplasia at 36 weeks' gestational age (13/63 [20.6%] vs. 10/65 [15.4%]; $P = 0.439$). The incidence of nasal trauma was significantly lower in HHHFNC infants compared to NCPAP (4/63 [6.3%] vs. 14/65 [21.5%]; $P < 0.02$) [11].

Oktem et al. recently compared four different non-invasive respiratory support techniques as primary respiratory support in preterm infants <32 weeks' gestational age ($n = 76$); infants were treated with HHHFNC, NCPAP, NIPPV, or NHFOV [12]. The need for intubation during non-invasive respiratory support was highest in the NCPAP (40%) and NHFOV (29.4%) groups compared to the NIPPV (10.5%) and HHHFNC (11.8%) groups [12]. The occurrence of nasal injury was highest in NIPPV (78.9%) and NHFOV (82.4%) groups compared to NCPAP (40%) and HHHFNC (35%) groups. No significant differences were reported between groups in the duration on non-invasive respiratory support or the incidence of bronchopulmonary dysplasia [12].

Overall, these studies suggest that HHHFNC may offer a safe alternative to other non-invasive methods, when applied immediately post-extubation or early as initial non-invasive respiratory support. This is supported by a recent meta-analysis examining the efficacy and safety of HHHFNC compared to standard treatments for preterm infants, where HHHFNC was used post-extubation following mechanical ventilation or as primary respiratory support [13]. The primary outcome was the need for re-intubation following extubation from mechanical ventilation (post-extubation analysis) or the need for intubation for infants not previously intubated (primary respiratory support analysis). The meta-analysis showed no statistically significant differences for outcomes measuring efficacy, including the primary outcome [13]. There were statistically significant differences favoring HHHFNC versus NCPAP for air leak (post-extubation, risk ratio [RR] 0.29, 95% CI 0.11–0.76, $I^2 = 0$) and nasal trauma (post-extubation, RR 0.35, 95% CI 0.27–0.46, $I^2 = 5\%$; primary respiratory support, RR 0.52, 95% CI 0.37–0.74, $I^2 = 27\%$) [13]. Although HHHFNC appears to offer an efficacious and safe alternative to NCPAP, there is still a need for further studies in very preterm infants ≤28 weeks' gestational age.

20.3 Summary

Humidification during non-invasive respiratory support in the delivery room, initial respiratory support, or post-extubation is a supportive strategy to support oxygenation, breathing, or thermoregulation.

References

1. Bahman-Bijari B, Malekiyan A, Niknafs P, Baneshi M-R. Bubble-CPAP vs. ventilatory-CPAP in preterm infants with respiratory distress. Iran J Pediatr. 2011;21:151–8.
2. Tagare A, Kadam S, Vaidya U, Pandit A, Patole S. Bubble CPAP versus ventilator CPAP in preterm neonates with early onset respiratory distress—a randomized controlled trial. J Trop Pediatr. 2013;59:113–9. https://doi.org/10.1093/tropej/fms061.
3. Bhatti A, Khan J, Murki S, Sundaram V, Saini SS, Kumar P. Nasal jet-CPAP (variable flow) versus bubble-CPAP in preterm infants with respiratory distress: an open label, randomized controlled trial. J Perinatol. 2015;35:935–40. https://doi.org/10.1038/jp.2015.98.
4. Bharadwaj SK, Alonazi A, Banfield L, Dutta S, Mukerji A. Bubble versus other continuous positive airway pressure forms: a systematic review and meta-analysis. Arch Dis Child Fetal Neonatal Ed. 2020;105:318165. https://doi.org/10.1136/archdischild-2019-318165.
5. Chao K-Y, Chen Y-L, Tsai L-Y, Chien Y-H, Mu S-C. The role of heated humidified high-flow nasal cannula as noninvasive respiratory support in neonates. Pediatr Neonatol. 2017;58:295–302. https://doi.org/10.1016/j.pedneo.2016.08.007.
6. Yoder BA, Stoddard RA, Li M, King J, Dirnberger DR, Abbasi S. Heated, humidified high-flow nasal cannula versus nasal CPAP for respiratory support in neonates. Pediatrics. 2013;131:1482–90. https://doi.org/10.1542/peds.2012-2742.
7. Manley BJ, Owen LS, Doyle LW, Andersen CC, Cartwright DW, Pritchard MA, et al. High-flow nasal cannulae in very preterm infants after extubation. N Engl J Med. 2013;369:1425–33. https://doi.org/10.1056/nejmoa1300071.
8. Roberts CT, Owen L, Manley BJ, Frøisland DH, Donath S, Dalziel KM, et al. Nasal high-flow therapy for primary respiratory support in preterm infants. N Engl J Med. 2016;375:1142–51. https://doi.org/10.1056/nejmoa1603694.
9. Collins CL, Holberton JR, Barfield C, Davis PG. A randomized controlled trial to compare heated humidified high-flow nasal cannulae with nasal continuous positive airway pressure postextubation in premature infants. J Pediatr. 2013;162:949–54. https://doi.org/10.1016/j.jpeds.2012.11.016.
10. Kugelman A, Riskin A, Said W, Shoris I, Mor F, Bader D. A randomized pilot study comparing heated humidified high-flow nasal cannulae with NIPPV for RDS. Pediatr Pulmonol. 2015;50:576–83. https://doi.org/10.1002/ppul.23022.
11. Yengkhom R, Suryawanshi P, Gupta B, Deshpande S. Heated humidified high-flow nasal cannula vs. nasal continuous positive airway pressure for post-extubation respiratory support in preterm infants: a randomized controlled trial. J Trop Pediatr. 2020;67:82. https://doi.org/10.1093/tropej/fmaa082.
12. Öktem A, Yiğit Ş, Çelik HT, Yurdakök M. Comparison of four different non-invasive respiratory support techniques as primary respiratory support in preterm infants. Turk J Pediatr. 2021;63:23. https://doi.org/10.24953/turkjped.2021.01.003.
13. Fleeman N, Dundar Y, Shah PS, Shaw BN. Heated humidified high-flow nasal cannula for preterm infants: an updated systematic review and meta-analysis. Int J Technol Assess. 2019;35:298–306. https://doi.org/10.1017/s0266462319000424.

Humidification in Neonatal-Pediatric Critical Care: Invasive Ventilation

21

M. O'Reilly and Georg M. Schmölzer

21.1 High-Frequency Ventilation

High-frequency ventilation (HFV) is a form of invasive mechanical ventilation that uses small tidal volumes and very fast ventilator rates. Compared to conventional mechanical ventilation (CMV), HFV can use lower peak alveolar pressures, can manage oxygenation and ventilation relatively independently in the recruited lung while using small tidal volumes, and can preserve normal lung architecture even while using high mean airway pressures [1]. Two types of HFV are routinely used in neonatal respiratory therapy: (1) high-frequency oscillatory ventilation (HFOV) and (2) high-frequency jet ventilation (HFJV). Although HFV has been used as respiratory support in neonates for more than 30 years, there is very limited available data on humidification during HFV.

21.2 High-Frequency Oscillatory Ventilation

High-frequency oscillatory ventilation (HFOV) is produced by ventilators that move gas back and forth at the airway opening, resulting in limited bulk gas flow [1]. Most HFOV ventilator devices can generate both CMV and HFOV, which prevents having to change machines according to the respiratory support requirement of the infant. An early study by Schiffmann et al. studied the performance and efficiency of a heated humidifier and a heat and moisture exchanger for airway humidification in HFOV using an artificial lung model [2]. Both the heated humidifier and heat and moisture exchanger were considered suitable devices for airway

M. O'Reilly · G. M. Schmölzer (✉)
Centre for the Studies of Asphyxia and Resuscitation, Neonatal Research Unit, Royal Alexandra Hospital, Edmonton, AB, Canada

Department of Pediatrics, University of Alberta, Edmonton, AB, Canada

© The Author(s), under exclusive license to Springer Nature Switzerland AG 2023
A. M. Esquinas (ed.), *Humidification in the Intensive Care Unit*,
https://doi.org/10.1007/978-3-031-23953-3_21

humidification in HFOV, with neither affecting the performance of the ventilator. Chikata et al. also investigated two different methods of providing airway humidification during HFOV in a neonatal lung model: a ventilator circuit with inner heating wire and another with an embedded heating element [3]. The circuit with an embedded heating element provided significantly higher absolute humidity and temperature than the ventilatory circuit with inner heating wire. A more recent study using an artificial lung model with a HFOV system (Babylog® 8000 plus) investigated temperature change in the endotracheal tube and compared it with the endotracheal tube temperature during conventional intermittent positive pressure ventilation (IPPV) [4]. The temperature change in the endotracheal tube was not dependent on the oscillatory frequency when the oscillatory volume was fixed. However, the temperature was dependent on the oscillatory volume when the oscillatory frequency was fixed. The authors suggest that there is a risk of higher temperatures and lower humidity gases being supplied to the respiratory circuit during HFOV than IPPV.

21.3 High-Frequency Jet Ventilation

High-frequency jet ventilation (HFJV) is produced by ventilators that deliver a high-velocity jet of gas directly into the airway and have passive exhalation [1]. Another type of HFV, called high-frequency flow interruption (HFFI), is also available albeit less commonly used in clinical practice. Like HFJV, HFFI generates a pulse of fresh gas and uses passive exhalation, but it does not produce a high-velocity jet of gas. An animal study by Todd et al. compared the degree of tracheobronchial damage following CMV and HFV (HFFI) at low and high humidity [5]. Newborn lambs were ventilated for 6 hours with CMV or HFFI ventilation, with a relative humidity of 30% or 90% (FiO$_2$ 0.21, 36.0 °C). Significant inflammation, erosion, necrosis, and blistering were reported following both CMV and HFFI ventilation when 30% humidity was used, compared to 90% humidity. These results show that, regardless of the mode of ventilation (CMV, HFV), endotracheal intubation and invasive ventilation can cause substantial damage to the tracheal mucosa when poorly humidified gases are inspired. A follow-up study by Todd et al. investigated the recovery of the tracheal epithelium following HFFI ventilation with 30% relative humidity inspired gas [6]. Deciliation of the tracheal mucosa was the greatest at 2 days post-ventilation, and the damaged mucosa has converted to non-ciliated epidermoid squamous metaplastic cells. However, recovery was not complete by 14 days post-ventilation, even though the squamous cells had differentiated into goblet and ciliated columnar epithelial cells. Data from these earlier animal studies highlight the importance of proper humidification of inspired gases during invasive mechanical ventilation.

References

1. Pillow JJ, Courtney S. High frequency ventilation. In: Keszler M, Gautham KS, editors. Assisted ventilation of the neonate. 7th ed. Amsterdam: Elsevier; 2021.
2. Schiffmann H, Singer S, Singer D, Richthofen EV, Rathgeber J, Züchner K. Determination of airway humidification in high-frequency oscillatory ventilation using an artificial neonatal lung model. Intensive Care Med. 1999;25:997–1002. https://doi.org/10.1007/s001340050995.
3. Chikata Y, Imanaka H, Onishi Y, Ueta M, Nishimura M. Humidification during high-frequency oscillation ventilation is affected by ventilator circuit and ventilatory setting. Pediatr Anesth. 2009;19:779–83. https://doi.org/10.1111/j.1460-9592.2009.03068.x.
4. Nagaya K, Tsuchida E, Nohara F, Okamoto T, Azuma H. The temperature change in an endotracheal tube during high frequency ventilation using an artificial neonatal lung model with Babylog® 8000 plus. Pediatr Pulmonol. 2015;50:173–8. https://doi.org/10.1002/ppul.22973.
5. Todd DA, John E, Osborn RA. Tracheal damage following conventional and high-frequency ventilation at low and high humidity. Crit Care Med. 1991;19:1310–6. https://doi.org/10.1097/00003246-199110000-00014.
6. Todd DA, John E, Osborn R. Recovery of tracheal epithelium following high frequency ventilation at low inspired humidity. Early Hum Dev. 1992;31:53–66. https://doi.org/10.1016/0378-3782(92)90014-8.

Technology, Complications, and Prevention

M. O'Reilly and Georg M. Schmölzer

22.1 Cold Passover, Bubble-Through, and Heated Water Humidifier

Cold passover are bubble-through humidification are used for low-flow supplemental oxygen therapy. Most importantly, the incoming gas flow does not cool the water reservoir below room temperature to allow for optimal water vapor saturation [1]. This is different from high flow, which comprised of three components, (1) a fixed oxygen concentration system, (2) a humidification system, and (3) a high-flow system [2], which enables high flow to constantly provide a prescribed FiO_2 while warming and humidifying the gas flow (37 °C, relative humidity 100%) that is delivered at a high-flow rate (usually 2–8 L/min) [2]. The heated and humidified gas is delivered through small binasal prongs, which are smaller than nasal continuous positive airway pressure prongs and are suggested to be more comfortable for the infant.

22.2 Heated Humidifier with Heated Wire Tubing Circuitry

Cold and dry gases pass through an unheated tube into the humidifier water-vaporizing chamber. The amount of water vaporized inside the chamber depends on the water temperature, water surface, and gas flow rate. At 37 °C water temperature, the gas could be saturated with a maximum of 44 mg/L of water vapor [3]. The water in the chamber is either automatically or manually refilled for a reservoir.

M. O'Reilly · G. M. Schmölzer (✉)
Centre for the Studies of Asphyxia and Resuscitation, Neonatal Research Unit, Royal Alexandra Hospital, Edmonton, AB, Canada

Department of Pediatrics, University of Alberta, Edmonton, AB, Canada

A. M. Esquinas (ed.), *Humidification in the Intensive Care Unit*, https://doi.org/10.1007/978-3-031-23953-3_22

The gas mixture is heated to ~39 °C by a heated wire inside the inspiratory limb of the circuit [3]. The main concerns in neonatal patients might include thermal injury and rainout. Within the humidifier, the inspiratory gas is heated to ~39 °C to allow for maximum saturated inspiratory gas. Although the inspiratory gas is heated to ~39 °C, the inspiratory gas slowly cools back to 37 °C prior to entering the airway system, which does not cause thermal injury [3]. Further rainout in the inspiratory limb, which could cause aspiration, indicates moisture loss rather than proper humidification. The condensation of water vapor indicates that the gas temperature decreased below the dew point [3].

22.3 Heat and Moisture Exchangers ("Artificial Noses")

Heat and moisture exchangers (HME) are intended to replace the normal warming [4–6], humidifying, and filtering functions of the upper airways and are most commonly used for short-term application including delivery room resuscitation, neonatal transport, and general anesthesia during neonatal surgery. Manufactures of HME provide performance specifications, which are based on in vitro measurements of moisture output using the International Organization for Standardization (ISO) 9360 method [4, 5]. There are five types of device available including (1) HME with no filter, (2) electrostatic filter only, (3) pleated filter only, (4) electrostatic filter with HME, and (5) pleated filter with HME [4, 5]. HME use different active mediums including hydrophobic filter membrane (e.g., water repelling condenser elements), microporous polymer foam, or hygroscopic materials (salts like $CaCl_2$, $MgCl_2$) and are expected to prevent microorganism (e.g., bacteria and viruses) from entering the airways [4, 5]. HME are used to provide humidification and warming of the inspiratory gases recovered as part of the heat and moisture from the expired air. The main concerns in neonatal patients include increased resistance to gas flow and ventilation, dead space, and potential blockage with liquids.

22.4 Summary

There are several different systems for respiratory gas conditioning for respiratory support of preterm and term infants available. Heated humidifier could cause rainout, while HME might increase resistance to gas flow and ventilation, dead space, and potential blockage with liquids.

References

1. Randerath WJ, Meier J, Genger H, Domanski U, Ruhle K-H. Efficiency of cold passover and heated humidification under continuous positive airway pressure. Eur Respir J. 2002;20:183–6. https://doi.org/10.1183/09031936.02.00267902.
2. Chao K-Y, Chen Y-L, Tsai L-Y, Chien Y-H, Mu S-C. The role of heated humidified high-flow nasal cannula as noninvasive respiratory support in neonates. Pediatr Neonatol. 2017;58:295–302. https://doi.org/10.1016/j.pedneo.2016.08.007.
3. Schulze A. Respiratory gas conditioning and humidification. Clin Perinatol. 2007;34:19–33. https://doi.org/10.1016/j.clp.2006.12.009.
4. Wilkes AR. Heat and moisture exchangers and breathing system filters: their use in anaesthesia and intensive care. Part 1 – history, principles and efficiency. Anaesthesia. 2011;66:31–9. https://doi.org/10.1111/j.1365-2044.2010.06563.x.
5. Wilkes AR. Heat and moisture exchangers and breathing system filters: their use in anaesthesia and intensive care. Part 2 – practical use, including problems, and their use with paediatric patients. Anaesthesia. 2011;66:40–51. https://doi.org/10.1111/j.1365-2044.2010.06564.x.
6. Gillies D, Todd DA, Foster JP, Batuwitage BT. Heat and moisture exchangers versus heated humidifiers for mechanically ventilated adults and children. Cochrane Database Syst Rev. 2017;9:CD004711. https://doi.org/10.1002/14651858.cd004711.pub3.

Part VIII

Humidification and Airways Clearance Secretions

Airway Clearance in Chronic Respiratory Disorders: Obstructive CF, COPD, and Asthma

Paolo Ruggeri, Claudia Profazio, and Francesco Nucera

Abbreviations

ACTs	Airway clearance techniques
AECOPD	Acute exacerbations of chronic obstructive pulmonary disease
BiPAP	Biphasic positive airway pressure
CF	Cystic fibrosis
CFTR	Cystic fibrosis transmembrane conductance regulator
COPD	Chronic obstructive pulmonary disease
CPAP	Continuous positive airway pressure
HFCWO	High-frequency chest wall oscillation
HFNC	High-flow nasal cannula
ICU	Intensive care unit
iPEEP	Intrinsic positive end-expiratory pressure
IPV	Intrapulmonary percussive ventilation
LTAE	Life-threatening asthma exacerbation
MCC	Mucociliary clearance
MI-E	Mechanical in-exsufflator
MODs	Muco-obstructive diseases
NIV	Noninvasive mechanical ventilation
oCF	Obstructive cystic fibrosis

P. Ruggeri (✉) · F. Nucera
Pneumology Unit, Pneumologia, Department BIOMORF, University of Messina, Messina, Italy
e-mail: plrugger@unime.it

C. Profazio
Pneumology Unit, Hospital "Papardo", Messina, Italy

A. M. Esquinas (ed.), *Humidification in the Intensive Care Unit*,
https://doi.org/10.1007/978-3-031-23953-3_23

PECF	Peak expiratory cough flow
PEF	Peak expiratory flow
PEP	Positive expiratory pressure
PIF	Peak inspiratory flow
PD	Postural drainage
VC	Vital capacity

23.1 Introduction

Several chronic lung diseases that affect the airways, including chronic obstructive pulmonary disease (COPD), obstructive cystic fibrosis (oCF), and bronchial asthma, can be defined from a pathophysiological point of view as muco-obstructive diseases (MODs) [1]. These diseases are characterized by exacerbations that when severe needed hospitalization and intensive care unit (ICU) admission [2]. MODs being part of all these diseases can be considered to be also characterized by episodic exacerbations, and their pathogenesis is generally correlated with an increase in bronchial secretions with a change in its rheology [3]. In these conditions, mucus in the small airways cannot be cleared by cough and accumulates, forming the nidus for airflow obstruction, infection, and inflammation which have a key role in respiratory failure development that need intensive care assistance [3]. Unfortunately, a large amount of bronchial secretions is a frequent cause of noninvasive mechanical ventilation (NIV) failure [4, 5]. The management of bronchial secretions is one of the main problems encountered during the intensive care management of patients with MODs. The early start of airway clearance techniques (ACTs) is a fundamental part of the management to reduce the negative impact on patients' prognosis. They aim to reduce airway obstruction induced by increased secretions occupying the airway lumen and so prevent respiratory tract infections and re-expand the collapsed areas of the lung, thus improving gas exchange and decreasing the pro-inflammatory response [6, 7]. A wide range of therapeutic options as techniques and devices are present on the market for managing bronchial encumbrance during ICU stay, but up to now, for all ACTs, there is an insufficient evidence to affirm the superiority of one technique over another [8]. A personalized tailored approach for a single patient is mandatory. Rarely is just one single technique used for a given pathological condition. The best approach is to combine the best effect on the clearance of the airways with the lowest possible incidence of side effects. A trained experienced staff is fundamental to achieving successful treatment.

23.2 Role of Airway Clearance in MODs

In healthy subjects, mucus secretion, hydration, and clearance play a key role in host defense against lower airway infections. The mucus secretion and hydration in distal airways are regulated by the transport of ions and fluids across the luminal membrane of the lining epithelial cells. In healthy subjects, a well-hydrated mucus layer is transported rapidly at a rate of approximately 50 μm/s from the distal airways toward the trachea [7]. In the MODs like oCF, COPD, and bronchial asthma, the mucus may be retained in the airways due to mucus hyper-concentration (like in oCF or asthma) or defective ciliary function (like in COPD). Retained secretions in the trachea can be expectorated in the form of sputum if there is adequate cough instead of mucus retained in the peripheral airways that cannot be expectorated [9]. MODs are characterized by acute exacerbations involving a vicious circle of airway inflammation, mucin hypersecretion, and mucus retention leading to the formation of mucus plugs. Retained secretions induce airway obstruction with increased airway resistance and thus work of breathing, lung hyperinflation, impaired ventilation/perfusion (V/P) ratio, and lung atelectasis formation, especially in the dependent lung areas. These factors contribute to respiratory failure development [1]. In such cases, the airway clearance techniques (ACTs) are useful in removing secretions from the lower airways of patients suffering from disorders that preclude normal secretion removal. Patients with MODs have both respiratory failure and secretion retention. The use of NIV for respiratory failure may be challenging in patients with retained secretions which necessitates the concurrent use of ACTs. Effective clearance of secretions is also essential for acute and chronic successful treatment with NIV. ACTs include proximal techniques (which help in clearing secretions from central airways) and peripheral techniques (which help in mobilizing secretions from peripheral airways) [8]. The proximal techniques help in augmenting the cough for the removal of secretions from the central airways, and it is generally used when patients have an impaired cough reflex. These are further sub-classified based on whether the inspiratory or expiratory muscles are supported. A mechanical in-exsufflator (MI-E) is the standard approach to treating a patient characterized by impaired cough reflex [10]. Patients with neuromuscular disorders are typical patients with impaired cough reflex that benefit from the use of this treatment [11]. Unfortunately, until now there are poor data about the benefits and risks of utilizing MI-E in patients with MODs because impaired cough reflex levels in this specific population during ICU stay have not been systematically evaluated. Investigating the presence of impaired cough reflex in patients with MODs admitted to ICU is mandatory to early start MI-E to help patients in clearing secretions from the large airways. The main objective is to select the best positive and negative pressure to achieve the best peak expiratory cough flow (PECF). However, only through monitoring ventilator pressure and flow waveform trends, we can achieve the best results [12]. The peripheral techniques assist in the proximal mobilization of the secretions from the small airways using oscillations that can be applied directly to the airways (intrapulmonary percussive ventilation [IPV]) or indirectly transmitted from the body surface (high-frequency chest wall oscillation [HFCWO], manual chest physiotherapy or postural drainage) [8]. A brief description of peripheral airway clearance techniques that can be used alone or in conjunction with NIV in intensive care unit is reported in Table 23.1. In addition, certain pharmacological treatments have been used to change the properties of the mucus to enable easier mobilization. Proper setting of NIV and ACTs is critical, and these represent the real challenges

Table 23.1 Lower airway clearance techniques

Technique	Aim	Methodic description
Ventilatory circuit humidification	Can prevent dry secretion induced by drying flow during ventilation	Use in NIV circuit a heated-humidifier attached
Chest wall percussion, vibration, and shaking	Manual techniques used to increase the peak expiratory flow and thus mobilize secretions	The therapist directly can deliver these techniques
Postural drainage	Can drain the secretions through gravity	Position the patients as lobes and segments of lungs are higher to the carina, and start breathing exercises
High-frequency chest wall oscillation	Through a chest wall compression (jacket mediated), an expiratory flow is generated that can mobilize lower airway secretions	Use of a jacket and air pulse generator device
Intrapulmonary percussive ventilation	Achieving secretion clearance through distal ventilation using high-frequency pulses	Using a device that mediates high-frequency inspiratory bursts superimposed on the patient's normal breath
Positive expiratory pressure	Increasing distal ventilation to obstruction mucus induced through a collateral ventilation	Use a specialized positive devices
Autogenic drainage	Technique based on an equal pressure point to induce clearance secretions	The breathing technique is characterized by three phases: unsticking, collection, and evacuation. The patient's breath at several vital capacity levels to obtain high expiratory flows in various generations of bronchi
Active cycle of breathing technique	To obtain distal ventilation to obstruction mucus mediated, inducing collateral ventilation	Breathing techniques characterized by breathing control, thoracic expansion exercises, and forced expiratory technique

shortly to improve the chances of success and minimize failures and adverse events. The complexity to understand the impact of ACT technologies on NIV is very high. Only poor studies have tried to analyze the best setting [13, 14]. Starting from a respiratory pathophysiology model to understand the impact of secretions retentions on NIV failure is mandatory. Lower airway mucus obstruction induced increased airway resistance which leads to a decrease in peak inspiratory and expiratory flow, while the time required for flow to reach zero during inspiration and expiration tends to increase. These mechanisms mediated a reduction of tidal volume and in MODs can enhance intrinsic positive end-expiratory pressure (iPEEP) that can mediate NIV asynchronies [15]. Another important aspect is to early detect the presence of secretion in the lower airway during NIV. In this case the flow waveform shows characteristic oscillations (Fig. 23.1). The most important determinants during ACTs are to achieve the best peak inspiratory flow (PIF) and peak expiratory flow (PEF) and to follow the best flow waveform changes and the trends in tidal

Fig. 23.1 Tracing corresponding to a patient with pressure support ventilation. Flow tracing shows oscillations characteristic of the presence of secretions in the airway. In some cases such as this case, the phenomenon can also be seen in pressure tracing

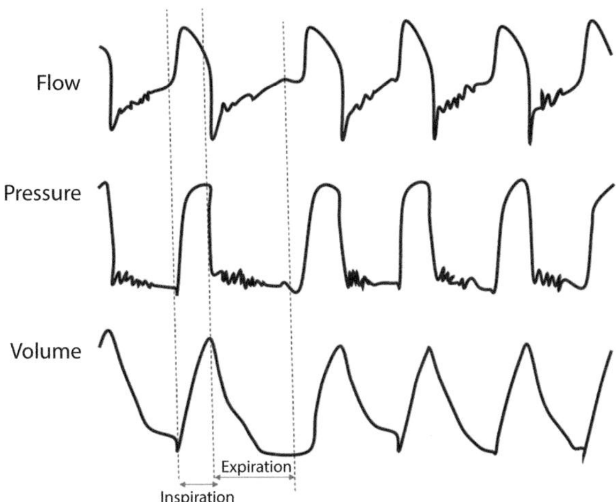

volume variation [12]. Another key element is to know the impact of the NIV interface used (nasal versus oro-facial or total face mask), its internal volume, and the leaks to predict the efficacy of the NIV-ACT combination treatment. A standardized protocol (to correctly select the best frequency, the best time, and the best period) to apply NIV and ACTs in patients with MODs during ICU stay is necessary [16]. It is mandatory to develop a specific clinical model of ACTs in adult and pediatric patients. Now poor data are showing how to incorporate ACTs to improve NIV because the rationale of this approach is to be sure that ACTs are an effective treatment. Today there is a great variability in the clinical practice between countries and health professionals on how to understand and try to resolve the problem of secretion retention [17, 18]. Airway clearance defects impact negatively on NIV and mechanical ventilation success during ICU stay. Multicenter randomized controlled trials should be well designed and conducted in this setting to try to resolve the many controversies that exist in this area. The main ACTs utilized in MODs during the ICU stay, oCF, COPD, and bronchial asthma, are reported below.

23.3   Airway Clearance in Acute Exacerbation of Bronchial Asthma

Asthma is a heterogeneous disease, characterized by chronic airway inflammation. It is defined by the history of respiratory symptoms such as wheeze, shortness of breath, chest tightness, and cough that vary over time and in intensity, together with variable expiratory airflow limitation [19]. Asthma exacerbations can be life-threatening, with 25,000–50,000 such patients per year requiring admission to an ICU in the United States [20]. Mucociliary clearance is altered in asthma, and mucus plugging of proximal and distal lower airways can mainly mediate death in patients during cases of fatal asthma [21]. Moreover, mucus plugging limits aerosol delivery, contributes to airway obstruction, and is one of the main causes of NIV failure. This notion by itself should set mucus hypersecretion among the most relevant therapeutic targets in severe asthma attacks that need ICU admission. Few studies have examined the effect of NIV (either biphasic positive airway pressure [BiPAP] ventilation or continuous positive airway pressure [CPAP]) in patients with life-threatening asthma exacerbation (LTAE). A Cochrane review concluded that the use of NIV with the standard of care may be beneficial but should be used cautiously [22]. Unfortunately, the usefulness of ACTs in LTAE alone or conjunction with NIV or CPAP is generally unknown. No randomized controlled trials are available, but only a few clinical cases report. Firstly Barach and Beck [23] used MI-E in 76 patients with "bronchopulmonary disease," including asthma, emphysema, and bronchiectasis. When using MI-E with bronchodilator aerosols, they found average vital capacity (VC) increases of 15% in 12 patients with bronchial asthma with reported marked improvement in dyspnea. This exceeded the VC improvements with the bronchodilator alone, but it is unclear whether the improvements were due to better distribution of aerosol during the insufflation phase (and, thus, better, relief of bronchoconstriction), lung recruitment, a reduction of obstructing airway secretions, or all of the above. Importantly, Barach and Beck reported no significant complications in their studies. Successful use of high-frequency percussive ventilation (HFPV) for a status asthmaticus in a patient failing conventional mechanical ventilation was reported in a single-case report, but larger studies are needed to verify its efficacy [24]. Finally, only one randomized, double-masked, controlled clinical trial investigated the role of HFCWO in the treatment of asthma exacerbation [25]. The authors concluded that HFCWO is feasible and may improve dyspnea during asthma exacerbations, but further research is needed to evaluate the role of HFCWO in improving clinical outcomes in this population.

23.4 Airway Clearance in Acute Exacerbation of Chronic Obstructive Pulmonary Disease (COPD)

Patients hospitalized for severe acute exacerbations of chronic obstructive pulmonary disease (AECOPD) with rapid clinical deterioration should be considered for NIV to prevent further deterioration in gas exchange and respiratory workload as well as the need for endotracheal intubation [26]. Airway inflammation, bronchospasm, and the increase in sputum volume are constant in these patients, and they are responsible for an increase in lower airways resistance and air trapping. In addition, increased secretions can lead to NIV failure and the need for intubation and invasive mechanical ventilation [27]. ACTs aim to remove sputum from the lower airways; however, literature data on their efficacy during AECOPD is unclear. Bellone et al. demonstrated that chest physiotherapy using a positive expiratory pressure mask in patients with mild acidosis requiring NIV with pressure support could produce benefits in sputum clearance and could reduce the amount of time that the patient requires NIV [28]. Several peripheral airway clearance techniques have been studied in AECOPD, but data on their use in conjunction with NIV is lacking [16]. Cough flows have value in predicting successful extubation and mortality rate in patients with COPD [29]. Cough augmentation with MI-E produces a significant increase in peak cough flow (PCF) and facilitates airway secretion clearance in NMDs [11]. Concerning COPD only early publications are available with controversial results [30]. Barach et al. describe some benefits [23], instead of Sivasothy et al. that reported that MI-E decreased PCF and did not induce significantly improvement, suggesting that it may even exacerbate hyperinflation [31]. Winck et al. in a prospective clinical trial demonstrated that MI-E improved oxygenation and breathlessness without a significant improvement in PCF, but also without any deterioration in breathing pattern or pulmonary parameters concluding that MI-E may be a potential complement to NIV, and may help reduce the frequency of pulmonary complications caused by retention of secretions with good tolerance and reduced adverse effects. However, further evaluation is warranted in a larger patient population [30]. IPV should be an interesting ACT to enhance intrabronchial secretion mobilization in conjunction or in association with NIV. A randomized controlled study was aimed to show that the use of IPV could prove effective in avoiding further deterioration in patients with AECOPD with mild respiratory acidosis. Exacerbation worsened in 6 of 17 patients in the control group versus 0 of 16 in the IPV group ($p < 0.05$). The hospital stay was also significantly shorter in the IPV group [32]. Antonaglia et al. evaluated in a randomized controlled trial the effect of IPV by mouthpiece during NIV with helmet in patients with AECOPD. A benefit in favor of the NIV-helmet plus IPV group was found in terms of reduction of the duration of ventilatory treatment and ICU stay and improvements in gas exchange at intensive care unit discharge. Improvement in gas exchange and other physiologic variables was found after the first IPV session [33]. Further studies are needed to confirm the advantage of adding IPV sessions to the strongly recommended practice of NIV and to improve the selection of the patients likely to benefit from IPV, beforc being able to adopt a "strength through unity for the non-invasive challenges" [34]. A systematic review evaluated the effect of ACTs in patients experiencing an AECOPD has shown that in patients with respiratory failure, techniques that apply positive pressure to the airways may reduce either the need for or duration of NIV and hospital length of stay [35]. It was notable that all other techniques were applied in the reviewed studies, including breathing exercises, postural drainage (PD), chest wall vibration, coughing, huffing, intermittent positive pressure breathing, positive expiratory pressure (PEP) mask therapy, and IPV, which were applied without any reported adverse effects. HFCWO was investigated in AECOPD with negative results [36]. Some of the issues that could have altered these negative results include that oscillation frequency is influenced by the degree of changes in expiratory flow and expiratory volume changes. Thus, a patient selection must be performed carefully in providing a patient-specific therapy. This is both a practical and physiologically relevant approach, due to variations in lung functions, airway resistance, and compliance among a heterogeneous group of acute COPD patients. It is also known that the frequency of HFCWO application must be personalized and should be set on parameters such as the severity of AECOPD and the extent of airway secretions. Further clinical studies focusing on the patient-specific parameters such as an airway secretion score and intrinsic predictive risk factors associated with AECOPD can be useful in understanding the influence of HFCWO on AECOPD during ICU stay [37]. Growing data show how also high-flow nasal cannula (HFNC) can represent a safe and effective therapeutic option in the management of AECOPD [38]. In addition, this device can provide to administer heated and humidified oxygen preventing oxidative damage and mucus drying. This can suggest the use of HFNC in COPD patient management with mucus hypersecretion/retention and impaired mucociliary clearance mechanism. However, there are no data about HFNC's effectiveness in preventing and treating muco-obstructive events.

23.5 Airway Clearance in Acute Exacerbation of Obstructive Cystic Fibrosis Bronchiectasis

Cystic fibrosis (CF), a single-gene disease, is characterized by autosomal recessive mutation (chemical change) in the CF gene-related termed as cystic fibrosis transmembrane conductance regulator (CFTR) protein [39]. The CFTR protein forms a chloride channel that has a key role in efficient mucus transport. Mutations in CFTR induce impaired chloride secretion, sodium reabsorption, and water transport, inducing a hyper mucus concentration and impaired mucociliary clearance [39]. Dehydrated and hyper viscous mucus secretions are correlated to lead endobronchial mucus stagnation and thus lower airway infection with a narrow spectrum of distinctive bacteria inducing a chronic inflammatory response that mediate the development of severe bronchiectasis [39]. Patients can develop acute or chronic respiratory failure that needs long-term oxygen therapy with or without NIV [40]. Literature data show several studies on airway clearance which have specifically recruited patients on long-term NIV instead of little scientific evidence of the role of ACTs alone or in conjunction with NIV during acute exacerbation of oCF [41–43]. These studies included patients who were not already on NIV for their management. The addition of NIV to chest physiotherapy in patients with acute exacerbation of oCF has been found to reduce muscle fatigue, dyspnea, and hypoxemia. MI-E has a potentially key role in CF patients with respiratory muscle weakness, especially in the presence of respiratory failure. In this setting, it has an advantage over NIV, as the latter is unable to provide active exsufflation. In a series of two CF patients with acute exacerbation, this approach proved a good profile in terms of safety and efficacy in achieving airway clearance [44]. However, patients must be monitored for dynamic airway compression or wheeze. In patients with cystic fibrosis, ACTs are the mainstay of secretion management. These include breathing manoeuvers (autogenic drainage and active cycle of breathing technique) and positive expiratory pressure devices. The choice of ACTs should be individualized based on the patient's clinical status, lung function, and local availability and expertise [45]. The use of peripheral ACTs in conjunction with NIV via a nasal mask in patients with both stable or acute exacerbation of cystic fibrosis is associated with reduced respiratory muscle fatigue. The use of ACTs in a combination with NIV may also result in reduced dyspnea and hypoxemia. The use of hydration such as hypertonic saline before ACT may improve patient satisfaction and lung function [16].

23.6   Conclusions

MODs like obstructive CF, COPD, and bronchial asthma are characterized by exacerbations that when severe needed hospitalization and intensive care unit (ICU) admission. The management of bronchial hypersecretion is one of the main problems encountered during the intensive care management and a frequent cause of noninvasive mechanical ventilation (NIV) failure. The early start of airway clearance techniques (ACTs) is a fundamental part of the management to reduce the negative impact on patients' prognosis. Data on their use in conjunction with NIV is lacking. A personalized tailored approach for a single patient is mandatory. Rarely is just one single technique used for a given pathological condition. The best approach is to combine the best effect on the clearance of the airways with the lowest possible incidence of side effects. It is mandatory to develop a specific clinical model of ACTs alone and in conjunction with NIV in adult and pediatric patients with MODs.

> **Key Messages**
> - Chronic lung diseases such as COPD, bronchial asthma, and CF are characterized during acute exacerbation by mucus hypersecretion/retention and impaired mucociliary clearance that can negatively impact patients' prognosis during ICU stay.
> - The management of bronchial hypersecretion is one of the main problems encountered during intensive care management and a frequent cause of NIV failure.
> - The early start of airway clearance techniques (ACTs) is a fundamental part of the management of these patients.
> - The best approach is to combine the best effect on the clearance of the airways with the lowest possible incidence of side effects. It is mandatory to develop a specific clinical model of ACTs alone and in conjunction with NIV in adult and pediatric patients with MODs.
> - Proper setting of NIV and ACTs is critical, and these represent the real challenges shortly to improve the chances of success and minimize failures and adverse events.
> - Multicenter randomized controlled trials should be well designed and conducted in this setting to try to resolve the many controversies that exist in this area.

References

1. Boucher RC. Muco-obstructive lung diseases. N Engl J Med. 2019;380(20):1941–53. https://doi.org/10.1056/NEJMra1813799.
2. Scala R. Respiratory high-dependency care units for the burden of acute respiratory failure. Eur J Intern Med. 2012;23(4):302–8. https://doi.org/10.1016/j.ejim.2011.11.002.
3. Fahy JV, Dickey BF. Airway mucus function and dysfunction. N Engl J Med. 2010;363(23):2233–47. https://doi.org/10.1056/NEJMra0910061.
4. Carlucci A, Richard JC, Wysocki M, Lepage E, Brochard L, Ventilation SCGoM. Noninvasive versus conventional mechanical ventilation. An epidemiologic survey. Am J Respir Crit Care Med. 2001;163(4):874–80. https://doi.org/10.1164/ajrccm.163.4.2006027.
5. Volsko TA. Airway clearance therapy: finding the evidence. Respir Care. 2013;58(10):1669–78. https://doi.org/10.4187/respcare.02590.
6. Randell SH, Boucher RC, University of North Carolina Virtual Lung G. Effective mucus clearance is essential for respiratory health. Am J Respir Cell Mol Biol. 2006;35(1):20–8. https://doi.org/10.1165/rcmb.2006-0082SF.
7. Wanner A, Salathe M, O'Riordan TG. Mucociliary clearance in the airways. Am J Respir Crit Care Med. 1996;154(6):1868–902. https://doi.org/10.1164/ajrccm.154.6.8970383.
8. Belli S, Prince I, Savio G, Paracchini E, Cattaneo D, Bianchi M, et al. Airway clearance techniques: the right choice for the right patient. Front Med. 2021;8:544826. https://doi.org/10.3389/fmed.2021.544826.
9. Button B, Goodell HP, Atieh E, Chen YC, Williams R, Shenoy S, et al. Roles of mucus adhesion and cohesion in cough clearance. Proc Natl Acad Sci U S A. 2018;115(49):12501–6. https://doi.org/10.1073/pnas.1811787115.
10. Homnick DN. Mechanical insufflation-exsufflation for airway mucus clearance. Respir Care. 2007;52(10):1296–305; discussion 306-7.
11. Auger C, Hernando V, Galmiche H. Use of mechanical insufflation-exsufflation devices for airway clearance in subjects with neuromuscular disease. Respir Care. 2017;62(2):236–45. https://doi.org/10.4187/respcare.04877.
12. Volpe MS, Guimaraes FS, Morais CC. Airway clearance techniques for mechanically ventilated patients: insights for optimization. Respir Care. 2020;65(8):1174–88. https://doi.org/10.4187/respcare.07904.
13. Nicolini A, Grecchi B, Ferrari-Bravo M, Barlascini C. Safety and effectiveness of the high-frequency chest wall oscillation vs intrapulmonary percussive ventilation in patients with severe COPD. Int J Chron Obstruct Pulmon Dis. 2018;13:617–25. https://doi.org/10.2147/COPD.S145440.
14. Longhini F, Bruni A, Garofalo E, Ronco C, Gusmano A, Cammarota G, et al. Chest physiotherapy improves lung aeration in hypersecretive critically ill patients: a pilot randomized physiological study. Crit Care. 2020;24(1):479. https://doi.org/10.1186/s13054-020-03198-6.
15. Vignaux L, Vargas F, Roeseler J, Tassaux D, Thille AW, Kossowsky MP, et al. Patient-ventilator asynchrony during non-invasive ventilation for acute respiratory failure: a multicenter study. Intensive Care Med. 2009;35(5):840–6. https://doi.org/10.1007/s00134-009-1416-5.
16. Hadda V, Suri TM, Pahuja S, El-Khatib M, Ciobanu LD, Cabrita B, et al. Secretion management in patients with ineffective airway clearance with non-invasive mechanical ventilation use: expert guidance for clinical practice. Monaldi Arch Chest Dis. 2021;91(4):1499. https://doi.org/10.4081/monaldi.2021.1499.
17. Ntoumenopoulos G, Hammond N, Watts NR, Thompson K, Hanlon G, Paratz JD, et al. Secretion clearance strategies in Australian and New Zealand intensive care units. Aust Crit Care. 2018;31(4):191–6. https://doi.org/10.1016/j.aucc.2017.06.002.
18. Connolly B, Barclay M, Blackwood B, Bradley J, Anand R, Borthwick M, et al. Airway clearance techniques and use of mucoactive agents for adult critically ill patients with acute respiratory failure: a qualitative study exploring UK physiotherapy practice. Physiotherapy. 2020;108:78–87. https://doi.org/10.1016/j.physio.2020.06.003.

19. Reddel HK, Bacharier LB, Bateman ED, Brightling CE, Brusselle GG, Buhl R, et al. Global initiative for asthma strategy 2021: executive summary and rationale for key changes. Eur Respir J. 2022;59(1):2102730. https://doi.org/10.1183/13993003.02730-2021.
20. Garner O, Ramey JS, Hanania NA. Management of life-threatening asthma: severe asthma series. Chest. 2022. https://doi.org/10.1016/j.chest.2022.02.029.
21. Kuyper LM, Pare PD, Hogg JC, Lambert RK, Ionescu D, Woods R, et al. Characterization of airway plugging in fatal asthma. Am J Med. 2003;115(1):6–11. https://doi.org/10.1016/s0002-9343(03)00241-9.
22. Ram FS, Wellington S, Rowe BH, Wedzicha JA. Non-invasive positive pressure ventilation for treatment of respiratory failure due to severe acute exacerbations of asthma. Cochrane Database Syst Rev. 2005;1:CD004360. https://doi.org/10.1002/14651858.CD004360.pub2.
23. Barach AL, Beck GJ. Exsufflation with negative pressure; physiologic and clinical studies in poliomyelitis, bronchial asthma, pulmonary emphysema, and bronchiectasis. AMA Arch Intern Med. 1954;93(6):825–41. https://doi.org/10.1001/archinte.1954.00240300019003.
24. Albecker D, Glen Bouder T, Franklin LB. High frequency percussive ventilation as a rescue mode for refractory status asthmaticus - a case study. J Asthma. 2021;58(3):340–3. https://doi.org/10.1080/02770903.2019.1687714.
25. Krishnan JS, Bilderback AL, Diette GB. Feasibility of high frequency chest wall oscillation (HFCWO) for treatment of asthma exacerbations. Chest. 2004;126:721. https://doi.org/10.1378/chest.126.4_MeetingAbstracts.721S-b.
26. American Thoracic Society. International consensus conferences in intensive care medicine: noninvasive positive pressure ventilation in acute respiratory failure. Am J Respir Crit Care Med. 2001;163(1):283–91. https://doi.org/10.1164/ajrccm.163.1.ats1000.
27. Plant PK, Owen JL, Elliott MW. Non-invasive ventilation in acute exacerbations of chronic obstructive pulmonary disease: long term survival and predictors of in-hospital outcome. Thorax. 2001;56(9):708–12. https://doi.org/10.1136/thorax.56.9.708.
28. Bellone A, Spagnolatti L, Massobrio M, Bellei E, Vinciguerra R, Barbieri A, et al. Short-term effects of expiration under positive pressure in patients with acute exacerbation of chronic obstructive pulmonary disease and mild acidosis requiring non-invasive positive pressure ventilation. Intensive Care Med. 2002;28(5):581–5. https://doi.org/10.1007/s00134-002-1210-0.
29. Bach JR, Saporito LR. Criteria for extubation and tracheostomy tube removal for patients with ventilatory failure. A different approach to weaning. Chest. 1996;110(6):1566–71. https://doi.org/10.1378/chest.110.6.1566.
30. Winck JC, Goncalves MR, Lourenco C, Viana P, Almeida J, Bach JR. Effects of mechanical insufflation-exsufflation on respiratory parameters for patients with chronic airway secretion encumbrance. Chest. 2004;126(3):774–80. https://doi.org/10.1378/chest.126.3.774.
31. Sivasothy P, Brown L, Smith IE, Shneerson JM. Effect of manually assisted cough and mechanical insufflation on cough flow of normal subjects, patients with chronic obstructive pulmonary disease (COPD), and patients with respiratory muscle weakness. Thorax. 2001;56(6):438–44. https://doi.org/10.1136/thorax.56.6.438.
32. Vargas FB, Boyer A, Salmi LR, Gbikpi-Benissan G, Guenard H, Gruson D, Hilbert G. Intrapulmonary percussive ventilation in acute exacerbations of COPD patients with mild respiratory acidosis: a randomized controlled trial. Crit Care Med. 2005;9(4):382–9. https://doi.org/10.1186/cc3724.
33. Antonaglia V, Lucangelo U, Zin WA, Peratoner A, De Simoni L, Capitanio G, et al. Intrapulmonary percussive ventilation improves the outcome of patients with acute exacerbation of chronic obstructive pulmonary disease using a helmet. Crit Care Med. 2006;34(12):2940–5. https://doi.org/10.1097/01.CCM.0000248725.15189.7D.
34. Vargas F, Hilbert G. Intrapulmonary percussive ventilation and noninvasive positive pressure ventilation in patients with chronic obstructive pulmonary disease: "strength through unity"? Crit Care Med. 2006;34(12):3043–5. https://doi.org/10.1097/01.CCM.0000248523.61864.D5.
35. Hill K, Patman S, Brooks D. Effect of airway clearance techniques in patients experiencing an acute exacerbation of chronic obstructive pulmonary disease: a systematic review. Chron Respir Dis. 2010;7(1):9–17. https://doi.org/10.1177/1479972309348659.

36. Goktalay T, Akdemir SE, Alpaydin AO, Coskun AS, Celik P, Yorgancioglu A. Does high-frequency chest wall oscillation therapy have any impact on the infective exacerbations of chronic obstructive pulmonary disease? A randomized controlled single-blind study. Clin Rehabil. 2013;27(8):710–8. https://doi.org/10.1177/0269215513478226.
37. Esquina AM, Patel B, Pravinkumar E. High-frequency chest wall oscillation in infective exacerbation of COPD: is airway secretion clearance the cornerstone? Clin Rehabil. 2014;28(2):206–7. https://doi.org/10.1177/0269215513508685.
38. Bruni A, Garofalo E, Procopio D, Corrado S, Caroleo A, Biamonte E, et al. Current practice of high flow through nasal cannula in exacerbated COPD patients. Healthcare. 2022;10(3):536. https://doi.org/10.3390/healthcare10030536.
39. Stoltz DA, Meyerholz DK, Welsh MJ. Origins of cystic fibrosis lung disease. N Engl J Med. 2015;372(4):351–62. https://doi.org/10.1056/NEJMra1300109.
40. Moran F, Bradley JM, Piper AJ. Non-invasive ventilation for cystic fibrosis. Cochrane Database Syst Rev. 2017;2:CD002769. https://doi.org/10.1002/14651858.CD002769.pub5.
41. Holland AE, Denehy L, Ntoumenopoulos G, Naughton MT, Wilson JW. Non-invasive ventilation assists chest physiotherapy in adults with acute exacerbations of cystic fibrosis. Thorax. 2003;58(10):880–4. https://doi.org/10.1136/thorax.58.10.880.
42. Placidi G, Cornacchia M, Polese G, Zanolla L, Assael BM, Braggion C. Chest physiotherapy with positive airway pressure: a pilot study of short-term effects on sputum clearance in patients with cystic fibrosis and severe airway obstruction. Respir Care. 2006;51(10):1145–53.
43. Dwyer TJ, Robbins L, Kelly P, Piper AJ, Bell SC, Bye PT. Non-invasive ventilation used as an adjunct to airway clearance treatments improves lung function during an acute exacerbation of cystic fibrosis: a randomised trial. J Physiother. 2015;61(3):142–7. https://doi.org/10.1016/j.jphys.2015.05.019.
44. Gaynor M, Wood J. Mechanical insufflation-exsufflation for airway clearance in adults with cystic fibrosis. Respirol Case Rep. 2018;6(4):e00307. https://doi.org/10.1002/rcr2.307.
45. Chaudary N, Balasa G. Airway clearance therapy in cystic fibrosis patients insights from a clinician providing cystic fibrosis care. Int J Gen Med. 2021;14:2513–21. https://doi.org/10.2147/IJGM.S274196.

Airway Clearance Neuromuscular Disorders: Chronic and Acute Conditions

24

Giuseppe Fiorentino, Antonio M. Esquinas, and Anna Annunziata

24.1 Introduction

Severe bulbar and glottic dysfunctions most commonly occur in patients with neuromuscular diseases (NMDs) as SMA type 1, ALS/MND and the pseudobulbar palsy of CNS aetiology.

A compromised upper airway function impacts on breathing, swallowing, coughing, and speech. Hypoventilation and managing secretions are amongst the most important problems from patients' perspectives and present the respiratory physiotherapist with unique management challenges in the care of people with NMD. In these patients, an ineffective cough together with severe bulbar dysfunction led to secretion retention and the possibility for successive lower respiratory tract infection, airway obstruction, hypoventilation, dyspnoea, and sleep disturbances that can unfavourably distress health-related quality of life morbidity and mortality.

Respiratory physiotherapy is an essential part of the multi-disciplinary management of these individuals, but, owing to the inherent heterogeneity of the condition and the growing number of available airway clearance techniques as well as associated technological developments, it is challenging for physiotherapists to understand what assessments are required and what treatment options are available and appropriate for people with NMD.

G. Fiorentino (✉) · A. Annunziata
Respiratory Unit AO Ospedali dei Colli Monaldi, Naples, Italy
e-mail: giuseppe.fiorentino@ospedalideicolli.it

A. M. Esquinas
Intensive Care Unit, Hospital General Universitario Morales Meseguer, Murcia, Spain

219

A. M. Esquinas (ed.), *Humidification in the Intensive Care Unit*,
https://doi.org/10.1007/978-3-031-23953-3_24

24.2 Respiratory Measurements for Patients with NMD

Respiratory function measurement is necessary for NMD evaluation, and it is preferable to make it with pneumotachographs due to their high sampling frequency and great accuracy. The VC is measured in standard pulmonary function tests. The absolute value of VC or its percentage predicted correlates with the severity of the restrictive disease and prognosis but does not correlate with cough impairment. The lung insufflation capacity (LIC), measured on exhalation, is the maximum, tolerable, externally assisted insufflation capacity that does not involve the patient holding their breath. The "lower-end" of the LIC is the residual volume (RV) as per VC.

The most used measurements to assess cough are vital capacity (VC), peak cough flow (PCF), maximal inspiratory pressure (MIP), and maximal expiratory pressure (MEP). PCF is measured using simple tools through a mouthpiece or face-mask while wearing nose clips linked to a peak flow meter or a pneumotachograph. MIP and MEP are also recommended for follow-up of respiratory strength. A MIP >35% of the baseline or a MIP <−80 cmH_2O and a MEP >60–90 cmH_2O indicate an effective cough and exclude significant muscle weakness [1].

In neuromuscular disease patients, PCF values of 160 L/min and below are considered ineffective airway clearance; hence, prompt cough augmentation therapy is demanded in this case. PCF measurements from MI-E devices should only be taken as a trend as measurements are not calibrated. PCF may be assisted (PCF assisted) or unassisted (PCF unassisted). During PCF alone, the patient is instructed to cough from their maximum, unassisted inspiratory lung volume (i.e. to take a deep breath before coughing). During PCF assisted, the patient is instructed to cough from their total aided inspiratory volume.

24.3 Management of Airway Clearance

Standard pre-cough inspiration ranges 85–90% of total lung capacity, and therefore assistance with inspiration can directly increase cough effectiveness. In patients with NMD, respiratory failure typically happens from incapability to successfully clear airway secretions, particularly during superficially mild upper or lower respiratory tract infections. An incapacity to cough efficiently and clear secretions during these events places patients at the possibility of ventilatory failure. Airway *clearance techniques* refer to various strategies used to eliminate excessive secretions. They aim to reduce airway obstruction caused by secretions occupying the airway lumen, prevent respiratory tract infections, and re-expand the collapsed areas of the lung, thus improving gas exchanges and decreasing the inflammatory response. Management of airway clearance can be applied during all cough phases. There is controversial data about if chest physiotherapy can strengthen and enhance the endurance of respiratory muscles with specific training programs. Still, some authors rely upon using the sitting position in both resistive breathing manoeuvres and maximal static inspiratory efforts against an almost occluded resistance to improve strength and endurance [2].

24.4 Postural Drainage (PD)

PD was one of the basic techniques used. Nelson was the first to describe the use of precise postures based on the anatomy of the bronchial tree. This technique exploits the force of gravity to enable the sliding of the mucus from the periphery towards the central airways where, with coughing, forced expiration technique or bronchial aspiration, it can be removed [3].

Assisted inspiration is usually used before coughing, and it is generally used in weak patients with NMD. Assisted inspiration is associated with increased PCF by improving inspiratory lung volumes. These techniques are relatively cheap methods of cough increasing. Assisted inspiration may be either a single or stacked breath inspiration. A single breath-assisted inspiration is where a bag valve mask increases the patient's inspiratory VC, NIV (in a preset pressure or volume mode) or IPPB device with a single breath by an oronasal mask or mouthpiece. This technique aims to reach LIC. The patient takes a long deep breath in by the chosen device and is then instructed to cough autonomously or with MAC. On the other hand, in *stacked breath-assisted inspiration*, the patient performs repeated inspirations without breathing out until they reach their MIC.

24.5 Chest Wall Strapping (CWS)

Chest wall restriction through applying chest wall strapping (CWS) with elastic material has been verified to be valid for lung secretion clearance, especially combined with NIV to maintain tidal volume. The principles and physiological effects of CWS are comparable to those of autogenic drainage. Strapping via CWS passively lowers the functional residual capacity (FRC) without using expiratory muscles. The strapped thorax diminishes pulmonary system compliance, while the work of breathing and dyspnoea increase. The latter is expected to dilate small airways, which may facilitate mucus transport. However, the benefits of these physiological changes may be overwhelmed in NMD as CWS has been associated with a significant decrease in tidal volume. There is no evidence regarding deflation and strapping to mimic breathing at a low lung volume as in the airway clearance technique, autogenic drainage.

24.6 Airway Clearance Techniques in NMD

The first three components involve peripheral and the latest proximal airway clearance techniques. Lannefors identified that for an adequate secretion clearance, physiotherapists first need to open up and get air behind secretions, mobilise and collect secretions from the peripheral airways, move secretions towards the central airways [4] and clear secretions. Proximal airway clearance techniques (also commonly known as cough augmentation techniques) aim to improve cough efficacy by augmenting inspiration, expiration or both. In contrast, peripheral airway techniques improve ventilation and mucus transport from the peripheral to the central airways [4].

24.7 Proximal Airway Clearance Techniques: Cough Augmentation Techniques

Inspiratory support may be delivered by devices and strategies that increase inspiratory volume and thus enhance expiratory flow prejudice during a spontaneous cough and therefore mobilise secretions. These inspiratory assistance manoeuvres and procedures are often called lung volume recruitment (LVR).

24.8 Assisted Inspiration in Patients Without Bulbar Dysfunction

Glossopharyngeal breathing (GPB) can assist inspiratory and, indirectly, expiratory muscle function. The technique includes using the glottis to improve an inspiratory effort by projecting (gulping) boluses of air into the lungs. One breath usually contains six to nine gulps of 40–200 mL each, through the nose or mouth. During the training period, the efficacy of GPB can be examined by a spirometer measuring the inspiratory volume of air per gulp and recording gulps per breath and breaths per minute. There is an improved cough efficacy and voice projection during this technique, and it maintains an external ventilator-free time electively, and it represents a short-term emergency strategy.

24.9 External Assisted Inspiratory Support

In patients with advanced NMDs, profound lung insufflation has become the central management of insufficient cough. Beyond GPB, weak inspiratory muscles can be supported by providing deep lung insufflations with positive pressure delivered through a "bagging (resuscitation/Ambu bag or other LVR) circuit" (a resuscitation bag with a one-way valve preventing expiration in the circuit) or a ventilator. The externally applied volume is typically pressure limited, and the expiratory control remains with the participant and their glottis. Breath-stacking is an LVR manoeuvre that uses the stacking of breaths by applying inspiratory pressure conducted to the airways through a hermetic facemask or mouthpiece. This results in lung inflation, followed by a spontaneous or assisted forced expiratory manoeuvre. The maximum inspiratory capacity (MIC) produced in this technique can overdo predicted inspiratory capacity (IC) in people with integral glottic function. Still, it only approaches predicted IC in patients with moderate to severe glottic dysfunction. The MIC can no longer exceed VC with complete loss of glottic closure, and the technique becomes ineffective. A single augmented breath to lung insufflation capacity (LIC) may be trained.

The aims of LVR are to increase alveolar recruitment, to maintain chest wall expansion and the range of motion and to enhance cough efficacy. Various aspects are important to different patients at different times in their disease progression, and their relative importance amongst patients also changes over time.

As with GPB, not all people with integral glottic function can successfully breath-stack.

In terms of security, there are case descriptions of difficulties with externally related lung insufflations such as gastric distension or discomfort and pneumothorax. Iperinsufflation at maximal lung volumes has been associated with barotrauma and volutrauma in the intensive care literature. Nevertheless, the relationships in the spontaneously breathing, non-intubated patients are not well established.

24.10 Manually Assisted Cough (MAC)

A MAC uses manual Heimlich/abdominal thrust manoeuvre and manual costphrenic compression to increase expiratory airflow. A self-induced thrust may also achieve expiratory assistance to the abdomen and/or chest. Compression of the abdomen causes a sudden increase in abdominal pressure; this causes the abdominal contents to push the diaphragm upwards, increasing expiratory airflow. Similarly, sudden thoracic compression causes air to be rapidly expelled, with an acceleration of airflow towards the mouth. The technique involves the patient taking a spontaneous or receiving an assisted inspiration, and, at the start of the cough, expiratory compression is applied. Care is taken to ensure that the compression direction is in line with the expiratory chest wall movement, i.e. down and in, except for the Heimlich-type assist techniques when the abdominal pressure is up and in.

MAC requires a cooperative patient, good coordination between the patient and caregiver, adequate physical effort and frequent application by the therapist or family caregiver. It may be ineffective in the presence of severe scoliosis. Abdominal compressions should not be used for 1–1.5 h following a meal. However, chest compressions can be used to augment PCF at this time. Chest compression techniques must be performed with caution in osteoporotic ribs. Unfortunately, since it is not widely taught to healthcare professionals, MAC is underutilised. Limits of effectiveness for the use of MAC in NMD have been reported when PCF unassisted $\geq$140 L/min, VC $\geq$1030 L or maximum expiratory pressure (MEP) $\geq$14cmH$_2$O, using MAC can augment PCF to >180 L/min. In patients with ALS, the predictor of ineffective MAC was a MAC PCF below 169 L/min.

Mechanical insufflation-exsufflation (MI-E) devices work simulating the usual cough by providing a profound inspiration to the lungs (insufflation) and, after 10 ms, a deep expiration (exsufflation), using sequentially positive and negative pressure by a full-face mask or catheter mount attached to an artificial airway. These techniques, by rapidly switching from positive to negative pressures, potentially assist secretion clearance. For instance, MI-E works both for weak inspiratory and expiratory capacities.

The implication for clinicians is that bulbar ALS patients are unlikely to benefit from high pressures as they are predisposed to upper airway collapse. This has not been reported in patients with other NMDs.

The usual set-up pressures are titrating up from ±15 to ±40 cmH$_2$O. Still, it should be personalised to each patient, as should the inspiratory, expiratory and pause times (s) and the inspiratory flow rate (L/min). High insufflation and exsufflation (+50 cmH$_2$O to −50 cmH$_2$O) pressures were required through endotracheal tubes and tracheostomies to produce high expiratory flows. The lesser the tube, the more excellent the resistance and the higher the pressures required to generate adequate expiratory flows. In a paediatric lung model, an insufflation time of >1 s was required for equilibration between insufflation and alveolar pressure. Longer exsufflation time did not significantly change mean expiratory flows. Higher insufflation and exsufflation pressures increased mean expiratory flows, but greater exsufflation pressures substantially increased mean expiratory flow. One study in an adult lung model showed set pressures of 40 to −40 cmH$_2$O with an insufflation time of 3 s, and an exsufflation time of 2 s was necessary to produce an exsufflation flow of 294 L/min. The authors concluded that increasing insufflation times might be more effective than exsufflation times in improving expiratory flows.

A recent study using direct visualisation of the upper airway during MI-E by flexible laryngoscopy showed that all patients developed laryngeal collapse during assisted inhalation despite the type of disease onset. They were occurring even before other bulbar symptoms in many patients.

MI-E increases PCF more when compared to other techniques, and the most significant change in PCF occurs in the weakest patients, except for Lacombe and co-workers. They found that MI-E did not produce the most remarkable shift in PCF in stronger patients. Sancho and co-workers reported airway closure in adults with bulbar ALS with exsufflation pressures of −40 cmH$_2$O evaluated with a CT scan. They did not examine what happens with insufflation. Andersen and co-workers recently showed the same phenomenon with video-recorded flexible trans-nasal fibre-optic laryngoscopy during MI-E in all ALS subjects regardless of bulbar symptoms. Still, in addition, they observed laryngeal collapse during insufflation in all subjects with bulbar symptoms.

One possible explanation for the difference in pressures reported could be related to the baseline strength of the patient groups. As spontaneous cough strength declines, there may be a need to increase pressures to improve expiratory flow. However, optimal MI-E dosage and frequency have not been determined.

Patient-reported complications of MI-E use in adults are rare, and MI-E treatments are usually well tolerated. However, side effects include abdominal bloating, pneumothorax, nausea, bradycardia, tachycardia and abdominal distention. Children have also reported thoracic wall discomfort, crying and agitation in response to treatment with MI-E. A significant limitation is the cost and/or reimbursement of the devices. There are also discrepancies in the availability in the acute and long-term settings. In some middle- and low-income countries, MI-E devices are not available. MI-E can be difficult to perform in very young infants who are not able to have minimal cooperation and who are not able to relax and accept being "insufflated" during the MIC manoeuvre. Should the technique be ineffective at this time, there is no reason not to try it as the child gets older. Lacombe et al. suggested that the combination of MI-E to MAC is useless in patients whose PCF assisted with an insufflation technique and MAC exceeds 5 L/s (300 L/min). In patients with ALS, the predictor of effective MI-E was MI-E-assisted PCF of 177 L/min. Andersen and co-workers evaluated upper-airway malfunction in patients with ALS during MI-E. Hypopharyngeal restriction during exsufflation was detected in all patients, especially those with ALS and bulbar symptoms. This severely obstructed the airflow and limited the efficacy of the treatment. They concluded that individually customised settings could prevent airway obstruction and thereby improve and extend the use of non-invasive MI-E. Settings that can help these patients can benefit from an optimized setting with a triggered insufflation, a decreasing the inspiratory flows and pressures and allowing a longer insufflation time to enable the equilibrium of pressure from the device to the lungs.

MI-E in a protocol with MAC, oximetry feedback and home use of NIV effectively decreased hospitalisations and respiratory complications and mortality in a program for patients with ALS. Because extubation failure can be a significant problem for patients with NMD, the use of MI-E in ICU has been evaluated.

24.11 High-Frequency Chest Wall Oscillations (HFCWO)/ High-Frequency Chest Wall Compression (HFCWC)

High-frequency oscillatory ventilation in ALS patients has been shown to reduce breathlessness and stabilise forced vital capacity (FVC) in patients with an FVC of 40–70% predicted. In patients with NMD, the total medical costs, hospitalisation and pneumonia after high-frequency oscillatory ventilation were reduced.

Peripheral airway clearance techniques' primary objective is to improve ventilation by clearing secretions, enhancing mucus transport from the peripheral airways to the central airways and creating higher expiratory than inspiratory airflows. Patients with NMD do not have excessive lung secretion production (sputum) because lung parenchyma, respiratory mucosa, mucociliary function and mucus rheology are not commonly affected. However, the patients could have difficulty in swallowing, hyper-secretion and pooling of oral secretions because of bulbar muscle dysfunction. Manual techniques and high-frequency chest wall oscillation are mainly used in these cases.

HFCWO or HFCWC is a strategy for secretion clearance based on an expandable vest linked to a compressor that can regulate rapid inflation and deflation of the vest. This oscillates with a 5–25 Hz frequency transmitted to the entire bronchial tree through the chest wall. The oscillations should upsurge the interaction between the airflow and the mucus, increasing the cutting forces and thus reducing the viscoelasticity of the excretions. Furthermore, according to Chang et al., the oscillations should increase ciliary activity. Studies showed a significant increase in the expectoration of secretions compared to baseline and control but no difference in other techniques [5]. Allan et al. in 2003 reported that the potential benefits of HFCWO could be obtained in various clinical conditions [6]. However, recent studies have evidence that this strategy removes a smaller amount of secretions than other unblocking techniques during an infectious exacerbation. It may even upsurge the occurrence of exacerbations related to PEP therapy. Nicolini et al. compared a large variety of unblocking techniques, including HFCWO, to a control group that did not receive the intervention [6].

All the techniques, including HFCWO, completed better results in all outcomes than the control, but it was impossible to affirm one technique's superiority over another.

HFCWO also provides compression of the chest wall at frequencies similar to the resonant frequency of the lungs via a negative pressure ventilator attached to a cuirass. As the ventilator delivers negative pressure, the air is sucked into the lungs. When the negative pressure ceases, the patient breathes out. The device can provide high-frequency intermittent negative pressure on the patient's spontaneous or NIV-supported breathing. This also produces a transient/oscillatory increase in airflow in the airways, vibrating the peripheral airways' secretions towards the mouth. Starting settings for this device are a frequency of 5 Hz building up to 10–15 Hz. There have been no studies evaluating treatment times or frequencies in NMD. Therefore, treatments are individualised or based on present manufacturer programs. Often treatments in NMD are around 5 min stages or until the patient feels the need to cough. There is no evidence regarding the physiological effects of chest wall oscillations. An intuitive explanation of the physiologic effects on mucus clearance relates to generating air-liquid shear forces. The eccentric flow pattern (higher expiratory flow than inspiratory flow) may centrally promote the transport of secretions. There is also some evidence that high-frequency oscillations reduce mucus viscosity.

Yuan and co-workers investigated HFCWC in patients with NMD. Data suggest safety, tolerability and better compliance with HFCWC than "standard chest physiotherapy" [7]. HFCWC is easy to use and accepted by patients with NMDs. HFCWC has been shown to decrease the work of breathing and decrease the sensation of breathlessness in ALS. A sub-group showed a reduced rate of FVC decline. More recently, Lechtzin and co-workers evaluated the impact of HFCWC on healthcare use in patients with NMD [8]. Total medical costs decreased after the initiation of HFCWC, along with inpatient admission costs and pneumonia costs.

24.12 Percussive Intrapulmonary Ventilation (IPV)

IPV has a role as an ACT in NMD because it improves airway clearance and lung function in patients with NMDs, but the data are limited.

IPV is delivered via an IPPB pneumatic device. IPV provides air to the lungs at frequencies of 100–300 cycles per minute at peak pressures from 10 to 40 cmH_2O. While the patient is breathing naturally, the device delivers high-frequency mini bursts of air (50–550 cycles/min), thus generating an internal vibration (or percussion) in the respiratory system. The vibration should stimulate clearance. This creates a global effect of internal percussion of the lungs, which promotes clearance from the peripheral bronchial tree. The high-frequency airflow pulsates to expand the lungs, vibrate and enlarge the airways. This potentially delivers air to the distal lung units beyond accumulated secretions. The physiological effects of IPV have been studied in vitro. Increasing frequency increases positive end-expiratory pressure (PEEP) and percussion (i.e. peak pressure) but decreases ventilation. Increasing inspiratory/expiratory (I/E) time increases PEEP and decreases percussion. Increasing pressure increases PEEP and ventilation. Higher expiratory than inspiratory flows are always produced by IPV, favouring proximal secretion mobilisation. The setting of IPV devices can be configured to obtain the highest-pressure peaks; increased frequency and short inspiration times are recommended.

However, lower frequencies and higher pressures are required when patients need assisted ventilation. Lower pressures and higher frequencies should be set for infants and children. Again, pressures may be increased to obtain normal oxygen saturation and carbon dioxide levels in ventilator-dependent patients, such as those with SMA type 1. The length of the IPV session is related to patient comfort. Patients cannot tolerate IPV ventilation longer than 1 or 2 consecutive minutes with face masks. However, using a nasal interface increases comfort and allows 15 min or longer sessions. Cooperation from the patient is not required with IPV. IPV is beneficial in patients with NMDs and acute respiratory failure. IPV is possible with artificial airways such as an endotracheal tube or tracheostomy. IPV is also possible in association with mechanical ventilation.

However, patients with neuromuscular weakness have reported that IPV is associated with improved airway clearance, less fatigue and absence of discomfort than chest physical therapy. There are also case reports of using IPV as a successful "rescue therapy" after other ACT forms have proven ineffective.

The fundamental limitation is that the devices may not be readily available in some countries and are expensive. Other significant limitations are the lack of evidence on adequate settings of parameters and the need for intensive training for professionals to build enough experience to be able to set parameters in different clinical conditions. Finally, IPV devices may hyperventilate patients with no arterial carbon dioxide control during titration, particularly children.

Preventive use of IPV has been suggested to prevent pulmonary infections in adolescents with NMDs who have impaired ability to clear secretions. IPV has also been shown to improve ongoing pulmonary consolidation and appears to be a safe and effective therapy for these patients who have difficulty mobilising sputum and who do not respond to conventional therapeutic techniques.

24.13 Vacuum Technique

Free Aspire is one device that employs the vacuum technique to clear the airways. The device uses expiratory flow accelerator technology (Venturi effect), which accelerates the expiratory flow, helping deep drainage and secretions elimination in patients with or without unproductive cough, without employing any pressure on the airways. The secretions securely reach the upper airways, where the patient can eject or swallow them physiologically through the mechanism of the mucociliary system. The air movement over the mucus layer acquires a cutting force on the surface itself. When the shear force exceeds the surface tension in the mucous layer, the mucus starts to be transported in the airflow direction, and secretions are "dragged" from peripheral to central areas. Garuti et al. described the use of Free Aspire in eight children with infantile cerebral palsy with the inability to collaborate [9].

The Free Aspire is safe and effective in reducing the impact of respiratory exacerbations in terms of visits to the paediatrician, days spent in hospital and days of antibiotic therapy. The regular use of the device maintains these effects over time.

There is a new generation of temporary positive expiratory pressure (TPEP) devices. At the beginning of the patient's expiratory phase, this machine produces a pulsed flow (about 42 Hz) opposing the exhaled air, resulting in a very low positive pressure of about 1 cmH_2O. This pulsed flow ends before the end of the exhalation so that the end of the expiratory phase is spontaneous, without any pressure support. The flow delivered is so slight that it does not generate a disproportionate capacity for the patient. The stoppage of resistance at the end of expiration produces a pressure gradient, which can support decreased pressure within the airways, thus improving the elasticity of the lung walls and consequently causing a decrease in excessive over-distention. The vibration produced by the pulsed flow is diffused throughout the respiratory tract, where its effect is to detach the secretions from the internal walls of the lungs. The shape of the mouthpiece is such that the patient has to carry out an active non-forced exhalation. The subsequent "open glottal exhalation", prolonging the expiratory phase, accelerates the expiratory flow. This effect makes UNIKO-TPEP a beneficial device for the drainage of secretions and decreasing air-trapping [10].

24.14 Conclusions

In patients without bulbar dysfunction, expiratory aids are techniques to improve cough efficiency and secretion clearance, by a supportive manual application during the expiratory phase of respiration or cough. Frequently expiratory supports can be used alone or after a supported inspiration. The manually assisted cough (MAC) and the exsufflation component of mechanical insufflation-exsufflation (MI-E) devices are the standard expiratory assistance techniques described in literature and used in clinical practice. The MAC can implicate a thoracic compression technique, abdominal push or a combination of both.

Various insufflation methods have been studied, namely, single breath insufflations (NIV, IPPB, insufflation component of an MI-E device) and stacked insufflations (GPB, breath-stacking via a volume-cycled ventilator and breath-stacking via an Ambu or lung volume recruitment bag). Regardless the insufflation method, peak cough flow achieved with combined techniques is consistently more significant than expiratory techniques alone. These data suggest that coughing from an increased inspiratory capacity is critical for improved cough effectiveness.

The "bulbar dysfunction" is a relatively non-specific term. It is also more likely to develop as neuromuscular disease progresses, and, as such, it requires modification of airway cleaning techniques. Similarly, there is substantial heterogeneity across individuals with NMDs. In a patient with NMDs, there may be excessive saliva production, combinations of upper and lower motor nerve impairment (with associated spastic and flaccid muscles), integrative neuromuscular control issues and mechanical upper airway dysfunction. This variability complicates clinical research and reinforces the need for an individualised approach to its management.

Conflict of Interest No.

References

1. Chatwin M, Toussaint M, Gonçalves MR, Sheers N, Mellies U, Gonzales-Bermejo J, Sancho J, Fauroux B, Andersen T, Hov B, Nygren-Bonnier M, Lacombe M, Pernet K, Kampelmacher M, Devaux C, Kinnett K, Sheehan D, Rao F, Villanova M, Berlowitz D, Morrow BM. Airway clearance techniques in neuromuscular disorders: a state of the art review. Respir Med. 2018;136:98–110. https://doi.org/10.1016/j.rmed.2018.01.012. Epub 2018 Feb 6. PMID: 29501255.
2. Silva IS, Pedrosa R, Azevedo IG, et al. Respiratory muscle training in children and adults with neuromuscular disease. Cochrane Database Syst Rev. 2019;9(9):CD011711. https://doi.org/10.1002/14651858.CD011711.pub2.
3. Belli S, Prince I, Savio G, et al. Airway clearance techniques: the right choice for the right patient. Front Med. 2021;8:544826. https://doi.org/10.3389/fmed.2021.544826.
4. Lannefors L, Button BM, McIlwaine M. Physiotherapy in infants and young children with cystic fibrosis: current practice and future developments. J R Soc Med. 2004;97(44):8–25. PMID: 15239290; PMCID: PMC1308795.
5. Chang HK, Weber ME, King M. Mucus transport by high-frequency nonsymmetrical oscillatory airflow. J Appl Physiol. 1988;65:1203–9. https://doi.org/10.1152/jappl.1988.65.3.1203.
6. Allan JS, Garrity JM, Donahue DM. The utility of high frequency chest wall oscillation therapy in the post-operative management of thoracic surgical patient. Chest. 2003;124:235. https://doi.org/10.1378/chest.124.4_MeetingAbstracts.235S-b.
7. Yuan N, Kane P, Shelton K, Matel J, Becker BC, Moss RB. Safety, tolerability, and efficacy of high-frequency chest wall oscillation in pediatric patients with cerebral palsy and neuromuscular diseases: an exploratory randomized controlled trial. J Child Neurol. 2010;25(7):815–21. https://doi.org/10.1177/0883073809350223.
8. Lechtzin N, Wolfe LF, Frick KD. The impact of high-frequency chest wall oscillation on healthcare use in patients with neuromuscular diseases. Ann Am Thorac Soc. 2016;13(6):904–9. https://doi.org/10.1513/AnnalsATS.201509-597OC. PMID: 26999271.
9. Garuti G, Verucchi E, Fanelli I, Giovannini M, Winck JC, Lusuardi M. Management of bronchial secretions with Free Aspire in children with cerebral palsy: impact on clinical outcomes and healthcare resources. Ital J Pediatr. 2016;42:7. https://doi.org/10.1186/s13052-016-0216-0.
10. D'Abrosca F, Garabelli B, Savio G, Barison A, Appendini L, Oliveira LV, et al. Comparing airways clearance techniques in chronic obstructive pulmonary disease and bronchiectasis: positive expiratory pressure or temporary positive expiratory pressure? A retrospective study. Braz J Phys Ther. 2017;21:15–23. https://doi.org/10.1016/j.bjpt.2016.12.001.

Weaning from Mechanical Ventilation, Extubation, and Airway Sections and Humidification Evaluation

25

Antonella Marotta, Maria Martino, and Eugenio Piscitelli

Invasive ventilation is a necessary procedure in various situations that cause acute respiratory failure. The orotracheal intubation is a life-saving maneuver for the patient used as a temporary solution to an acute problem.

In most patients, mechanical ventilation (MV) can be discontinued as soon as the underlying reason for ARF has been resolved. However 20–30% of patients are considered difficult to wean from MV.

Successful weaning is defined as the ability to maintain spontaneous ventilation without the need for reintubation and invasive mechanical ventilation for 48 h after extubation.

Weaning process, evaluated with spontaneous breathing test (SBT), can be conducted in protocols such as T-piece, CPAP, or pressure support ventilation:

- T-piece consists in administration of only supplemental oxygen through a T-shaped tube connected to an endotracheal tube.
- Continuous positive airway pressure (CPAP): the weaning protocol involves using a continuous pressure, equal to the previous positive end-expiratory pressure level used before.
- Pressure support: the use of progressive lower levels of inspiratory pressure support until it reaches 5–8 cmH_2O [1].

There is no current evidence suggesting that one of these approaches is better than the others; however it's suggested that T-piece technique may be used if there

A. Marotta · M. Martino
Department of Respiratory Pathophysiology and Rehabilitation,
V. Monaldi Hospital – A.O. Dei Colli, Naples, Italy

E. Piscitelli (✉)
Department of Critical Care – Intensive Care and ECMO Unit,
V. Monaldi Hospital – A.O. Dei Colli, Naples, Italy

A. M. Esquinas (ed.), *Humidification in the Intensive Care Unit*,
https://doi.org/10.1007/978-3-031-23953-3_25

are unsatisfactory results with the other approaches or the PEEP removal could make patent lung or cardiac dysfunction [2]. Having a well-defined protocol for SBT is also demonstrated to lead to a total shorter duration of the mechanical ventilation without extra side effects.

The SBT should last between 30 and 120 min to evaluate correctly the tolerance of the test and the early appearance of respiratory muscle fatigue. Another important factor to be properly assessed for successful weaning is the optimization of sedation therapy. Excessive sedation can result in poor performance in SBT and prolong the duration of mechanical ventilation. Anyhow these trials are not always necessary prerequisites for successful extubation to continuous MV.

The International Consensus Conference in 2005 defined three categories of weaning outcome: *simple* if it is successful at first attempt, *difficult* if it requires up to three trials or <7 days to reach SBT, and *prolonged* if more than 7 days are needed.

Although not recommended by the International Consensus Conference in 2005, there are some useful parameters that help in the prediction whether weaning attempts will be successful or not. These parameters can facilitate the detection of signs indicating that the patient is not ready yet for extubation such as:

- Reduced heart rate variability
- Impaired mental status
- Poor quality of sleep
- Patient inability to manage respiratory tract secretions
- Muscle weakness assessed with handgrip strength test
- Acquired diaphragmatic dysfunction defined as a difference equal or greater than 30% of the diaphragm thickness at the end of inspiration and expiration measured with ultrasonography (US)
- High plasma level of oxidative stress markers as malondialdehyde and ascorbic acid [1]

Weaning can be considered *unsuccessful* when present at least two of these criteria: respiratory acidosis (pH <7.35; $PaCO_2$ >45 mmHg); SpO2 <90% or PaO_2 <60 mmHg with FiO_2 >50%; i > 35 rpm; decreased level of consciousness, restlessness, or excessive sweating; or signs suggestive of respiratory muscle fatigue, such as the use of accessory muscles or paradoxical movement of the abdomen [3]. The chances of extubation greatly decrease if pCO_2 is >35–40 mmHg, if pO_2 in ambient air is <95%, and if airway secretions aren't correctly swiped out neither using mechanical insufflation-exsufflation.

If SBT is unsuccessful, it is advisable to search removable underlying cause of respiratory failure, to replace the respiratory support in use with another one more comfortable, well synchronized with the patient's breathing acts to not cause fatigue and finally try again the SBT every 24 h.

It is advisable to avoid the extubation failure as this factor is independently associated with prolonged hospitalization, increased use of tracheotomy, and higher mortality [4].

In the cases of intubated patients in which ventilator weaning or spontaneous breathing trial fails, the only option is tracheotomy.

High-flow nasal cannula (HFNC) is a high-flow delivery system [5]. Heated and humidified oxygen is delivered at fixed FiO_2 and has many beneficial physiological effects, such as better clearing of the airway secretions [6], positive end-expiratory pressure (PEEP) effect [7], and flushing out carbon dioxide effectively [8]. In critically ill patients, HFNC is being put to innovative usage in patients with respiratory failures [5, 9].

A prospective pilot monocentric study in acute respiratory failures (majority hypercapnic respiratory failures) [10] revealed that the use of HFNC was associated with significant improvement in respiratory rate, thoracic-abdominal compliance and oxygenation. A study on an Indian group [11] has shown, in two cases, that high-flow tracheal oxygenation (HFTO) involves a progressive improvement of the P/F ratio until reaching a plateau. The two patients reached different levels of the plateau. A subnormal level of the plateau, as in case 2, was an indicator that the patient was not ready to be weaned directly from HFTO.

In a study incidence of post-extubation respiratory failure after 72 h was significantly less in the HFNC group ($n = 264$) as compared to the conventional oxygen therapy (COT) group ($n = 263$) (4.9 vs 12.2%; *p-value* = 0.004), but overall ICU stay and mortality were similar in both the groups [12]. In this study, a crossover was not allowed, and the patients who were at low risk of extubation failure were included. Another study compared HFNC ($n = 290$) with noninvasive ventilation (NIV) ($n = 304$) in patients with a high risk of extubation failure [13] concluded that HFNC is non-inferior to NIV when used as prophylactic respiratory support in planned extubated patients with regard to the incidence of reintubation, ICU stays, and mortality in both the groups. However, HFNC offered better comfort to the patients. Similar favorable results with HFNC have been reported in the pediatric age group too [14].

There are few data on the use of HFNC facilitated weaning of tracheostomy patients [15]. In tracheostomized patients, HFTO may have different physiological effects from HFNC because of the different interface. No improvement in the neuro-ventilatory drive, work of breathing, respiratory rate, and the gas exchange was observed with HFTO compared with COT after disconnection from the ventilator in tracheostomized patients at high risk of weaning failure from mechanical ventilation [16].

In a study by Natalini et al., 17 tracheostomized patients were enrolled with the aim of weaning them with HFTO at different gas flows (10, 30, and 50 L/min), evaluating the effects on oxygenation, respiratory rate, and tracheal pressures [17], and it was shown that with increasing gas flows, there was a significant improvement in oxygenation (p-value <0.001) and also a modest increase in tracheal pressure (p-value = 0.01), with no significant changes in respiratory rate and $PaCO_2$.

The tracheostomy patient must pay particular attention to the inadequate humidification of the inhaled gases since the tracheostomy path bypasses the natural humidification process; this could lead to the drying of secretions and atelectasis, resulting in failure to wean patients with PMV. The use of HFTO cancels this detrimental effect by providing oxygen heated to more than 30 mg/L absolute humidity (AH), which is 100% relative humidity (RH) [18]. Hence, the heated and humidified delivery of oxygen to the tracheostomy patient via HFTO closely matches physiological humidification in contrast to suboptimal humidification by NIV.

The HFTO is considered an open circuit, but the high inspiratory flow gives a "PEEP effect" throughout the respiratory cycle. A PEEP of nearly 4–6 mmHg is created with inspiratory flows of 40–60 L/min [15]. This effect could balance the "dynamic hyperinflation" of the lungs in very severe obstructive airway disease when they are tested for spontaneous breathing (SBT) while also neutralizing the backward failure commonly seen in these right-sided heart failure patients associated.

Corley et al. in their randomized crossover study of 20 tracheostomized patients compared the physiological advantages of HFTO ventilation versus low-flow T-piece ventilation [19]. They found significantly better oxygenation of the HFTO group at 5 min (p-value = 0.002) and 15 min (p-value = 0.001) and a noticeable increase in their positive airway pressures compared to the T-piece (mean difference of +0.7 cm H_2O, p-value = 0.001) but no impact on end-expiratory lung volume (EELV).

Lately, Mitaka et al. reported successful weaning of two PMV patients with restrictive pulmonary function [20]. He observed that high inspiratory oxygen flow facilitates weaning by improving the tidal volume and decreasing their inspiratory efforts and work of breathing. He further suggested that in contrast to their study, Corley et al. failed to exhibit an increase in EELV as their patients were more generalized and lacked any restrictive pulmonary dysfunction.

Future randomized controlled trials are needed to verify the role of HFNC in weaning IMV patients with various types of respiratory diseases in prolonged mechanical ventilation with difficult weaning.

References

1. Zein H, Baratloo A, Negida A, et al. Ventilator weaning and spontaneous breathing trials; an educational review. Emergency. 2016;4:65–71.
2. MacIntyre NR. The ventilator discontinuation process: an expanding evidence base. Respir Care. 2013;58(6):1074–86.
3. Kim SM, Kang S-W, Choi Y-C, et al. Successful extubation after weaning failure by noninvasive ventilation in patients with neuromuscular disease: case series. Ann Rehabil Med. 2017;41:450–5.
4. Epstein SK. Extubation failure: an out come to be avoided. Crit Care. 2004;8:310–2.
5. Nishimura M. High-flow nasal cannula oxygen therapy in adults. J Intensive Care. 2015;3(1):15. https://doi.org/10.1186/s40560-015-0084-5.
6. Salah B, Dinh Xuan AT, Fouilladieu JL, Lockhart A, Regnard J. Nasal mucociliary transport in healthy subjects is slower when breathing dry air. Eur Respir J. 1988;1(9):852–5.
7. Parke R, McGuinness S, Eccleston M. Nasal high-flow therapy delivers low level positive airway pressure. Br J Anaesth. 2009;103(6):886–90. https://doi.org/10.1093/bja/aep280.

8. Frizzola M, Miller TL, Rodriguez ME, Zhu Y, Rojas J, Hesek A, et al. High-flow nasal cannula: impact on oxygenation and ventilation in an acute lung injury model. Pediatr Pulmonol. 2011;46(1):67–74. https://doi.org/10.1002/ppul.21326.

9. Maury E, Alves M, Bige N. High-flow nasal cannula oxygen therapy: more than a higher amount of oxygen delivery. J Thorac Dis. 2016;8(10):E1296–300. https://doi.org/10.21037/jtd.2016.10.86.

10. Sztrymf B, Messika J, Mayot T, Lenglet H, Dreyfuss D, Ricard JD. Impact of high-flow nasal cannula oxygen therapy on intensive care unit patients with acute respiratory failure: a prospective observational study. J Crit Care. 2012;27(3):324.e9–324.e13. https://doi.org/10.1016/j.jcrc.2011.07.075.

11. Ramachandran L, Jha OK, Sircar M. High-flow tracheal oxygenation: a new tool for difficult weaning. Indian J Crit Care Med. 2021;25(2):224–7. https://doi.org/10.5005/jp-journals-10071-23724. PMID: 33707904; PMCID: PMC7922460.

12. Hernandez G, Vaquero C, Gonzalez P, Subira C, Frutos-Vivar F, Rialp G, et al. Effect of postextubation high-flow nasal cannula vs conventional oxygen therapy on reintubation in low-risk patients: a randomized clinical trial. JAMA. 2016;315(13):1354–61. https://doi.org/10.1001/jama.2016.2711.

13. Hernandez G, Vaquero C, Colinas L, Cuena R, Gonzalez P, Canabal A, et al. Effect of postextubation high-flow nasal cannula vs conventional oxygen therapy on reintubation in high-risk patients: a randomized clinical trial. JAMA. 2016;316(15):1565–74. https://doi.org/10.1001/jama.2016.14194.

14. Shioji N, Kanazawa T, Iwasaki T, Shimizu K, Suemori T, Kuroe Y, et al. High-flow nasal cannula versus noninvasive ventilation for postextubation acute respiratory failure after pediatric cardiac surgery. Acta Med Okayama. 2019;73(1):15–20. https://doi.org/10.18926/AMO/56454.

15. Schwabbauer N, Berg B, Blumenstock G, Haap M, Hetzel J, Riessen R. Nasal high-flow oxygen therapy in patients with hypoxic respiratory failure: effect on functional and subjective respiratory parameters compared to conventional oxygen therapy and non-invasive ventilation (NIV). BMC Anesthesiol. 2014;14:66. https://doi.org/10.1186/1471-2253-14-66.

16. Stripoli T, Spadaro S, Di Mussi R, Volta CA, Trerotoli P, De Carlo F, et al. High-flow oxygen therapy in tracheostomized patients at high risk of weaning failure. Ann Intensive Care. 2019;9(1):4. https://doi.org/10.1186/s13613-019-0482-2.

17. Natalini D, Grieco DL, Santantonio MT, Mincione L, Toni F, Anzellotti GM, et al. Physiological effects of high-flow oxygen in tracheostomized patients. Ann Intensive Care. 2019;9(1):114. https://doi.org/10.1186/s13613-019-0591-y.

18. Chikata Y, Oto J, Onodera M, Nishimura M. Humidification performance of humidifying devices for tracheostomized patients with spontaneous breathing: a bench study. Respir Care. 2013;58(9):1442–8. https://doi.org/10.4187/respcare.02093.

19. Corley A, Edwards M, Spooner AJ, Dunster KR, Anstey C, Fraser JF. High-flow oxygen via tracheostomy improves oxygenation in patients weaning from mechanical ventilation: a randomised crossover study. Intensive Care Med. 2017;43(3):465–7. https://doi.org/10.1007/s00134-016-4634-7.

20. Mitaka C, Odoh M, Satoh D, Hashiguchi T, Inada E. High-flow oxygen via tracheostomy facilitates weaning from prolonged mechanical ventilation in patients with restrictive pulmonary dysfunction: two case reports. J Med Case Rep. 2018;12(1):292. https://doi.org/10.1186/s13256-018-1832-7.

Airway Clearance Disorders (Hypoxemic): ARDS, Pneumonia, and Cardiac Pulmonary Edema

Rosana Mara da Silva and Thales Cantelle Baggio

26.1 Introduction

In the mechanically ventilated patient, the primary mechanisms of secretion clearance (such as mucociliary transport and coughing) are impaired. In addition to the presence of an artificial airway, poor humidification of inspired gases and relative immobility are the main causes of retention of pulmonary secretions in this population [1].

The secretion accumulated in the airways, when increased, initiates a self-sustaining cycle of ventilation/perfusion mismatch [1], causing impaired gas exchange, increased respiratory effort, and subsequent increased risk of dependence on mechanical ventilation, which in turn closes a positive cycle predisposing to greater retention of secretions, increasing the risk for infections.

26.2 Changes in Mucociliary Clearance and Intensive Care Unit

Airway care interventions can prevent the accumulation of secretions and promote hygiene [2].

The management of bronchial secretions is one of the main problems encountered in the intensive care unit [3], in addition to respiratory disorders, neuromuscular disorders, and patients undergoing thoracic or abdominal surgery, among others.

R. M. da Silva (✉)
Municipal Health Department, Estácio de Sá University – Medical School, Jaraguá do Sul, SC, Brazil

T. C. Baggio
Intensive Care Physician, Hospital Jaraguá and Hospital São José, Estácio de Sá University – Medical School, Jaraguá do Sul, SC, Brazil

© The Author(s), under exclusive license to Springer Nature Switzerland AG 2023
A. M. Esquinas (ed.), *Humidification in the Intensive Care Unit*,
https://doi.org/10.1007/978-3-031-23953-3_26

Mechanically ventilated patients with respiratory failure often require adjunctive therapies to achieve special needs, such as administering inhaled drugs to relieve airway obstruction, treat lung infections, stabilize gas exchange, and provide therapies that improve lung hygiene [4].

Mechanically ventilated patients tend to accumulate a large amount of secretions due to ineffective coughing, non-closing of the glottis, prolonged recumbency, neurodegenerative conditions, advanced age, smoking history, and decreased mucus transport due to the existence of the tracheal tube. This mucus retention contributes to the appearance of atelectasis, hypoxemia, and pneumonia associated with invasive ventilatory support [5, 6]. Thus, the accumulation of secretions in the airways results from the combination of the underlying disease and abnormal mucociliary activity, due to changes in mucus production and composition, changes in ciliary structure and function, and changes in the coughing mechanism [6, 7].

These factors are related to the increased risk of secretion retention and the development of atelectasis due to airway obstruction, which can cause impaired gas exchange, pulmonary infection, and fibrosis, in addition to a progressive reduction in lung compliance [6, 8].

Airway clearance techniques have been developed to aid in the removal of secretions from the lungs and airways [1, 9]. Non-invasive airway clearance strategies aim to [1]:

1. Increase inspired lung volume to reach maximum insufflation capacity (MIC) through lung volume recruitment (LVR) or "breath-stacking."
2. Increase expiratory force in the expulsive phase of coughing with manually assisted coughing by applying abdominal pressure.
3. Acceleration of expiratory airflow through the application of positive and negative airway pressures with mechanical in-exsufflation (MI-E).

Other important issues within the management are the physical therapy techniques that help in the mobilization of secretions from the distal airways and agents that change the viscosity of secretions, which can help clear the airways. Finally, aspiration is also often applied to clear secretions from the large airways of tracheostomy patients [1, 9].

26.3   Airway Clearance Hipomexic Disorders

Promoting bronchial hygiene is one of the main problems encountered in the intensive care unit, so there is a need for adequate management for therapeutic support. In many cases of hypoxemic disorders (ARDS, pneumonia, cardiac pulmonary edema), immediate management occurs through tracheal intubation and the use of invasive mechanical ventilation (IMV) as life support in patients with ventilatory distress [10], requiring adequate airway, bronchial clearance techniques, and pharmacological management.

26.3.1 Acute Respiratory Distress Syndrome (ARDS)

Acute respiratory distress syndrome (ARDS) is defined as the rapid onset of noncardiogenic pulmonary edema, resulting in respiratory failure and hypoxemia [11]. It is pathologically characterized by diffuse alveolar damage and, pathophysiologically, by the development of noncardiogenic pulmonary edema due to increased permeability of the pulmonary alveolar-capillary membrane [11, 12].

Etiologic risk factors for ARDS) include direct and indirect lung injuries [11], such as pneumonia, sepsis, noncardiogenic shock, aspiration, trauma, contusion, transfusion, and inhalation injuries. ARDS is still a leading cause of death in critically ill patients, with reported mortality rates consistently around 30–40% [12].

Among the best-established guidelines in the management of patients with ARDS is the use of small tidal volumes during mechanical ventilation. In an investigator-directed study of the ARDSNet Lower Tidal Volume Trial (ARMA), significantly reduced mortality rates (31.0% vs. 39.8%) were reported in ARDS patients ventilated with tidal volumes of 6 ml/kg of predicted body weight (kg) versus those ventilated with 12 ml/kg [11, 13].

Another referenced issue in the literature is the use of PEEP, which is administered to reduce atelectrauma (repetitive opening and closing of alveoli) through the recruitment of collapsed alveoli. Studies reporting trials that controlled for low tidal volumes (6 ml/kg), including the 2004 ARDS) Network ALVEOLI trial, failed to demonstrate a survival benefit for higher PEEP [11, 13, 14].

To achieve a more uniform distribution of gravitational force in pleural pressure, allowing better ventilation of the dorsal lung space and limiting alveoli overdistension, the prone position is used with mechanical ventilation [11, 15].

Guérin et al. [11, 15] reported the results of the Proning Severe ARDS Patients (PROSEVA) study, in which patients) with severe ARDS (PaO_2/FiO_2 ratio less than 150, with FiO_2 of at least 0.6) were randomized for prone positioning for a minimum of 16 h/day. Patients randomized to prone positioning had a 50% reduction in mortality (16% vs. 32.8%) at 28 days. Munshi et al. [11, 16] performed a meta-analysis which corroborates these results and reiterates the survival benefits of prolonged prone positioning (greater than 12 h) in patients with severe ARDS.

Another reference in the literature is the physical therapy intervention in patients undergoing MV, through bronchial hygiene maneuvers, improving the rheological profile of the mucus, pushing it more easily, which significantly reduces the clinical scores of pulmonary infection and the mortality rates [17, 18].

26.3.2 Pneumonia

The accumulation of bronchial secretion is observed in patients submitted to MV, causing episodes of atelectasis and greater risk of mechanical ventilation-related pneumonia, increasing the morbidity and mortality of these patients [5]. The need for mechanical ventilation (MV) in the intensive care unit increases the risk of pneumonia by three to ten times. This risk is also related to the duration of MV, increasing by 3% per day during the first 5 days, by 2% between 5 and 10 days, and by 1% after the 10th day [5], while more than 7 days of MV is considered one of the most common risk factors.

Physiotherapy can help remove excess secretions using active exercises to increase mucociliary clearance. In addition to encouraging coughing, active breathing, body positioning, and vibration techniques (i.e., manual percussion, chest wall shaking, and high-frequency vibration of the airways with asymmetrical flow patterns) can be used to release secretions and thus provide easier expectoration. Other devices that manipulate the airway with positive pressure, including positive expiratory pressure masks, intermittent positive pressure breathing, and insufflation-exsufflation (assisted cough) may also be used [19, 20]. Manual hyperinflation techniques may be necessary in some intubated patients.

26.3.3 Cardiac Pulmonary Edema

Cardiogenic pulmonary edema is a common and potentially fatal cause of acute respiratory failure. Cardiogenic pulmonary edema is most often the result of acute decompensated heart failure (ADHF). The clinical presentation is characterized by the development of dyspnea associated with rapid accumulation of fluid in the interstitial and/or alveolar spaces of the lung as a result of acutely elevated cardiac filling pressures [21].

A variety of conditions or events can cause cardiogenic pulmonary edema in the absence of heart disease [21], including primary fluid overload (e.g., due to excessive blood transfusion), severe hypertension, renal artery stenosis, and severe kidney disease.

Noncardiogenic pulmonary edema is a distinct clinical syndrome associated with diffuse filling of alveolar spaces in the absence of elevated pulmonary capillary occlusion pressure. As a support in the treatment, the use of respiratory physiotherapy works to improve respiratory function and promote and maintain adequate levels of oxygenation and carbon dioxide in the circulation, preserving lung function. Two aspects characterize respiratory physiotherapy: bronchial hygiene (removal of retained secretions, also used in the treatment of diseases of the respiratory system) and maintenance of lung expansion [7, 18, 19].

26.4 Conclusion

The immediate treatment of acute respiratory failure is tracheal intubation and the use of invasive mechanical ventilation (IMV) as life support in patients with ventilatory distress. Although IMV is commonly used in intensive care units, it can cause complications to the patient, which can cause tracheal injury, barotrauma and/or volutrauma, decreased cardiac output, and toxicity from inadequate oxygen use.

It is also important to consider the damage caused by the accumulation of respiratory secretions due to ineffective coughing, impossibility of closing the glottis, and impaired mucus transport due to the presence of the tracheal tube. Secretion retention contributes to episodes of hypoxemia, atelectasis, cardiogenic pulmonary edema, and ventilator-associated pneumonia.

The management of adequate parameters in IMV and the indication of respiratory physiotherapy (RP) techniques provide an improvement in airway permeability and prevention of the accumulation of bronchial secretions, aiming to improve respiratory mechanics by increasing dynamic lung compliance and decreased resistance of the respiratory system.

References

1. Katz SL, CTS Pediatric, Home Ventilation Guidelines Panel. Section 5: airway clearance. Can J Resp Crit Care Sleep Med. 2018;2(Suppl 1):32–40. https://doi.org/10.1080/24745332.201 8.1494979.
2. Stilma W, Van der Hoeven SM, Scholte Reimer WJM, Schultz MJ, Rose L, Paulus F. Intervenções de Cuidados nas Vias Aéreas para Adultos Criticamente Doentes Invasivamente Ventilados—Uma Pesquisa Nacional Holandesa. Rev Med Clín. 2021;10(15):3381. https://doi.org/10.3390/jcms10153381.
3. Belli S, Prince I, Savio G, et al. Técnicas de desobstrução das vias aéreas: a escolha certa para o paciente certo. Front Med. 2021;8:544826. https://doi.org/10.3389/fmed.2021.544826.
4. Kallet RH. Terapias adjuntas durante a ventilação mecânica: técnicas de desobstrução das vias aéreas, aerossóis terapêuticos e gases. Cuid Resp. 2013;58(6):1053–73. https://doi.org/10.4187/respcare.02217.
5. Judson MA, Sahn SA. Mobilization of secretions in ICU patients. Respir Care. 1994;39:213–26.
6. Chicayban LM. Efeitos agudos da hiperinsuflação com o ventilador com aumento do tempo inspiratório sobre a mecânica respiratória: ensaio clínico cruzado randomizado. Rev Bras Ter Intensiva. 2019;31(3):289–95. https://doi.org/10.5935/0103-507X.20190052.
7. Macchione M, Guimarães ET, Saldiva PH, Lorenzi-Filho G. Methods for studying respiratory mucus and mucus clearance. Braz J Med Biol Res. 1995;28(11-12):1347–55.
8. Konrad F, Brecht-Kraus D, Schreiber T, Georgieff M. Mucociliary transport in ICU patients. Chest. 1994;105(1):237–41.
9. Kravitz RM. Desobstrução das vias aéreas na distrofia muscular de Duchenne. Pediatria. 2009;123(4):231–5.
10. Brower RG, Matthay MA, Morris A, Schoenfeld D, Thompson BT, Wheeler A, Network ARDS. Ventilação com volumes correntes mais baixos em comparação com volumes correntes tradicionais para lesão pulmonar aguda e síndrome do desconforto respiratório agudo. N Engl J Med. 2000;342:1301–8.
11. Williams GW, Berg NK, Reskallah A, Yuan X, Eltzschig HK. Acute respiratory distress syndrome. Anesthesiology. 2021;134(2):270–82. https://doi.org/10.1097/ALN.0000000000003571.
12. Bellani G, Laffey JG, Pham T, Fan E, Brochard L, Esteban A, Gattinoni L, van Haren F, Larsson A, McAuley DF, Ranieri M, Rubenfeld G, Thompson BT, Wrigge H, Slutsky AS, Pesenti A, Investigadores LS, Grupo ET. Epidemiologia, Padrões de Atendimento e Mortalidade para Pacientes com Síndrome do Desconforto Respiratório Agudo em Unidades de Terapia Intensiva em 50 Países. JAMA. 2016;315:788–800.
13. Amato MB, Barbas CS, Medeiros DM, Magaldi RB, Schettino GP, Lorenzi-Filho G, Kairalla RA, Deheinzelin D, Munoz C, Oliveira R, Takagaki TY, Carvalho CR. Efeito de uma estratégia de ventilação protetora na mortalidade em mortalidade a síndrome do desconforto agudo. N Engl J Med. 1998;338:347–54.
14. Villar J, Kacmarek RM, Pérez-Méndez L, Aguirre-Jaime A. Uma estratégia ventilatória de alta pressão expiratória final positiva, baixo volume corrente melhora o resultado na síndrome do

desconforto respiratório agudo persistente: um estudo randomizado e controlado. Med Cuid Int. 2006;34:1311–8.

15. Guérin C, Reignier J, Richard JC, Beuret P, Gacouin A, Boulain T, Mercier E, Badet M, Mercat A, Baudin O, Clavel M, Chatellier D, Jaber S, Rosselli S, Mancebo J, Sirodot M, Hilbert G, Bengler C, Richecoeur J, Gainnier M, Bayle F, Bourdin G, Leray V, Girard R, Baboi L, Ayzac L, Grupo PS. Poscionamento prono na síndrome do desconforto agudo grave. N Engl J Med. 2013;368:2159–68.

16. Munshi L, Del Sorbo L, Adhikari NKJ, Hodgson CL, Wunsch H, Meade MO, Uleryk E, Mancebo J, Pesenti A, Ranieri VM, Fan E. Posição Prona para Síndrome do Desconforto Respiratório Agudo. Ann Am Thorac Soc. 2017;14:280–8.

17. Pattanshetty RB, Gaube S. Effect of multimodality chest physiotherapy in prevention of ventilator-associated pneumonia: a randomized clinical trial. Indian J Crit Care Med. 2010;14(2):70–6.

18. Matilde INE, et al. Bronchial hygiene techniques in patients on mechanical ventilation: what are used and why? Einstein. 2018;16(1):3856. https://doi.org/10.1590/S1679-45082018AO3856.

19. Branson RD. Umidificação dos gases respirados durante a ventilação mecânica: considerações mecânicas. Respir Care Clin N Am. 2006;12(2):253–61.

20. Marini JJ, Formenti P. Fisiopatologia e prevenção da retenção de escarro. In: Oxford textbook of critical care. 2nd ed. Oxford: Oxford University Press; 2016. https://doi.org/10.1093/med/9780199600830.001.0001/med-9780199600830-chapter-119.

21. Ware LB, Matthay MA. Prática clínica. Edema pulmonar agudo. N Engl J Med. 2005;353:2788.

Airway Clearance in Conditions of High-Risk Infections: COVID-19 and Other Conditions

Giuseppe Fiorentino, Maurizia Lanza, Anna Annunziata, and Antonio M. Esquinas

Abbreviations

ICU	Intensive care unit
VAP	Ventilator-associated pneumonia
CPT	Chest physiotherapy techniques
MCC	Muco-ciliary clearance
ARDS	Acute respiratory distress syndrome
NAC	N-acetylcysteine

27.1 Introduction

Airway clearance therapy targets to decrease airway infections and inflammation due to mucus stasis on the airways and lung parenchyma and the consequent effects of the obstruction it causes. Maintaining airway secretion clearance, or airway hygiene, is essential for maintaining a patent airway and preventing respiratory tract infections [1]. Impaired airway clearance often requires hospitalization in an intensive care unit (ICU) and is maybe a cause and contributor to acute respiratory failure. The improved secretion volume in the setting of a respiratory infection makes secretion removal a critical aspect of care. However, given the potential for increased aerosolization of secretions with these therapies, it is essential to

G. Fiorentino (✉)
Monaldi Hospital, Naples, Italy

M. Lanza · A. Annunziata
AO dei Colli PO Monaldi Hospital, Naples, Italy

A. M. Esquinas
Intensive Care Unit, Hospital General Universitario Morales Meseguer, Murcia, Spain

A. M. Esquinas (ed.), *Humidification in the Intensive Care Unit*,
https://doi.org/10.1007/978-3-031-23953-3_27

understand the necessary precautions when delivering this cure. In postmortem studies of COVID-19 patients, copious viscous secretions were observed throughout the respiratory tract, indicating the need for recurrent pulmonary hygiene [2]. Therefore, the practice of the usual CPT techniques, such as manual techniques, cough assistance, and nebulizers with positive pressure breathing devices and intra-/extrapulmonary high-frequency oscillation devices, can be helpful in high-risk infections. Physical methods of increasing airway clearance are often used in ICU, but clinical data confirm few. Although there are challenges to present clinical trials evaluating the effectiveness of airway clearance therapeutic strategies, resources are presented in the literature. In adding to device evaluations and clinical research, you will discover expert opinions, systematic reviews, and evidence-based practice guidelines.

27.2 Infection Consideration

Infectious diseases are caused by the transmission and dissemination of droplets that remain infectious when suspended in the air over long distances (>1 m) and for a particular time. Any procedure that generates aerosols is known to have the highest risks of viral transmission. Droplet spread is caused by viral particles within tiny droplets of body fluids. The droplets are generated by a person (source) who infects mainly during coughing, sneezing, and conversation. Transmission occurs when these droplets, containing microorganisms, are pushed a short distance (usually <1 m) [3].

27.3 Role of Mucosal Hydration

The nasal cavity is wetted, while the condensate of the warm breath, coming from the lungs, moves to the nasal epithelial surface during exhalation. Reduced ciliary and reduced muco-ciliary clearance (MCC) function is correlated with the drying of the respiratory mucus and excessive dryness of the nose [4]. For example, the passage of dry cold air current or freshening reduces the temperature of the mucous membrane of the nose and the ciliary movement, which happens in the nasopharynx which represents a greater surface than the post-nasal areas. The rate of heating of the inhaled air differs on the respiratory frequency and the volume of the inhaled air; therefore, hyperventilation leads to more rapid drying of the mucosa and a reduced clearance from the lungs. Polyphonic patients with lung infections may suffer more frequently from a dehydrated mucosa while exhibiting altered eyelashes, slower ciliary beat, modified mucus properties, and slower MCC. Nasal dryness is also induced by body temperature; the temperature of the nose varies straight with the interior body temperature. Thus, even during elevated fever, earlier dehydrating of the respiratory mucosa can happen, making patients with fever even more vulnerable to viral aggression and bacterial infections. In addition, extended use of face masks is associated with dehydrated mucosa of the oro-nasal cavity. This is not surprising, as the training mechanism, comprising of the cooling of the mucosa during inhalation and the condensation of saturated, warm, and exhaled air, is drastically reduced [5].

27.4 Clearing the Airways

Effective airway cleansing requires an equilibrium between production and elimination of respiratory secretions via the muco-ciliary escalator. In ICU patients, both sides of balance can be compromised. Infections, aspiration, or swallowing disorders can increase the number of respiratory secretions. The removal of respiratory secretions may be reduced by upper airway dysfunction and weakness of the respiratory muscles resulting in ineffective or abolished coughing for sedation. Many pre-existing or ICU-acquired situations, such as chronic neuromuscular disease, ICU-acquired neuromuscular weakness, sepsis, delirium, or decreased level of consciousness due to brain damage, can impair optimal functioning of the glottis or the strength of the respiratory muscles and, therefore, promote the imbalance between production and removal of respiratory secretions [6].

However, lung infections mainly manifest with dry cough early on, and sputum is rarely produced. As the disease progresses, sputum may gradually increase and is relatively sticky and challenging to expectorate without assistance, thus requiring sputum aspiration. Sputum viscosity can be measured with a sputum rheometer, but mainly subjective determination is used in the clinic [7]. An outbreak of novel coronavirus-induced pneumonia occurred in Wuhan City, Hubei province, China, in December 2019. This disease was officially named coronavirus disease 2019 (COVID-19), has become a global pandemic, and has overwhelmed health systems globally [8]. The death of critically ill patients with COVID-19 has essentially elevated, and changes in sputum characteristics may be one of the first warning signs that COVID-19 is critical. Cases of COVID-19 are classified into mild, moderate, severe, and critical types. Ninety percent of patients who are cured and discharged from the hospital have mild, self-limiting cases, and patients recover on their own. The cases that led to the death toll applied severe and critical COVID-19 [9]. Some of the patients had yellow, purulent sputum, which could occur even before patients progressed from severe to critical illness and was accompanied by increased neutrophil counts and the possibility of secondary bacterial infection. These findings suggested that changes in sputum features may be one of the first warning signs of the criticality of COVID-19. This imbalance's significant pathophysiological consequences include increased airway resistance and respiratory work, hypoxemia, atelectasis, and superinfection.

Respiratory therapy for lower respiratory tract infections, which mainly involves breathing practices, physical training, and education, can increase SpO_2 value, lung capacity, and dyspnea [10]. Based on recent studies, some patients show fever, nucleic acid positive for SARS-CoV-2, and virus in the oropharyngeal swab after becoming afebrile and recovering from respiratory syndrome. In these cases, eradicating the virus is not achieved successfully, while the clinical symptoms disappear. Patients with comorbidities, comprising cardiovascular disease and diabetes mellitus, and the elderly seem to be more prone to degeneration due to being in hospital for more extended periods.

27.5 Oral/Pharyngeal Hygiene

Accurate upper airway hygiene, which often obtains little consideration from intensivists, aims to reduce colonization of the oropharyngeal cavity of critically ill patients with consequent reduction of lower respiratory tract infections. We know that hospital-acquired pneumonia and ventilator-associated pneumonia (VAP) are always preceded by lower respiratory tract infections that are preceded by colonization or upper respiratory infection [11]. Therefore, most nosocomial pneumonia results from the micro- or macro-aspiration of infected secretions from the upper airways. Many risk factors have been correlated to airway colonization, comprising disease severity, length of hospitalization, previous or connected antibiotic use, malnutrition, endotracheal intubation, and underlying lung disease. Thus, oral rinsing with chlorhexidine gluconate, an inexpensive and easy-to-apply agent, is recommended to avoid lower respiratory tract infections and should be a routine aspect of critical patient care.

27.6 Tracheal Aspiration

In critically ill patients, airway hygiene is poor for reduced cough reflex and unproductive muco-ciliary cleaning secondary to sedation and high inspired oxygen concentrations but also high pressure exerted by the endotracheal tube cuff and inflammation and injury to the tracheal mucosa. In intubated patients, tracheal aspiration is therefore especially suggested to support the removal of airway secretions, which is necessary to support airway clearance and control lung infections. However, tracheal aspiration often causes mucosal lesions, thus allowing bacterial adhesion. It is also related to a reduction in arterial oxygen tension (12–20 mmHg), which may be clearer in cardiac surgery and hypoxemic respiratory failure necessitating high levels of positivity at the end of expiratory pressure, in patients with cardiac arrhythmias (7–81%) and cardiac arrest in patients with acute spinal cord injury [12]. To bypass these side consequences, aspiration is often preceded by manual hyperinflation, preoxygenation, sedation, and optimal aspiration technique. But also decreasing the frequency and length of tracheal aspiration and the use of saline installation can avoid its adverse effects without affecting the duration of mechanical ventilation, ICU length of stay, ICU mortality, and incidence of lung infections [13]. Tracheal aspiration of intubated patients should be conducted firstly on the amount of secretions present and not at predetermined intervals. Therefore, it should be performed as needed, defined by the number of secretions found, not at set intervals. Repeated use of closed (in-line) endotracheal suction devices reduces the need for suspension from mechanical ventilation and does not demand sterile one-handed technique as open suction methods have become conventional in ICUs. Recently, endotracheal tubes have been developed with a dorsal suction channel that opens immediately before the inflatable cuff in the subglottic area. Suction is applied through this port either constantly or intermittently to remove secretions from the subglottic space. A recent meta-analysis reported that these endotracheal tubes reduce early-onset VAP in patients who are expected to require more than 72 h of mechanical ventilation [14]. But the continuous aspiration of subglottic secretions can cause severe damage to the tracheal mucosa. Endotracheal tubes with a dorsal suction channel are significantly more expensive than standard endotracheal tubes, increase the nursing workload, and therefore have the potential to increase ICU costs. They are currently not preferable to closed endotracheal suction devices.

27.7 Therapy Kinetics

The immobility of bedridden patients is known to impair cough and muco-ciliary clearance, resulting in stagnation of secretions. A modest number in the literature there are a modest number of studies in general on the use of kinetic beds for serial lateral rotation therapy. These are beds that perform periodic or continuous rotations along their longitudinal axis of 40, which have thus obtained tolerance in the care of sick patients to facilitate airway hygiene. Kinetic beds for serial lateral rotation therapy decrease the incidence of pneumonia and the length of ICU stay in diverse groups of critically ill patients obtaining mechanical ventilation [15].

27.8 Chest Physiotherapy

Thoracic physiotherapy techniques that focus on decreasing respiratory work and promoting alveolar recruitment could help alleviate the frequency and severity of pulmonary complications, thereby decreasing the risk of recurrence. Although manual physiotherapy techniques to clear the airways are often integrated into the sputum induction procedure, their effectiveness in this context is unexplored [16]. Airway cleaning techniques have been shown to accelerate mucus reduction in diseases such as cystic fibrosis and bronchiectasis, where there is substantial retention of mucus with abnormal rheological properties. As a consequence, airway cleaning techniques are designed to remove sticky mucus and use airflow to move it more centrally, from where it can be cleared with coughing or forced exhalation techniques. Chest physiotherapy, including exclusion techniques and positioning primarily in the prone position, aids oxygenation in ICU patients. In certainly, techniques such as percussion and vibration are advantageous for moving aggregate secretions from the airways. Active breathing cycle techniques performed by patients independently may also support the removal of lung secretions, improvement in lung function, and effective cough improvement in these patients [17]. Respiratory physiotherapy is one of the helpful possibilities for alleviating symptoms in several respiratory viral infections. In particular, studies in patients with influenza support the utility of prone positioning on airway clearance and oxygenation. Breathing exercises, combined with other interventions, may increase total lung capacity in patients with influenza-related acute respiratory distress syndrome (ARDS) [18]. In infants with respiratory syncytial virus bronchitis, thoracic physiotherapy techniques comprising of protracted slow exhalation have been shown to rapidly recuperate respiratory parameters, but no modifications in the length of hospitalization have been reported. Several randomized control studies have considered the consequence of respiratory therapy on children hospitalized with acute viral bronchiolitis. An increase in SpO_2, reduction in respiratory rate, and chest retraction, as well as decrease of wheezing, have been demonstrated. Respiratory physiotherapy techniques, particularly active techniques, could help improve airway clearance and lung capacity as well as reduce respiratory effort during active disease [19].

In parallel, it could lead to the prevention of disabilities resulting from infection and prolonged hospitalization in patients recovered from COVID-19. This supports physiotherapy as both a prophylactic and therapeutic strategy for COVID-19. Chest physiotherapy, including gravity-assisted drainage, chest wall percussion, chest wall vibrations, and manual lung hyperinflation, supports re-expansion of the atelectatic lung and increase peak expiratory flow. Chest physiotherapy is as efficient as early bronchoscopy in patients with acute atelectasis. In addition, chest physiotherapy can cause cardiac arrhythmias, bronchospasm, and transient hypoxemia and can extend the duration of mechanical ventilation [20]. These difficulties, as well as the increased utilization and costs of personnel, together with the paucity of data on the advantageous effects on the prevention of nosocomial pneumonia, should limit the use of chest physiotherapy to ICU patients with acute atelectasis, exacerbations of bronchiectasis, and conditions that are described by excessive sputum production and impaired cough. There are limited data on flutter valves, handset devices, or intrapulmonary percussive ventilation in ICU patients. Cough assist devices, which generate strong expiratory flow through the application of positive pressure followed by the application of negative pressure, have been demonstrated to aid in the elimination of secretions and can avoid intubation in patients with neuromuscular diseases [21]. However, the long-term benefit of these devices in other ICU populations is unclear. A small study of high-frequency pneumatic chest compression in long-term mechanically ventilated patients found it as effective as percussion and postural drainage, and additional studies in patients directly following cardiopulmonary bypass surgery described a decrease in pain from sternotomy with cough.

27.9　Thoracic Physiotherapy Techniques

Airway clearance indicates two separate but related mechanisms: muco-ciliary clearance and increased cough. Methods to avoid airway secretion retention in critically ill patients with mechanical ventilation comprise pharmacotherapy to decrease mucus production or to liquefy secretions and chest physiotherapy techniques (CPT). The intratracheal physiological solution or with bicarbonate and inhaled β2-agonists are unconfirmed but commonly used pharmacological interventions. CPT can be very efficient in the prevention of pulmonary complications in critically ill adult patients with an increase in broncho-pulmonary secretion. The principles of manual CPT consist of the application of manual or mechanical external forces on the rib cage that has a direct effect on expiratory flow and mucus mobilization. In one study conventional CPT for secretion management failed to increase weaning and extubating success, which had some limitations [22], but improved patient outcomes in a prospective cohort study [23]. Assessment of cough strength remains a challenge in ICU patients, and its assistance has a major impact on effective secretion clearance as it can decrease the incidence of post-extubating respiratory failure and provide early extubating, thus avoiding tracheostomy provided that the glottic function is sufficient to avoid aspiration of secretion. The use of MI-E can avoid intubation or rapidly extubate patients with acute respiratory failure without respiratory acceptance and copious airway secretions due to associated chest infections. Mechanical insufflation-exsufflation (MI-E) is a cough assistance therapy in which the device gradually expands the lungs followed by an instantaneous change to negative pressure, which creates a rapid exhalation aimed at stimulating changes in the flow of air that occurs during coughing and aids to sputum elimination [24]. Positive intermittent percussion ventilation is another means of increasing secretion clearance. Although there is a lack of evidence to support the use of MI-E in critically ill patients, Goncalves et al. found that secretion management with MI-E is a useful complementary technique to avoid reintubation in patients who develop acute respiratory failure in the first 48 h after extubating [25]. There are reduced data on the efficacy of CPT) in the acute phase of the disease COVID-19, and it may be useful during the recovery phase [20]. To date, the biggest challenge in implementing CPT in these patients is the debate on the risk of aerosolization with these procedures. CPT includes several procedures that can generate each aerosol but must be evaluated individually. Contrary to the perceived risk of aerosolization, many CPT techniques do not substantially generate aerosols. For example, the aerosol generated by nebulizers ceases to be airborne once it encounters the mucous secretions of patients due to the increase in particle size, corroborated by the pooled risk analysis of three cohort studies evaluating the risk of infection in healthcare professionals during the SARS outbreak [26]. Metered dose inhalers are considered safer alternatives to nebulizers since the drug is administered in a closed chamber with a relatively shorter treatment time and lower total aerosol mass than nebulizers. Manual chest physiotherapy, comprising of cycles of deep breathing with percussion or vibration followed by an assisted cough, generates droplets >10 microns, which are more concentrated within 1 m closest to the patient [27]. In contrast, positive pressure devices, such as cough assist, can theoretically generate more bioaerosol that travels a greater distance than other CPT techniques, although the lack of studies makes it difficult to extrapolate data from manual CPT.

Given the uncertainty surrounding the risk of aerosol generation, most national and international guidelines approve the provision of CPT) and airway remediation in hospital settings with appropriate personal protective equipment, in negative pressure rooms and with viral-bacterial filters, when possible. For patients at home, we encourage self-management or supervised telemedicine to assist with the implementation of chest physiotherapy as needed. Care should be taken for adequate handling and disposal of secretions with the expectoration of secretions in a closed bag/chamber with strict hand hygiene [28].

27.10 Mucus Control Agents

Distilled water, normal saline, and hypertonic and hypotonic saline have long been utilized to "loosen" thick airway secretions and promote airway hygiene. Regardless, the mucus created does not readily integrate locally applied water. The raised sputum production and clearance attributed to mild aerosols, especially hypertonic saline, may be due to the irritating nature of the aerosol, which may cause bronchoconstriction preferably than mucolytic [29]. The saline solution achieves better diffusion of the alveolar lining fluid and has been shown to decrease bioaerosols and viral load. The saline solution hydrates the respiratory epithelia, gels the mucus, stimulates the ciliary beat, and improves muco-ciliary clearance. Coronavirus and SARS-CoV-2 damage the ciliated epithelium in the nose and airways. Saline inhibits SARS-CoV-2 replication; potential interactions involve the entry mechanism of viral ACE2 (ACE2 chloride-dependent configuration) and the sodium channel ENaC. Saline shifts myeloperoxidase activity in epithelial or phagocytic cells to produce hypochlorous acid [30]. Clinically, saline nasal or respiratory airway therapy reduces seasonal coronaviruses and other common cold viruses. Its use as an aerosol reduces hospitalization rates for bronchiolitis in children. Preliminary data suggest a decrease in symptoms in symptomatic patients with COVID-19 if saline is started within 48 h of symptom onset. The saline solution interacts at various levels relevant to nasal or respiratory hygiene (nasal irrigation, gargle, or aerosol). When used from the onset of common cold symptoms, it can be a valuable complement to first-line interventions for COVID-19. A formal evaluation in mild COVID-19 is desirable to establish efficacy and optimal treatment regimens. Respiratory secretions from COVID-19 infection can behave similarly to those of severe bronchitis or bronchiolitis; the cough may be dry, but the secretions may be clear and mucopurulent and thus must be mobilized to be cleared from the airways. For the mucolytic property that breaks the disulfide bonds reducing the elasticity and viscosity of the mucus, and for the anti-inflammatory properties of N-acetylcysteine (NAC), many professionals recommend its use in intensive care to facilitate the removal of secretions from the airways [31]. Although there are limited data on the use of NAC in ICU patients, physicians must recognize the potentially deleterious effects of this practice. There is evidence for and against the use of NAC. In vitro, it can antagonize aminoglycoside and β-lactam antibiotics, but concentrations below 10% inhibit the growth of *Pseudomonas* strains in vitro with false-negative aspirate cultures [32, 33]. NAC can also cause bronchoconstriction and inhibit ciliary function. Tracheal instillation of NAC through an endotracheal tube or bronchoscope can induce the rapid accumulation of liquefied secretions, which must be aspirated instantly to prevent asphyxia. However, direct tracheal instillation of NAC is shown to be effective in treating atelectasis caused by mucoid occlusion. Therefore, despite its widespread use, few data are available to support NAC as a mucolytic agent. Salbutamol increases muco-ciliary clearance of the large airways, both in stable patients with chronic obstructive pulmonary disease and healthy subjects [34]. There are no data from ICU patients. Therefore, despite the simplicity and attractiveness of this approach, there are no data to support the use of inhaled β2-adrenergic agonists as airway hygiene adjuvants in ICU patients.

27.11 Bronchoscopy for Atelectasis

Fiber-optic bronchoscopy is frequently required and often managed for "pulmonary toilet" or the remedy of atelectasis in critically ill patients; regardless, its effectiveness in improving gas exchange and preventing nosocomial pneumonia is incomplete. Atelectasis happens when the volume of alveolar closure exceeds the functional residual capacity. Critically ill patients have high closure volumes due to low residual functional capacity due to respiratory muscle weakness, sedation, and supine positioning [35]. Only one randomized study matched the effectiveness of fiber-optic bronchoscopy with chest physiotherapy for treating acute atelectasis [36]. Thirty-one patients with acute lobar atelectasis were randomly allocated to obtain urgent fiber-optic bronchoscopy with airway flush followed by chest physiotherapy every 4 hours for 48 hours or to receive chest physiotherapy alone. This study indicated that bronchoscopy in patients with acute or emerging respiratory failure is not deprived of adverse effects. Decreased gas exchange, high airway pressure barotrauma, augmented myocardial oxygen demand, and intracranial pressure have been reported [37]. However, subgroup analysis, case series, and clinical experience support the role of bronchoscopy for some patients with atelectasis: in particular, critically ill patients with acute whole-lung atelectasis, lobar, or segmental without bronchograms that cannot support airway hygiene independently and persist symptomatic after 24 h of aggressive thoracic physiotherapy (every 4 h). Clinical experience denotes that atelectasis frequently persists after bronchoscopy because the cause of decreased airway hygiene persists. Therefore, failure to resolve the primary problem should not indicate repeated invasive airway surgery. There is no role for empirical "airway cleaning" with a bronchoscope. Furthermore, bronchoscopy in patients with acute or incipient respiratory failure is not without adverse effects. Impaired gas exchange, high airway pressure barotrauma, increased myocardial oxygen demand, and intracranial pressure have been reported. However, subgroup analysis, case series, and clinical experience support the role of bronchoscopy for some patients with atelectasis: in particular, critically ill patients with whole acute lung, lobar, or segmental atelectasis without air bronchograms who are not able to maintain airway hygiene independently and remain symptomatic after 24 h of aggressive chest physiotherapy (every 4 h). Clinical experience indicates that atelectasis frequently recurs after bronchoscopy because the cause of impaired airway hygiene perseveres [1]. Therefore, failure to resolve the primary problem should not indicate repeated invasive airway surgery. There is no role for empirical "airway cleaning" with a bronchoscope.

27.12 Discussion and Conclusion

As we look to the future to understand the best use and precautions needed for CPT and airway cleaning in SARS-CoV-2 infection, experts are examining the feasibility of home-based high-frequency chest wall oscillation devices for respiratory patients to reduce the hospitalization burden during the COVID-19 pandemic. We understand that the motivation for airway hygiene is the deterrence of pneumonia and respiratory failure. The recent practice considers the clinical experience, not the results of controlled clinical trials. Several evidence-based suggestions can be made on airway hygiene in critically ill patients. Preferably, oropharyngeal decontamination with oral solutions drops the frequency of nosocomial pneumonia and should be a measure of the routine care of the mechanically ventilated patient. Second, tracheal aspiration should only be done "as needed." Closed (in-line) suction catheter devices must be used, and no routine changes of these devices are required. Third, aerosolized mucus regulator agents, such as NAC and routine saline installation, have no demonstrable outcomes on airway secretion clearance and should not be used regularly in critically ill patients. Fourth, kinetic therapy decreases the percentage of nosocomial pneumonia and can shorten the length of stay in the ICU and hospital. Fifth, chest physiotherapy should be limited to patients with acute atelectasis and/or excessive sputum production who cannot manage airway hygiene on their own. Sixth, the beneficial role of bronchoscopy in acute atelectasis is incomplete and short-term and should be reserved primarily for patients with acute atelectasis concerning more than a single lung segment in the absence of air bronchograms that persist symptomatic after 24 hours of chest physiotherapy. Effective airway cleansing requires an equilibrium between production and removal of respiratory secretions via the muco-ciliary escalator. In ICU patients, both sides of balance can be compromised. Infections, aspiration, or swallowing disorders can increase the number of respiratory secretions. The removal of respiratory secretions can be reduced by upper airway dysfunction and/or weakness of the respiratory muscles. Many pre-existing or ICU-acquired situations, such as chronic neuromuscular disease, ICU-acquired neuromuscular weakness, sepsis, delirium, or decreased level of consciousness due to brain damage, can impair optimal glottal functioning or muscle strength respiratory, therefore favoring the imbalance between production and removal of respiratory secretions. This imbalance's important pathophysiological consequences include increased airway resistance and respiratory work, hypoxemia, atelectasis, and superinfection. To date, we have various treatment methods based on the sputum characteristics of COVID-19 patients attempting to modify prognosis. We know that the use of oxygen flow or invasive procedures results in the formation of virus-laden bioaerosols, which deliver air to the surface of the respiratory tract containing infected surfactants. The saline aerosol instead leads to the suppression and reduction of the exhaled bioaerosol. It is recommended to combine saline aerosols and irrigation with basic hygiene measures for COVID-19, with disposable or washable handkerchiefs to collect unnecessary rinses and mucus, with hand washing and adequate ventilation of the rooms. Nor is there evidence that nasal rinsing would lead to worsening of smell. Nasal irrigation with saline does not affect the normal sense of smell, and its use in nasal diseases has not led to adverse outcomes. There were no significant differences in the various types of oxygen inhalation, antiviral treatments, and early-stage antibacterial treatments between groups of patients with or without progression from severe to critical illness. Before the patient undergoes invasive mechanical ventilation, humidification and nebulizer therapy are recommended, which may not act effectively on the lower respiratory tract. The latest consensus on diagnosing and managing severe COVID-19 [29] recommends intravenous administration of 300 mg of ambroxol daily for airway protection and repair. However, more research is needed to confirm the role of high-dose ambroxol in sputum removal and airway protection in patients with COVID-19 [38]. According to the respiratory rehabilitation guidelines for patients with COVID-19 [39], techniques, such as postural drainage clap on patients' backs to facilitate expectoration and disruption of sputum with machine vibrations, can be used to improve sputum retention and sputum difficulty in expectoration among patients. Furthermore, the pathophysiological feature of ARDS due to severe and critical COVID-19 is the heterogeneity of lung damage. Prone ventilation is a very important rescue therapy for critically ill COVID-19 patients [40]. This study showed no differences in applying mechanical or manual sputum removal in the two groups of severely ill and severely ill COVID-19 patients. However, as a sputum drainage measure, prone positioning of patients without mechanical ventilation has been applied in clinical practice in COVID-19. The rate of drainage application in the prone position is relatively high in COVID-19 patients with a good prognosis, suggesting that early application of drainage in the prone position in patients with COVID-19 may prevent progression to critical illness and improve health prognosis. In existing relevant COVID-19 publications, there is not much information describing critically ill COVID-19 patients. Controlling the progress of the disease in seriously ill COVID-19 patients to avoid the development of severe to critical COVID-19 is the most important goal in treating COVID-19. In clinical practice, the central link is still closely monitoring respiration, especially changes in oxygenation and heart rate of COVID-19 patients. Furthermore, the monitoring of related biomarkers is also very important. However, the latest autopsy results of COVID-19 patients have shown many viscous secretions in the airways. Therefore, effective and early removal of mucus in the airways is critical to the prognosis of seriously ill COVID-19 patients.

References

1. Jelic S, Cunningham JA, Factor P. Clinical review: airway hygiene in the intensive care unit. Crit Care. 2008;12:209.
2. Liu Q, Wang RS, Qu GQ, et al. Gross examination report of a COVID-19 death autopsy. Fa Yi Xue Za Zhi. 2020;36:21–3.
3. Judson SD, Munster VJ. Nosocomial transmission of emerging viruses via aerosol-generating medical procedures. Viruses. 2019;11:10.
4. Ximena M. Bustamante-Marin and Lawrence E. Ostrowski cilia and mucociliary clearance. Cold Spring Harb Perspect Biol 2017; 9(4): a028241

5. Workman AD, Cohen NA. The effect of drugs and other compounds on the ciliary beat frequency of human respiratory epithelium. Am J Rhinol Allergy. 2014;28(6):454–64.

6. Demoule A, Jung B, Prodanovic H, et al. Diaphragm dysfunction on admission to the intensive care unit. Prevalence, risk factors, and prognostic impact—a prospective study. Am J Respir Crit Care Med. 2013;188:213–9.

7. Patarin J, Ghiringhelli É, Darsy G, et al. Rheological analysis of sputum from patients with chronic bronchial diseases. Sci Rep. 2020;10:15685.

8. Zhu H, Wei L, Niu P. The novel coronavirus outbreak in Wuhan, China. Glob Health Res Policy. 2020;5:6.

9. Contour D, Cally R, Sarfati F, et al. Causes and timing of death in critically ill COVID-19 patients. Crit Care. 2021;25:79.

10. Narges S, Razieh M, Niloofar R, et al. Potential prophylactic and therapeutic effects of respiratory physiotherapy for COVID-19. Acta Biomed. 2021;92(1):e2021020.

11. Garrouste-Orgeas M, Chevret S, Arlet G, Marie O, Rouveau M, Popoff N, Schlemmer B. Oropharyngeal or gastric colonization and nosocomial pneumonia in adult intensive care unit patients. Am J Respir Crit Care Med. 1997;156:1647–55.

12. Van de Leur JP, Zwaveling JH, Loef BG, et al. Endotracheal suctioning versus minimally invasive airway suctioning in intubated patients: a prospective randomised controlled trial. Intensive Care Med. 2003;29:426–32.

13. Overend TJ, Anderson CM, Brooks D, et al. Updating the evidence base for suctioning adult patients: a systematic review. Can Respir J. 2009;16(3):e6–e17.

14. Dezfulian C, Shojania K, Collard HR, Kim HM, Matthay MA, Saint S. Subglottic secretion drainage for preventing ventilator-associated pneumonia: a meta-analysis. Am J Med. 2005;118:11–8. https://doi.org/10.1016/j.amjmed.2004.07.051.

15. Kirschenbaum L, Azzi E, Sfeir T, et al. Effect of continuous lateral rotational therapy on the prevalence of ventilator-associated pneumonia in patients requiring long-term ventilatory care. Crit Care Med. 2002;30:1983–6.

16. Nici L, Donner C, Wouters E, et al. American Thoracic Society/European Respiratory Society statement on pulmonary rehabilitation. AMJ Respir Crit Care Med. 2006;173:1390–413.

17. Mckoy NA, Saldanha IJ, Odelola OA, et al. Active cycle of breathing technique for cystic fibrosis. Cochrane Database Syst Rev. 2012;7(7):CD007862.

18. Tse GMK, To KF, Chan PKS, et al. Pulmonary pathological features in coronavirus associated severe acute respiratory syndrome (SARS). J Clin Pathol. 2004;57(3):260–5.

19. Dalziel SR, Haskell L, O'Brien S, Borland ML, Plint AC, Babl FE, Oakley E. Bronchiolitis. Lancet. 2022;400(10349):392–406. https://doi.org/10.1016/S0140-6736(22)01016-9. Epub 2022 Jul 1. PMID: 35785792.

20. Abdullahi A. Safety and efficacy of chest physiotherapy in patients with COVID-19: a critical review. Front Med. 2020;7:454. https://doi.org/10.3389/fmed.2020.00454.

21. Kang S-W. Pulmonary rehabilitation in patients with neuromuscular disease. Yonsei Med J. 2006;47(3):307–14.

22. Templeton M, Palazzo MG. Chest physiotherapy prolongs duration of ventilation in the critically ill ventilated for more than 48 hours. Intensive Care Med. 2007;33:1938–45.

23. Castro AA, Calil SR, Freitas SA, et al. Chest physiotherapy effectiveness to reduce hospitalization and mechanical ventilation length of stay, pulmonary infection rate and mortality in ICU patients. Respir Med. 2013;107:68–74.

24. Homnick DN. Mechanical insufflation-exsufflation for airway mucus clearance. Respir Care. 2007;52(10):1296–305.

25. Goncalves MR, Honrado T, Winck JC, Paiva JA. Effects of mechanical insufflation-exsufflation in preventing respiratory failure after extubation: a randomized controlled trial. Crit Care. 2012;16:R48.

26. Ari A. Practical strategies for a safe and effective delivery of aerosol medications to patients with COVID-19. Respir Med. 2020;167:105987.

27. Lazzeri M, Lanza A, Bellini R, et al. Respiratory physiotherapy in patients with COVID-19 infection in acute setting: a Position Paper of the Italian Association of Respiratory Physiotherapists (ARIR). Monaldi Arch Chest Dis. 2020;90:1285.
28. Wang TJ, Chau B, Lui M, et al. Physical medicine and rehabilitation and pulmonary rehabilitation for COVID-19. Am J Phys Med Rehabil. 2020;99(9):769–74.
29. Rau JL. Mucus-controlling agents. In: Rau JL, editor. Respiratory care pharmacology. St Louis: Mosby; 1994. p. 195–222.
30. Huijghebaert S, Hoste L, Vanham G. Essentials in saline pharmacology for nasal or respiratory hygiene in times of COVID-19. Eur J Clin Pharmacol. 2021;77(9):1275–93.
31. Aldini G, Altomare A, Baron G, et al. N-Acetylcysteine as an antioxidant and disulphide breaking agent: the reasons why. Free Radic Res. 2018;52(7):751–62.
32. Di Landini G, Maggio T, Blasi F, et al. Effect of N-acetylcysteine on the activity of antibiotics against relevant respiratory pathogens. Eur Respir J. 2016;48:2631.
33. Boogaard R, de Jongste JC, Merkus PJ. Pharmacotherapy of impaired mucociliary clearance in non-CF pediatric lung disease. A review of the literature. Pediatr Pulmonol. 2007;42:989–1001. https://doi.org/10.1002/ppul.20693.
34. Frohock JI, Wijkstrom-Frei C, Salathe M. Effects of albuterol enantiomers on ciliary beat frequency in ovine tracheal epithelial cells. J Appl Physiol. 2002;92:2396–240.
35. Tobin M. Principles and practices of mechanical ventilation. New York: McGraw Hill; 2006.
36. Marini JJ, Pierson DJ, Hudson LD. Acute lobar atelectasis: a prospective comparison of fiberoptic bronchoscopy and respiratory therapy. Am Rev Respir Dis. 1979;119:971–8.
37. Kreider ME, Lipson DA. Bronchoscopy for atelectasis in the ICU: a case report and review of the literature. Chest. 2003;124:344–50. https://doi.org/10.1378/chest.124.1.344.
38. Wei P-F. Diagnosis and treatment protocols of severe pneumonia caused by a novel coronavirus. J Intern Intens Med. 2020;26:1–5.
39. Wang C, Xie YX, Zhao HM. Recommendations for respiratory rehabilitation of coronavirus disease 2019 in adult. Chin J Tuberc Respir Dis. 2020;43:308–14.
40. Pan C, Chen L, Lu C, et al. Lung recruitability in SARS-CoV-2 associated acute respiratory distress syndrome: a single-center, observational study. Am J Respir Crit Care Med. 2020;201:1294–7.

Humidification, Airway Secretion Management, and Aerosol Therapy

28

Giuseppe Fiorentino, Maurizia Lanza, and Anna Annunziata

Abbreviations

NIV/NIMV   Noninvasive mechanical ventilation
VT   Tidal volume
HME   Heat and moisture exchangers
HH   Active humidifiers
pMDI   Pressurized metered dose inhalers
VHC   Valved holding chambers
VMN   Vibrating network nebulizer
ICU   intensive care unit

28.1 Introduction

28.1.1 Concept Humidity and Physiology and Role of the Upper Airway

Humidity is the amount of water vapor contained in the gas and is usually defined as absolute or relative humidity. The gas temperature is critical because its water vapor content depends on the gas temperature. The corresponding humidity is the percentage (%) of water vapor in the gas near its maximum carrying capacity. Absolute humidity is the total amount of water vapor in the gas, expressed in milligrams of suspended water in liters of gas (mg/L). Absolute humidity is directly related to the gas temperature. It is necessary in terms of humidification as, at low temperatures, the relative humidity can be 100%, while the total humidity can be

G. Fiorentino (✉) · M. Lanza · A. Annunziata
Monaldi Hospital, Naples, Italy

A. M. Esquinas (ed.), *Humidification in the Intensive Care Unit*,
https://doi.org/10.1007/978-3-031-23953-3_28

far below the recommended value [1]. Inspired air conditioning occurs when a gas is heated and hydrated as it passes through the airways to reach the alveolar level in optimal conditions. Although the gas acquires temperature and humidity during its path inside of the airways, the main area in which takes place the heating of the air breathed in is the nose. The temperature of the nasal mucosa is relatively 32 °C, and although the contact time between inspired air and nasal mucosa is short, this time it is sufficient to give heat. In extension, the nose has a high potential to control blood perfusion and thus balance the loss of heat during inspiration. The respiratory mucosa is lined by ciliated columnar epithelium and pseudostratified numerous goblet cells. These cells and submucosal glands support the mucosal layer that serves as a trap for the pathogens and as an interface for moisture exchange. At the level of the concluding bronchioles, the epithelium becomes a simple cubic type with minimum few goblet cells and submucosal glands. Therefore, the capacity of these pathways to perform the same level of humidification as the upper airway is limited. In addition, the air circulates through a narrow conduit by generating a turbulent flow that optimizes the heating, humidifying, and filtering. The exhaled air humidity is partially preserved by condensation on the mucosa during exhalation due to temperature differences approximately 25% of the heat, and humidity increases during exhalation [2]. The eyelash movement is called metachronal ciliary; the pulse frequency is directly proportional to the temperature (t °). It is expected that at 37°C the ciliary beat is 750 b/min and at 40°C it rises to 1100 b/min. Excessive moisture affects the ciliary function since it increases the volume of secretions due to its low viscosity and the risk of atelectasis obstructing the airway. This explains the motivation of gas condensation at a temperature higher than 37 °C and 100% of the gas saturation, thus causing a reduction in mucus viscosity and an increase in the pericellular liquid thickness, which may be too liquid to be adequately coupled to the tips of the eyelashes, thereby influencing the mucociliary transport. Considering the temperature of the inspired air rises throughout its passage through the airway, at the level of the alveolar-capillary interface, it is at body temperature (37 °C), with 100% relative humidity and 44 mg/L absolute humidity. The feature where the gas acquires these conditions is the isothermal saturation limit; this limit is ordinarily close to the fourth or fifth bronchial generation. It is crucial to reaching the isothermal saturation limit to bypass injury to the mucosa and the ciliary epithelium. An artificial airway prevents inspired air from contacting the mucosa of the upper airway affecting conditioning gas. The normal physiology of conditioning gas is altered when the patient requires an artificial airway; intubation eliminates the natural filtration mechanisms, humidification, and warming of inspired air. The humidification of inspired gas is necessary for all mechanically ventilated patients; however, the discussion about the fitting humidification continues today [3].

NIMV provides dry and cold gas through the upper airway, causing dryness of the mucosa and respiratory dysfunction. Leakage compensation used by NIMV creates high flow during the respiratory cycle, which leads to the lack of heat and humidity [4]. Although in NIMV the upper airway is saved, humidification during NIMV might not be optimal due to the higher flow delivered, thus producing increased mucous viscosity and secretion recognition. These conditions improve the danger of obstruction of the upper airways.

28.2 Humidification Devices

Two prototypes of devices for conditioning inspired gases in the presence or inadequacy of an artificial airway are possible: heat and moisture exchangers (HME) and active humidifiers (HH) [5].

Despite of which device is chosen, it should infallibly coincide the minimum conditions to reinstate the role of the upper airway, which, according to the American Association for Respiratory Care, are [1]:

- 30 mg/L absolute humidity, 34 °C, and 100% related humidity for HME
- Within 33 and 44 mg/L absolute humidity, between 34 °C and 41 °C, 100% relative humidity for HH

28.3 Active Humidifiers

The active humidifiers are devices formed of an electric heater placed a plastic casing with a metal base in which is stored sterile water. When the base is heated, the water temperature rises by convection. Some active humidifiers are self-regulated by a mechanism consisting of a heating wire (a wire-heated breathing circuit) that keeps constant the temperature of the gas during its passage in the circuit and a wire with two temperature sensors connected to the output of the heater (distal) and to a part of the circuit (near the patient) to control the system temperature.

28.3.1 Assembly

Active humidifiers are positioned in line in the inspiratory leg of the respirator. The circuit leaving the inhalation valve is connected to the inlet hole of the plastic casing, which must always be filled to the level indicated by the manufacturer. Subsequently, a second section of the circuit (of standard length) is connected to the outlet hole of the casing and to the "Y" of the circuit responsible for supplying gas to the patient. With this type of humidification device, it is necessary to use siphons, tanks with unidirectional circulation systems that allow the excess condensate to be deposited without air leaks. Among other problems, excessive accumulation of water in the circuit can lead to self-activation, misreading of the ventilator monitor, or even the drainage of contaminated material into the patient's airways. The output circuit from the inhalation valve is connected to the casing inlet hole in plastic, which must always be filled to the level indicated by the manufacturer. Subsequently, a second section of the (standard length circuit) is connected to the casing output hole and the "Y" of the charge circuit to provide gas to the patient. With this type of humidification device, it is required to use siphons, tanks with unidirectional circulation systems that deposit the excess condensate without air leakage. Among other problems, the excessive accumulation of water in the circuit can lead to autotrigger, the misreading of the fan, or even to monitor drainage of contaminated material in the patient's airway. These humidifier varieties are separated into several categories: bubble humidifiers, waterfall humidifiers, bypass humidifiers, and shirt humidifiers [6]. Of the active humidification systems, the bypass is the most generally used now in the ICU, and they are utilized in mechanical ventilation and noninvasive ventilation. The gas that goes to the patient moves across the heated water surface, which creates the humidification to come close to 100% RH and can deliver up to 44 mg/L of AH [7]. The water is heated via heating base, which transfers heat by convection from the metal of the bases. It is self-regulating by a servomechanism and consists of a heating cable (which controls the temperature of the gas in the circuit, thus limiting condensation in the piping and the possibility of bacterial colonization), a cable with two temperature sensors, which are secured at the output of the humidifier, and a Y-piece (near the patient) to servo-control the temperature of the system. In most current devices, the temperature is preset at 37 °C. This system manages control of the gas temperature to the patient, despite of differences in the gas flow or water level in the reservoir, notwithstanding having an average time of reaction. The water that condenses the pipes is supposed to be contaminated and should not be returned to the humidifier. The main obstacle with this device is that it does not filter particles [8].

28.3.2 Precautions and Monitoring for Active Humidifiers

- Recognize that the tubing drains the water downward and not near the artificial airway or the ventilator.
- Place the water traps accurately to receive drained water.
- Regularly monitor the active humidifier device (water level and temperature level indicate the presence of condensation).
- Never fill above the suggested level.
- Comply with the manufacturer's terms.
- Do not remove the condensation toward the humidifier chamber.

28.4 Passive Humidifiers

They are economical and simple to use with conventional connectors for IMV. They include a high communication surface of paper, with compressed metallic parts which attract particles of expired water vapor and heat, pressing and releasing it in the next inspiration. The dispositive without a particle filter is used only for disposable heat and moisture exchangers (HME). To fulfill this purpose, the HME can be hydrophobic (HMEF, heat and moisture exchanger filter), hygroscopic (HHME, hygroscopy heat and moisture exchanger), or both with filter (HHMEF, hygroscopy heat and moisture exchanger and filter). Hygroscopic is an attribute of a compound chemical material, which absorbs condensation from the air. The aluminum element of this device immediately exchanges temperatures during expiration condensation created between the layers of this material. The preserved heat and moisture are replaced during inspiration. Adding a fibrous component helps retain moisture and decreases the accumulation of condensation in the secondary position of the device. Hydrophobic is an adjunct for those substances or elements that resist water and cannot combine or absorb. They utilize a paper or polypropylene treated with calcium or lithium chloride, to improve moisture maintenance and repel water that is not absorbed. It is essential to consider that these devices additionally perform as a bacterial filter. The HME are situated between the Y-piece of the patient, which can increase the resistance to airflow, not only during inspiration but also when expiration. The minimum resistance to the flow is 0.5–3.6 cmH$_2$O/L/s. It is essential to record the dead space produced by these devices, which can be mutable. Among separate devices, according to some measurements, it can reach 95 mL. Passive humidifiers should never be used in conjunction with active humidifiers [9].

28.4.1 Dead Space

The working system of passive humidifiers means that a higher volume of condenser material will produce better device performance. For this reason, the "ideal" dead space for a humidifier is approximately 50 mL. This dead space does not describe a problem for patients with invasive mechanical ventilation (iMV) because the dead space can be counterbalanced for the ventilator's programming. However, in patients with artificial airways, without the necessity of iMV, the increase in the ventilatory minute volume as a compensatory mechanism for the dead space could generate a hard-to-tolerate load in patients with low ventilatory reserve. Consequently, passive humidifiers with a "small volume" were produced. Although they can be more "tolerable," they produce a low humidification capacity that worsens when the tidal volume (VT) increases and supplementary O$_2$ [10]. The necessary dead space added by the passive humidifiers during iMV becomes essential when the pathology requires strategies for lung protection (low VT). Studies conducted by Prat [11] and Hinkson [12] account for this, showing significant changes in arterial carbon dioxide partial pressure (PaCO$_2$) (and in pH) under these circumstances.

28.4.2 Resistance

Although the resistance of an additional device could be judged negligible (5 cmH$_2$O/L/s assessed as "dry"), resistance can vary under differences in the conditions (presence of condensation, impaction due to secretions, changes in ventilatory parameters, increases in the VT, and the flow). Although some studies [13] have registered that the presence of "humidity" in a device does not lead to essential changes in resistance, redundant condensation or impaction (due to secretions or blood) can alter it.

28.4.3 Active or Passive Humidification?

In utilizing NIMV, the type of ventilators assumes a vital role in the decision of the humidifier to be used. For a single-branch turbine ventilator and with leakage compensation, the use of HH in patients undergoing times more significant than 24 h of NIMV to enhance the feeling of oral dehydration and tolerance as recommended by Oto in 2014 would be recognized [4]. It is also essential to examine the testimonials of Esquinas et al. [14] in terms of the factors involved in choosing the type of humidification to use, such as air leakage, interface type, type of ventilator, ambient temperature, and inhaled gas temperature, among others. Considering when using HME in single-branch NIMV, there must be a description of where the exhalatory port is in the system. Current recommendations favor the use of heated humidifiers (HH) during NIMV [15], decreasing nasal resistance, helping expectoration, and increasing adhesion and comfort, especially in patients with bronchial secretions [15]. HME is not supported in NIMV because the dead space of the device harms CO_2 removal and minute ventilation in patients managed with NIMV in ICU; this is more evident in hypercapnic patients [15]. *Also*, it has been seen that it increases work in breathing. In Table 28.1 the main advantages and disadvantages on the use of HME and HH are reported.

Table 28.1 Advantages and disadvantages of HH and HME

Devices	Advantages	Disadvantages
Active	Universal application	Cost
	Reliability	Using water
	Alarms	Condensation
	Wide ranges of temperature and humidity	Risk of contamination
	Temperature monitoring	Low possibility of electrical shock and burns
	Reaches the maximum absolute humidity	No filter
Passive	Cost	Does not apply all patients
	Passive operation	Increase dead space
	User-friendly	Increase resistance
	Removal of condensation	Potential occlusion
	Portable	Misting problems

28.4.4 Background of Aerosol Therapy

The drug concentrations in lung tissue are affected by the aerosol dose administered, patient factors, device factors, and drug formulation. The productiveness of the aerosolized drug depends on the dose accumulated at the target site of action and its distribution in the lungs.

The overall efficiency of the aerosol system is a compound of the emitted dose (ED), the dose delivered to the lung (PSF as a surrogate marker), and lung bioavailability. The ED and the PSF are generally determined in vitro and are regulated by the characteristics of the particles and the composition of the device. The bioavailability of the drug is influenced by patient factors, such as the anatomy of the airways and lungs, the permeability of the drug through the membranes, the drug metabolism, and the clearance of phagocytes in the lung [16]. We know that the airflow is not homogeneous in all lungs, even in health. The apical portions of the lungs receive a lung deposition of the order of a 2:1 ratio higher than the basal regions. This difference is significantly decreased in the supine position. Among the factors that affect the administration of aerosolized drugs in critically ill patients include the position of the patient, the formulation, the temperature, the size of the endotracheal tube, the obstruction of the airways or the ventilatory asynchrony, the flow pattern, the respiratory rate, the dose, and the applied frequency or the nebulizer position in the circuit.

28.4.5 Fundamentals of Aerosol Therapy

The size of the drug particles (measured in microns) used in an aerosol for respiratory diseases determines in which the airways will be deposited. The ideal size of the particles for respiratory drugs is from 1 to 8 microns. At these dimensions, the particles can reach the walls of the distal airways via sedimentation and diffusion. In contrast, the microscopic particles of the drug (<1 micron) have a poor transportability and high probability of being exhale. In contrast, very large particles (> 8 microns) tend to agglomerate and settle rapidly in the upper airways (oropharynx and language), from where they can be swallowed and absorbed, finally causing systemic side effects. It should be noted that the nebulizers, devices that generate aerosols of drugs, do not allow a uniform particle size; instead, they produce a wide range of particle sizes.

The pressurized metered dose inhalers (pMDIs) with valved holding chambers (VHC) have demonstrated efficacy superior deposition compared to nebulizers in various studies. However, VHC cannot be used for mechanical ventilators due to the inability to synchronize with the inspiratory delivery. The DPI (Dry-Powder Inhalers) have no fuel; they are inherently synchronized/activated with the breath and produce small variations in particle size. The deposition in the airways may occur by inertial impaction, gravitational settling, or diffusion (Brownian motion). Due to the turbulence and high air velocities associated with aerosol, the inertial impact method is predominant in the first ten ramifications of the airways. However, in five to six generations, distal airway predominates sedimentation due to the lower air velocity [16]. At the alveolar level, a minimum air velocity means that there will be no effect of impact. A combination of sedimentation and diffusion will affect the deposition of the drug. The inspiratory flow of the patient influences the amount and type of deposited particles and the deposition mechanism. The scope of preferred aerosol is from 30 to 60 L/min. Elevated inspiratory flow (>100 L/min) favors the deposition to provide high impact and penetration speed. On the contrary, low inspiratory flow (<30 L/min) favored the sedimentation but involved the risk that the patient inhales only a tiny amount of the drug. The deposition of particles in the lower airways of children is hampered by the combination of high flow rates and decreasing diameter (from top to bottom) of the airways. The affinity of the particles for the water determines the extent to which they can change the size. For the aerosol successfully you must consider the aerosol system. The aerosol system includes the drug, the aerosol device, the disease (which is the target site), and the patient's respiratory system. The ventilator is an additional factor in mechanically ventilated patients.

28.4.6 Device Effects

Nebulizers are several devices that are used to transform liquid formulations and suspensions in the form of aerosols. These devices can be used to produce larger volumes of a drug in aerosol form, intermittently or continuously, to the purpose of prevention or treatment. Depending on their development mechanism, there are three types of nebulizers: jet, ultrasonic, and SMN. The subsequent development of "new-generation" devices such as the ultrasonic nebulizer and vibrating network nebulizer (VMN) has encouraged further studies and applications of aerosol therapy in the ICU because of the ability of these devices to constantly generate the particle size of aerosol desired, which considered to be optimal for deep lung penetration. The jet nebulizers are the cheapest and simple, although they are inefficient in administering drugs. Their disadvantages are the noise, the lack of control of the dosage, and the need to modify the ventilator settings such as the airflow and the tidal volume. The ultrasonic nebulizers are rarely used and also have limitations. They are expensive and large in size, increase the concentration of the drug during nebulization, and can cause thermal inactivation of the nebulized drug. A significant fraction of the aerosolized drug is trapped in the mucous membranes of the conducting airways. Conditions such as pneumonia and other inflammatory lung diseases cause lung surfactant deficiencies in both content and effect. Drugs with high solubility are likely to have a uniform dispersion than insoluble drugs. Inferential, soluble drugs are likely to have longer and more effective lung residence times, thereby improving drug potency. Surfactant deficiency is associated with atelectasis, which in turn reduces drug deposition [17]. Where possible, pMDI with spacers should be used. The use of PPE is likely to be limited in the ICU. The device should be selected for nebulizers based on the formulation used and the desired deposition site and effect. The rate and extent of absorption of aerosolized substances depend on molecular weight, pH, electric charge, solubility, and stability.

28.4.7 The Heliox Effect

A mixture of helium and oxygen (heliox) reduces the density of the gas and increases the deposition of aerosols, in particular in the peripheral lung. With pMDI, it was reported that heliox administration of aerosolized medications during mechanical ventilation increases [18]. However, with the jet nebulizers, heliox also increases the nebulization time, requiring higher gas flows to compensate for the low-density gas.

28.4.8 Type of Aerosol Generator in the Circuit

Currently, nebulizers and pMDIs, with and without spacers, are two types of devices prepared for use in mechanically ventilated patients. Depending on the site of action, they should be used in devices that produce one of the appropriate particle sizes. Nebulizers take much longer to deliver a standard dose compared to other devices. There is also a variation of efficiency between the nebulizer types and between different batches in nebulizers. This effect is accentuated if associated with the impact of different modes of ventilation and pulmonary mechanics. Thorough cleaning and disinfection of the nebulizer inadequately increase the risk of nosocomial pneumonia. The pMDIs are easy to administer, require less time for staff, provide a reliable dosage, and have a minimum of bacterial contamination risk than nebulizers. When used with a collapsible spacer into the circuit, it is not necessary to disconnect the circuit. The pMDIs are also cheaper nebulizers. Furthermore, the optimal location for the aerosol source connection 1 is approximately 15 cm from the wye in the inspiratory line, although there are no in vivo studies to draw definitive conclusions [19].

Humidification is believed to have a significant effect on aerosol drug delivery. Due to the hygroscopic effects of humidification, there may be a two to three times growth in particle size as they pass through the airways. This increase in size can reduce drug deposition in the peripheral lungs and hence pharmacological efficacy. The particulate air filter in the expiratory tract protects the ventilator, and the flowmeter may become saturated, causing the airflow to be blocked. It is supported to replace the filter after each nebulization treatment.

28.4.9 Features of Breath

The aspects of the ventilator breath have an influential effect on the efficacy of the administration of aerosol. Slower inspiratory flows, inspiratory time consumption, and tidal volumes >500 ml (using a pMDI) correlate well with improved aerosol dispensing. The common effective mixture of tidal volume, flow, and other parameters of the fan for the aerosol dispensing can be calibrated on the drug and on the dispensing device using in vitro models [20].

The positive end-expiratory pressure (PEEP) is a setting of usually used ventilation as part of the lung protective ventilation strategy in severe lung disease. PEEP has significant effects on regional ventilation and perfusion and may affect the pharmacokinetics of aerosolized medication. In an animal model that used radiotracers, it was discovered that the PEEP improves the aerosol removal [20]. This could be due to the alveolar epithelium stretching and improving the aerosol distribution in the bloodstream. Meaning: PEEP is potentially advantageous, although further data to quantify the effect on the administration of aerosolized medications are necessary.

Optimization of ventilator parameters required for antibiotic aerosol modified by Lu et al. [21] as as follows:

- Positioning of the nebulizer: in the inspiratory limb 10 cm proximal to the Y fitting.
- Diluted in 10 ml of physiological solution.
- Remove the HME filter.
- Ventilation mode—volume control.
- Airflow pattern: constant inspiratory flow.
- Ventilator settings: RR 12/minute, 50% I:E ratio, VT 8 ml/kg.
- End of inspiration pause, 20% duty cycle.
- Expired aerosol particles collected in a filter.

28.4.10 Dose Effect and the Time

Despite the administration of inhaled medicines, significant extrapulmonary drug losses can mean that the actual amount of drug delivered may be less than the set. The doses should be different in patients with colonization, tracheobronchitis, or pneumonia. Increasing doses require longer nebulization times that are not well tolerated by patients with ARDS or other serious lung diseases. Most of the loss of drug occurs in the expiratory phase of ventilation. To minimize this loss, the activation of the inhaler or nebulizer may be coupled to inhalation.

28.5 High-Flow Nasal Cannula Effect

High-flow nasal oxygen therapy is growing in use in various care settings including in intensive care units (ICU). A number of factors influence nebulization therapy in patients using high flow, which has recently been studied in an in vitro model [22].

1. Nebulizer location: A location away from the humidifier (closer to the patient) improves drug delivery upstream.

2. Nebulizer type: VMNs have demonstrated better delivery than jet nebulizers, although the choice of nebulizer depends on the formulation and desired site of action.
3. Airflow: Breathing mass delivery is lower with higher airflow and improves with lower airflow.
4. Patient efforts: Talking about the effect of airflow with a high-flow oxygen system, in situations mimicking respiratory distress (i.e., an increase in the patient's inspiratory airflow), delivery was indeed best. An open mouth, in contrast, had no significant differences from a closed mouth with respect to drug administration.

28.5.1 Contemporary Applications of Aerosol Therapy in Critical Care: Focus on Antibiotics

Despite these developments, the best evidence for the administration is not enforced, particularly for aerosolized antibiotics. Data from clinical and experimental studies to aminoglycosides and colistin are perhaps the most numerous to antibiotics in intensive care. The aminoglycosides are concentration-dependent antibiotics for which the Cmax/MIC ratio describes the most of the bactericidal effect. Studies have shown that aminoglycosides intravenously penetrate evil in the epithelial lining fluid [23].

In a model of pneumonia inoculation of *Escherichia coli*, it was observed that the aerosolized amikacin lung reaches significant concentrations.

On the other hand, there was no accumulation effect with repeated administration and therefore no toxicity problem with the aerosolized amikacin. In experimental studies, serum concentrations of amikacin were higher when the aerosolized amikacin was used in a pneumonia model compared to healthy lungs. In addition, a combination of intravenous aminoglycosides and aerosols has not been shown to increase cure rates compared to only aerosol antibiotics [24]. Therefore, for the treatment of ventilator-associated pneumonia, aerosol therapy alone may be adequate without the need for an intravenous therapy, decreasing the risk of systemic toxicity.

28.5.2 Limits of Aerosol Therapy in Intensive Care

In fact, there is a possibility of causing systemic toxicity (e.g., aminoglycoside nephrotoxicity) or local toxicity in the form of irritation of the airways, cough, and often bronchospasm, worsening hypoxemia (and secondary arrhythmias) and lung lesions during the use of aerosol therapy [25]. There have been reports of the fan malfunctions and obstruction of expiratory filters, contraindicated for the use of drugs with lipid components or sugar lactose in the formulation (such as zanamivir or formulations of lipid-based amphotericin). You need close monitoring of the potential increase in airway pressure and oxygen saturation to anticipate serious adverse events. Tolerance aerosol is different when medications are nebulized for various periods of time. This may limit the use of the aerosol in patients with ARDS or severe hypoxemia, such as severe pneumonia (in contrast with the ventilator-associated tracheobronchitis), which often have poor tolerance [26]. The environmental contamination caused by aerosols of drugs in an open-loop system represents a small but significant risk to healthcare workers. The use of expiratory filters with valves in the aerosol dispensing devices could minimize this problem. This exposure to the occupational hazard should be evaluated, and interventions should be implemented to mitigate the risks. When using aerosolized antibiotics, it is recommended to change the filter after each therapy.

28.6 Conclusion

During the use of NIMV, inadequate air humidification is related to structural and functional impairment of the nasal mucosa. It suggests the use of active humidification (evidence 2B), while it is not recommended to use passive humidification (evidence 2C). However, recent publications using ICU ventilators disagree with these recommendations. We believe that to choose the type of humidifier for use during NIMV, there are certain aspects that must be taken into consideration as the fan type, the type of interface, and losses, among others, which could favor the use of HH compared to HME to improve tolerance and patient comfort. Aerosol drug delivery in NIV is affected by several factors, including the type of ventilator, mode of ventilation, circuit conditions, type of interface, type of aerosol generator, breathing parameters, drug-related factors, and patient-related factors. Aerosol drug delivery during NIV has gained popularity over the years. Due to many factors that impact drug delivery to patients receiving NIV, aerosol therapy in this patient population can be extremely complex. However, if clinicians know what to use, how to use it, and why, aerosol therapy can be feasible and effective during NIV.

References

1. Restrepo RD, Walsh BK. Humidification during invasive and noninvasive mechanical ventilation: 2012. American Association for Respiratory Care. Respir Care. 2012;57(5):782–8.
2. Keck T, Leiacker R, Heinrich A, et al. Humidity and temperature profile in the nasal cavity. Rhinology. 2000;38(4):167–71.
3. Gross JL, Park GR. Review humidification of inspired gases during mechanical ventilation. Minerva Anestesiol. 2012;78(4):496–502.
4. Oto J, Nakataki E, Okuda N, et al. Hygrometric properties of inspired gas and oral dryness in patients with acute respiratory failure during noninvasive ventilation. Respir Care. 2014;59(1):39–45.
5. Uchiyama A, Yoshida T, Yamanaka H, et al. Estimation of tracheal pressure and imposed expiratory work of breathing by the endotracheal tube, heat and moisture exchanger, and ventilator during mechanical ventilation. Respir Care. 2013;58(7):1157–69.
6. Al Ashry HS, Modrykamien AM. Review humidification during mechanical ventilation in the adult patient. Biomed Res Int. 2014;2014:715434.

7. Schena E, Saccomandi P, Cappelli S, et al. Mechanical ventilation with heated humidifiers: measurements of condensed water mass within the breathing circuit according to ventilatory setting. Physiol Meas. 2013;34(7):813–21.
8. Nishida T, Nishimura M, Fujino Y, et al. Performance of heated humidifiers with a heated wire according to ventilatory settings. J Aerosol Med. 2001;14(1):43–51.
9. Branson RD. Review humidification of respired gases during mechanical ventilation: mechanical considerations. Respir Care Clin N Am. 2006;12(2):253–61.
10. Brusasco C, Corradi F, Vargas M, et al. In vitro evaluation of heat and moisture exchangers designed for spontaneously breathing tracheostomized patients. Respir Care. 2013;58(11): 1878–85.
11. Prat G, Renault A, Tonnelier JM, et al. Influence of the humidification device during acute respiratory distress syndrome. Intensive Care Med. 2003;29(12):2211–5.
12. Hinkson CR, Benson MS, Stephens LM, et al. The effects of apparatus dead space on P(aCO2) in patients receiving lung-protective ventilation. Respir Care. 2006;51(10):1140–4.
13. Lucato JJ, Tucci MR, Schettino GP, et al. Evaluation of resistance in 8 different heat-and-moisture exchangers: effects of saturation and flow rate/profile. Respir Care. 2005;50(5):636–43.
14. Esquinas Rodriguez AM, Scala R, Soroksky A, et al. Review clinical review: humidifiers during non-invasive ventilation–key topics and practical implications. Crit Care. 2012;16(1):203.
15. Mas A, Masip J. Review noninvasive ventilation in acute respiratory failure. Int J Chron Obstruct Pulmon Dis. 2014;9:837–52.
16. Laube BL, Janssens HM, de Jongh FH, et al. What the pulmonary specialist should know about the new inhalation therapies. European Respiratory Society, International Society for Aerosols in Medicine. Eur Respir J. 2011;37(6):1308–31.
17. Ari A, Fink JB. Review guidelines for aerosol devices in infants, children and adults: which to choose, why and how to achieve effective aerosol therapy. Expert Rev Respir Med. 2011;5(4):561–72.
18. Goode ML, Fink JB, Dhand R, et al. Improvement in aerosol delivery with helium-oxygen mixtures during mechanical ventilation. Am J Respir Crit Care Med. 2001;163(1):109–14.
19. Dugernier J, Wittebole X, Roeseler, et al. Influence of inspiratory flow pattern and nebulizer position on aerosol delivery with a vibrating-mesh nebulizer during invasive mechanical ventilation: an in vitro analysis. J Aerosol Med Pulm Drug Deliv. 2015;28(3):229–36.
20. Bayat S, Porra L, Albu G, et al. Effect of positive end-expiratory pressure on regional ventilation distribution during mechanical ventilation after surfactant depletion. Anesthesiology. 2013;119(1):89–100.
21. Lu Q, Luo R, Bodin L, et al. Efficacy of high-dose nebulized colistin in ventilator-associated pneumonia caused by multidrug-resistant Pseudomonas aeruginosa and Acinetobacter baumannii. Anesthesiology. 2012;117(6):1335–47.
22. Réminiac F, Vecellio L, Heuzé-Vourc'h N, et al. Aerosol therapy in adults receiving high flow nasal cannula oxygen therapy. J Aerosol Med Pulm Drug Deliv. 2016;29(2):134–41.
23. Solé-Lleonart C, Rouby JJ, Chastre J, et al. Intratracheal administration of antimicrobial agents in mechanically ventilated adults: an international survey on delivery practices and safety. Respir Care. 2016;61(8):1008–14.
24. Goldstein I, Wallet F, Nicolas-Robin A, et al. Lung deposition and efficiency of nebulized amikacin during Escherichia coli pneumonia in ventilated piglets. Am J Respir Crit Care Med. 2002;166(10):1375–81.
25. Van Heerden PV, Caterina P, Filion P, et al. Pulmonary toxicity of inhaled aerosolized prostacyclin therapy–an observational study. Anaesth Intensive Care. 2000;28(2):161–6.
26. Lu Q, Yang J, Liu Z, Gutierrez C, Aymard G, Rouby JJ, Nebulized Antibiotics Study Group. Nebulized ceftazidime and amikacin in ventilator-associated pneumonia caused by Pseudomonas aeruginosa. Am J Respir Crit Care Med. 2011;184(1):106–15.

Airway Clearance in Neonatology-Pediatric Critical Care

Erennur Tufan, Selman Kesici, and Benan Bayrakci

The primary objective of airway clearance therapy is to reduce or eliminate the mechanical consequences of obstructing secretions and possibly also to remove infective materials and toxic substances such as proteolytic enzymes, oxidative agents, and other mediators of inflammation [1].

Many acute and chronic respiratory diseases are associated with retained airway secretions due to increased mucus production, impaired mucociliary transport, and weak cough [2].

Airflow obstruction secondary to retained secretions increases the work of breathing, produces ventilation-perfusion mismatch, and can result in gas exchange abnormalities. Retained secretions can serve as a source of infection and inflammation.

29.1 Physiology

Airway mucus and its biophysical and biochemical properties are related to the effectiveness of airway clearance therapy [3]. Submucosal glands, which are present wherever there is cartilage, are located mainly in the submucosa, between the cartilage and the surface epithelium, and are responsible for producing most of the mucus in the large airways [3]. In a normal adult, the area occupied by gland constitutes about 12% of the wall, whereas in children that area is about 17%. The importance of this is unclear, but it suggests that mucus hypersecretory states might be of greater consequence in children than adults [4]. Mucus viscoelasticity is determined primarily by mucins, and the mucin content of infantile pulmonary secretions is different than adults. Adult mucus contains sialomucins and sulfomucins.

E. Tufan · S. Kesici (✉) · B. Bayrakci
Department of Pediatric Critical Care Medicine, Life Support Center, Faculty of Medicine, Hacettepe University, Ankara, Turkey

© The Author(s), under exclusive license to Springer Nature Switzerland AG 2023
A. M. Esquinas (ed.), *Humidification in the Intensive Care Unit*,
https://doi.org/10.1007/978-3-031-23953-3_29

Sulfomucins are prevalent at birth, and sialomucins become evident over the first 2 years of life [4, 5]. Mucus viscoelasticity is determined primarily by mucins. The mucin gene products (MUC2, MUC5AC, MUC5B, and MUC7) in infantile pulmonary secretions are different than those in adults. Respiratory tract secretions in children are also more acidic, which may lead to greater viscosity [5].

When there is excessive mucus secretion from the airway and the amount of mucus produced is abnormal, this physiological protective mechanism becomes harmful. During mucus hypersecretion, there are submucosal gland hypertrophy, goblet cell hyperplasia, and increased mucin synthesis. There are also plasma exudation, decreased mucociliary transport, mucostasis, and mucus plugs. Inducers of airway mucus secretion/hypersecretion include inflammatory mediators, cellular-derived mediators, plasma-derived mediators, neural mechanisms, proteinases, bacterial products, irritant gases, reactive gas species, mechanical strain, pH, and ovalbumin sensitization mucus production [6]. Cough is important for airway defense and protection of the lower respiratory tract against inhaled irritations [6].

Ciliary movement and cough are the two chief mechanisms by which the bronchopulmonary airway clears mucus. Expulsion of mucus via cough depends upon the upstream movement of the equal pressure point from the trachea toward the bronchial periphery, and the resulting dynamic compression of the airways creates a moving choke point that catches mucus and facilitates expiratory airflow to propel it downstream [7]. With this mechanism, the airway narrows locally. For these reasons, infants and children may develop atelectasis with partial or complete narrowing of the airway.

The bronchus will collapse when the pleural pressure reaches or exceeds the local airway pressure. This collapse is opposed by the rigidity of the airway. In infants, airway cartilage is more compliant than that of older children and adults [8]. Furthermore, peripheral airway smooth muscle mass increases during the first 8 months of life, and central airway smooth muscle mass continues to develop into adulthood so infants and children have less airway strength [8]. This greater compliance of airway walls leads to dynamic airway collapse with lower-pressure differences between pleural and airway pressures. This tendency can be worsened by aggressive chest percussion that leads to excessive pleural pressure and also by the administration of beta adrenergic medications (bronchodilators), which decrease smooth muscle tone, leading to increased floppiness of the airway wall and increased collapsibility of the airway [9].

Infants and children have high chest wall compliance because they have less musculature and less stiffness of the bony ribcage [10], and their lungs have greater elasticity and lower compliance compared to adults [11]. Thus, functional residual capacity equilibrates at a lower volume, relative to the total lung capacity, than in older patients, which increases the tendency to airway closure [3].

According to Poiseuille's law, resistance to flow through a cylinder is inversely proportional to the fourth power of the radius of that cylinder. Thus, even at baseline the airway resistance is disproportionately high in children compared to adults [12], and to further compound the problem, small compromises in airway diameter due to edema or airway secretions lead to an even greater disproportionate increase in airway resistance and decrease in airflow. Furthermore, in contrast to the case in adults and older children, the nose causes important additional resistance to airflow [12], and nasal congestion can significantly increase the work of breathing. Thus, the nose and upper airway cannot be neglected from discussions of airway clearance therapies in infancy.

Collateral ventilation channels (the interalveolar pores of Kohn and bronchiolar-alveolar channels of Lambert) can contribute to the aeration of alveoli distal to obstructed airways in older children and adults. However, this compensatory mechanism is missing in infants, in whom collateral ventilation channels are not well developed.

29.2 Pharmacology

Pharmacologic approaches to airway clearance have high-level evidence of benefit. Dornase alfa (recombinant human deoxyribonuclease) reduces the viscosity and tenacity of cystic fibrosis (CF) sputum by enzymatically cleaving extracellular deoxyribonucleic acid released from necrotic neutrophils. Dornase alfa reduces the frequency of pulmonary exacerbations and improves pulmonary function in CF patients. It is safe and effective across the severity spectrum from mild to severe lung disease and seems to reduce airway inflammation. It has not, however, been shown to be effective in any non-CF conditions [13].

Hypertonic saline, which appears to work primarily by increasing airway surface liquid, also improves forced expiratory volume in the first second (FEV1) and decreases the number of pulmonary exacerbations [14]. Hypertonic saline is thought to improve mucociliary clearance by changing the osmotic gradient in the airways, increasing the movement of water from the cells to the airway, increasing the airway surface fluid layer, and providing hydration to thick and viscous secretions [15]. Several other drugs, such as mannitol, denufosol, and nebulized N-acetylcysteine, which were frequently used in the past, have important toxicity and no clinical evidence of efficacy.

Sympathomimetics have been shown that they improve mucociliary clearance in several species, several diseases, and with several formulations. Increased mucociliary clearance may require greater doses than those used for bronchodilatation.

Overall, the clinical importance of sympathomimetic on airway clearance is unclear. Moreover, sympathomimetic may also be counterproductive in some conditions, such as tracheomalacia. The effects of anticholinergics on mucociliary clearance has also been studied in several species, several diseases, and with several formulations. Commonly used inhaled anticholinergics do not retard mucus clearance in a clinically important manner.

There are four groups of medicine: expectorants (which increase volume and/or hydration of secretions and may induce cough), mucolytics (which reduce viscosity of mucus), mucokinetics (which increase kinesis of mucus by cough), and mucoregulators (which reduce the process of chronic mucus hypersecretion).

A thin mucus layer, increased elasticity, and decreased viscosity favor mucociliary clearance. A thick mucus layer, lower elasticity, and higher viscosity induce cough. A Cochrane review suggests that mucolytics may be of benefit in COPD [16]. However, it is unclear whether the mechanism was indeed airway clearance or some other effect, such as antioxidant effects. Although affecting mucus would seem a reasonable goal, the usefulness of mucolytics is essentially unproven. This continues to be an area of active scientific inquiry, and new agents are being explored.

29.3 Techniques

Conventional chest physiotherapy technique (CPT) is the traditional technique used to enhance airway clearance. CPT is any combination of postural drainage, percussion, chest shaking, huffing, and directed coughing; it does not include the use of exercise, forced expiration technique, positive expiratory pressure (PEP), or other mechanical devices.

Also forced expiration technique, directed cough, and autogenic drainage are the other techniques. This includes techniques such as directed cough, breathing maneuvers, and positive airway pressure. High-frequency oscillation of the airway and chest wall more directly support normal mucus transport mechanisms than postural drainage. This is supported by the observations that gravity is not a major mechanism for airway clearance in health, and the viscosity of normal mucus resists flow into gravity-dependent terminal bronchioles. The definitions for directed cough, active cycle of breathing, and autogenic drainage were appropriately clarified, as these are often confused in clinical usage. A meta-analysis showed that, although standard CPT resulted in a significantly greater sputum expectoration than no treatment, there were no differences between conventional CPT, PEP, forced expiration technique, and autogenic drainage [17].

PEP was first developed as an airway clearance technique in Denmark in the 1970s. PEP devices can be categorized as low-pressure devices (5–20 cmH$_2$O at mid-exhalation) and high-pressure devices (26–102 cmH$_2$O via forced expiratory maneuvers after maximal inspiration). Oscillatory PEP was first developed in Switzerland as the Flutter device, but there are now similar devices from other manufacturers, such as Acapella and Quake. Proposed mechanisms of action of these devices include a decrease in the viscoelastic properties of mucus and the creation of short bursts of increased expiratory flow acceleration that assist mucus clearance. In a Cochrane review [17], it was reported that, in patients with CF, there is no advantage of conventional CPT over other airway clearance techniques in terms of respiratory function. Moreover, there was a trend reported for participants to prefer self-administered airway clearance techniques. In relation to PEP for airway clearance in people with CF, another Cochrane review [6] reported no clear evidence that PEP was a more or less effective intervention overall than other forms of CPT. There was limited evidence that PEP was preferred by participants, compared to other techniques.

Airway clearance is an essential part of the care of patients receiving mechanical ventilation. Airway humidification in intubated patients is crucial, and inadequate humidity can partially or completely occlude the artificial airway with dried secretions. Generally, heated humidity is superior to passive humidity, such as that from a heat-and-moisture exchanger. Recent innovations intended to decrease mucus adherence to the inside of the endotracheal tube include the Mucus Slurper, Mucus Shaver, and silver-impregnated endotracheal tubes. However, the utility of these devices in usual practice is yet to be determined. Suctioning should be done as needed, not routinely, with caution for complications. Evidence does not support manual hyperinflation as an airway clearance technique or the use of saline instillation. From the perspective of secretion removal, open suctioning may be superior to closed suctioning, because disconnection stimulates a cough, and it prevents the inspired gas flow from moving secretions away from the distal suction catheter. Continuous lateral rotation and kinetic therapy may improve resolution of atelectasis, but studies on secretion removal are scant. If percussion and postural drainage are used in the mechanically ventilated patient, care must be taken to avoid adverse effects.

Although somewhat controversial, it is generally accepted that gastroesophageal reflux can be problematic in children with airway disease. Chest physical therapy (CPT) performed in a head-down position for postural drainage aggravates reflux [18], whereas CPT without a head-down tilt does not, so the latter approach should be used in infants and children, the majority of whom have a tendency to reflux [16].

Chest physical therapy entails the application of substantial and potentially traumatic forces, and the newborn infant, particularly the premature infant, does not always have adequate musculoskeletal support to resist injury. Thus, there have been reports of substantial neurologic injury [19] and rib fractures [20] following CPT in the neonatal intensive care unit (ICU).

An important consideration is the lack of interaction and cooperation from the child, which can be problematic in the context of airway clearance therapy. It was concluded that airway clearance techniques appear to be of [21] proven benefit in routine care of CF (specific technique is probably less important than adherence) [22]; likely benefit in routine care of neuromuscular disease, cerebral palsy, and the ventilated child with atelectasis [17] possible benefit in routine care of the neonate immediately post-extubation; and [17] minimal benefit in routine care of acute asthma (without atelectasis), bronchiolitis, the intubated infant with respiratory distress syndrome, the intubated child with respiratory failure, and the postoperative child.

A number of approaches to airway clearance in the patient with neuromuscular disease have been described. These include respiratory muscle training, manually assisted cough (quad-cough), mechanical cough assist, high-frequency chest wall compression/oscillation, and intrapulmonary percussive ventilation. Each of these may be helpful and appear not to be harmful in the patient with neuromuscular disease, but this is not based on strong evidence.

Respiratory disease is an important cause of morbidity in the newborn and particularly in premature infants. The most important respiratory conditions cared for in the neonatal ICU are [7] hyaline membrane disease, caused primarily by surfactant deficiency, which leads to alveolar collapse and decreased airway compliance [4]; bronchopulmonary dysplasia, which is the iatrogenic sequela of hyaline membrane disease, in which inflammation and airway obstruction may supervene, and which is often complicated by asthma, tracheobronchomalacia, and gastroesophageal reflux/aspiration; and [4] less commonly, congenital anomalies of the lung.

Routine use of CPT for intubated neonates with hyaline membrane disease has been evaluated in several clinical trials. Older studies (from 1978) suggested benefit in regard to secretion clearance and arterial oxygenation [23], but others failed to show that and emphasized the risks of hypoxia, rib fractures, and neurologic damage [24, 25].

Another potential application of CPT in the neonatal ICU is in the newly extubated neonate, to prevent atelectasis and other morbidity. A Cochrane collaboration analysis evaluated four published clinical trials and found no clear benefit from peri-extubation CPT. There was no effect on the rate of post-extubation atelectasis, but there was a reduction in the rate of re-intubation. The latter conclusion was driven by the findings of the oldest studies (published in 1978 and 1989), which suggests that newer approaches to neonatal care might eliminate the benefit of CPT [26].

Most of the important airway diseases of childhood are associated with mucus hypersecretion; the classic example is CF. Airway collapse and obstruction are more likely in young children. Compared to adults, children have decreased stiffness of airway walls, decreased functional residual capacity and relative lung volumes, decreased airway diameter, and decreased alveolar collateral channels. Self- and assisted airway cleaning techniques are important to prevent worsening of children's respiratory diseases.

References

1. Hess DR. The evidence for secretion clearance techniques. Respir Care. 2001;46(11):1276–93.
2. Hess DR. Airway clearance: physiology, pharmacology, techniques, and practice. Respir Care. 2007;52(10):1392–6.
3. Schechter MS. Airway clearance applications in infants and children. Respir Care. 2007;52(10):1382–90; discussion 90-1.
4. Jeffrey PK. The development of large and small airways. Am J Respir Crit Care Med. 1998;157(5):174–80.
5. Rogers DF. Pulmonary mucus: pediatric perspective. Pediatr Pulmonol. 2003;36(3):178–88.
6. Rogers DF. Physiology of airway mucus secretion and pathophysiology of hypersecretion. Respir Care. 2007;52(9):1134–46; discussion 46-9.
7. Oberwaldner B. Physiotherapy for airway clearance in paediatrics. Eur Respir J. 2000;15(1):196–204.
8. Shaffer TH, Bhutani VK, Wolfson MR, Penn RB, Tran NN. In vivo mechanical properties of the developing airway. Pediatr Res. 1989;25(2):143–6.
9. Panitch HB, Keklikian EN, Motley RA, Wolfson MR, Schidlow DV. Effect of altering smooth muscle tone on maximal expiratory flows in patients with tracheomalacia. Pediatr Pulmonol. 1990;9(3):170–6.

10. Papastamelos C, Panitch HB, England SE, Allen JL. Developmental changes in chest wall compliance in infancy and early childhood. J Appl Physiol. 1995;78(1):179–84.
11. Lai-Fook SJ, Hyatt RE. Effects of age on elastic moduli of human lungs. J Appl Physiol. 2000;89(1):163–8.
12. von der Hardt H, Leben M. Bodyplethysmography in healthy children. Measurement of intra-thoracic gas volume and airway resistance. Eur J Pediatr. 1976;124(1):13–21.
13. Henke MO, Ratjen F. Mucolytics in cystic fibrosis. Paediatr Respir Rev. 2007;8(1):24–9.
14. Bye PT, Elkins MR. Other mucoactive agents for cystic fibrosis. Paediatr Respir Rev. 2007;8(1):30–9.
15. Amin R, Ratjen F. Emerging drugs for cystic fibrosis. Expert Opin Emerg Drugs. 2014;19(1):143–55.
16. Button BM, Heine RG, Catto-Smith AG, Phelan PD, Olinsky A. Chest physiotherapy, gastro-oesophageal reflux, and arousal in infants with cystic fibrosis. Arch Dis Child. 2004;89(5):435–9.
17. Main E, Prasad A, Schans C. Conventional chest physiotherapy compared to other airway clearance techniques for cystic fibrosis. Cochrane Database Syst Rev. 2005;1:Cd002011.
18. Button BM, Heine RG, Catto-Smith AG, Phelan PD. Postural drainage in cystic fibrosis: is there a link with gastro-oesophageal reflux? J Paediatr Child Health. 1998;34(4):330–4.
19. Harding JE, Miles FK, Becroft DM, Allen BC, Knight DB. Chest physiotherapy may be associated with brain damage in extremely premature infants. J Pediatr. 1998;132(3 Pt 1):440–4.
20. Chalumeau M, Foix-L'Helias L, Scheinmann P, Zuani P, Gendrel D, Ducou-le-Pointe H. Rib fractures after chest physiotherapy for bronchiolitis or pneumonia in infants. Pediatr Radiol. 2002;32(9):644–7.
21. Poole PJ, Black PN. Mucolytic agents for chronic bronchitis or chronic obstructive pulmonary disease. Cochrane Database Syst Rev. 2003;2:Cd001287.
22. van der Schans C, Prasad A, Main E. Chest physiotherapy compared to no chest physiotherapy for cystic fibrosis. Cochrane Database Syst Rev. 2000;2:Cd001401.
23. Finer NN, Boyd J. Chest physiotherapy in the neonate: a controlled study. Pediatrics. 1978;61(2):282–5.
24. Raval D, Yeh TF, Mora A, Cuevas D, Pyati S, Pildes RS. Chest physiotherapy in preterm infants with RDS in the first 24 hours of life. J Perinatol. 1987;7(4):301–4.
25. Fox WW, Schwartz JG, Shaffer TH. Pulmonary physiotherapy in neonates: physiologic changes and respiratory management. J Pediatr. 1978;92(6):977–81.
26. Flenady VJ, Gray PH. Chest physiotherapy for preventing morbidity in babies being extubated from mechanical ventilation. Cochrane Database Syst Rev. 2002;2:Cd000283.

Part IX

Technology and Methodology Airway Clearance Techniques, Cough Assisted and Oscillation

Non-assisted Airway Clearance Techniques

Rosana Mara da Silva and Thales Cantelle Baggio

30.1 Introduction

Airway clearance techniques (ACTs) refer to a variety of different strategies used to clear excess secretions. Its goal is to reduce airway obstruction caused by secretions that occupy the airway lumen and thus prevent respiratory tract infections, re-expanding collapsed areas of the lung, improving gas exchange, and decreasing the inflammatory response [1–3].

Physiotherapy maneuvers related to the respiratory system consist of manual, postural, and kinetic techniques of the thoracoabdominal components, which can be applied alone or in association with other techniques, which generally have the following objectives: to mobilize and eliminate pulmonary secretions, improve lung ventilation, promote lung re-expansion, improve oxygenation and gas exchange, decrease respiratory effort and oxygen consumption, prevent complications, and accelerate patient recovery [4].

Among the main alternatives are bronchial hygiene maneuvers, postural drainage, percussion, vibration and manual hyperinflation, vibrocompression, acceleration of expiratory flow (AEF), passive manual expiratory therapy (PMET), instrumental therapy (Flutter®, Acapella®), PEP mask, assisted cough, tracheobronchial aspiration, and ZEEP (zero end-expiratory pressure) [2, 3].

R. M. da Silva (✉)
Municipal Health Department, Jaraguá do Sul, SC, Brazil

T. C. Baggio
Intensive Care Physician, Hospital Jaraguá and Hospital São José, Jaraguá do Sul, SC, Brazil

© The Author(s), under exclusive license to Springer Nature Switzerland AG 2023
A. M. Esquinas (ed.), *Humidification in the Intensive Care Unit*,
https://doi.org/10.1007/978-3-031-23953-3_30

30.2 Non-assisted Airway Clearance Techniques

The treatment of bronchial obstruction through unassisted techniques, that is, techniques that involve the active participation of the patient, can allow some independence in its performance. The maneuvers that the patient performs voluntarily are defined as active secretion removal techniques. Therefore, they encompass the techniques that involve voluntary alteration of the respiratory flow with the objective of displacing and eliminating secretions [2, 3].

30.2.1 Manual-Assisted Techniques

These are techniques that involve applying certain forces to the patient's chest using the hands. Vibration is one of the most used techniques, which consists of the application, during the entire expiratory phase, of fine oscillatory movements combined with a compression of the chest wall. The force that the therapist uses must be sufficient to compress the rib cage and increase the expiratory flow, but, at the same time, it must not generate discomfort for the patient [2, 5]. Main et al. described the association of the technique with postural drainage as clearing strategies, together with forced expiration techniques [2, 6, 7].

30.2.2 Active Breathing Cycle

The technique consists of three distinct respiratory cycles performed in sequence: breath control, chest expansion exercises, and forced exhalation technique (FET) [2, 8].

The technique is based on three to four respiratory acts characterized by a slow and deep inspiration (volumes greater than the tidal volume) through the nose, followed by a passive expiration [2]. This deep inspiration should facilitate collateral ventilation and then airflow through Martin's intrabronchial canals, Lambert's bronchoalveolar canals, and Kohn's interalveolar pores [8, 9]. At the end, the patient must perform the FET, which consists of a combination of one or two forced expirations (called "Huff") and a tidal volume respiratory act. The main benefit is the alveolar expansion, which makes the airway homogeneous, and through aeration of the distal air spaces, it can promote the removal of mucous plugs from the peripheral airway [8].

30.2.3 PEP Mask

PEP mask therapy is an expansive technique based on increasing ventilation through collateral ventilation pathways, expanding the alveoli compromised by atelectasis, and leading to an increase in functional residual capacity (FRC) [8].

Fig. 30.1 PEP mask.
Source: Rand et al. [11]

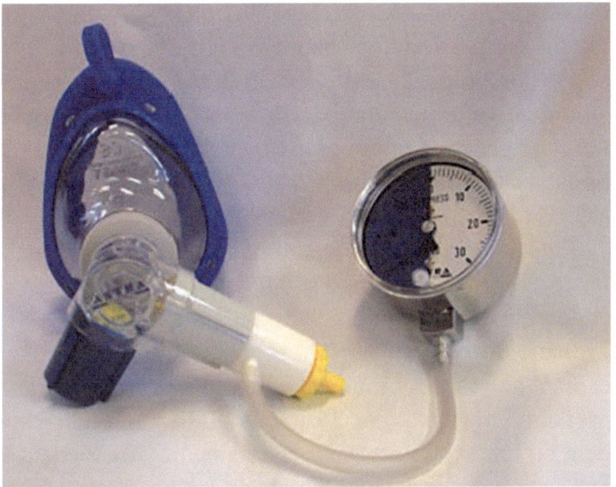

The technique consists of exhaling against an airflow or threshold resistance to produce positive airway pressure throughout the expiratory phase. The most commonly used PEP therapy in clinical practice is low pressure (also called "low PEP"). It consists of maintaining a relatively low expiratory pressure in the mouth, between 5 and 20 cmH$_2$O [2, 8]. Inspiration is required for a volume of air slightly greater than tidal volume, with a pause at the end of inspiration (to allow the physiological flow mechanisms, interdependence, and collateral ventilation) and then a slightly active expiration against resistance [2].

PEP can be associated with high-frequency airflow oscillations, called oscillatory PEP (OPEP). Among the devices used in OPEP are the Flutter®, Acapella®, RC-Cornet®, Lung Flute®, and the PEP Bottle® [2]. All of these devices are characterized by intermittent breathing against expiratory resistance to induce oscillations of variable frequency (depending on the device or use), which are transmitted to the respiratory tract during the expiratory cycle [2, 8, 10] (Fig. 30.1).

30.2.4 Instrumental Therapy: Acapella® and Flutter®

It consists in a device that produces vibrating positive expiratory pressure (PEP) therapy through a plug used as a counterweight. The oscillation produced by this device is transmitted to the airway wall to release and mobilize secretions, allowing expectoration [11]. It is indicated for the treatment of chronic obstructive pulmonary disease and lung diseases that progress with hypersecretion, also useful in the prevention and reversal of atelectasis [12, 13].

There are several types of OOAF devices, including Flutter®, Shaker®, and Acapella®. All devices are based on the same principle: to promote intrathoracic oscillations that reduce the viscoelasticity of the mucus, facilitating lung clearance, associated with an expiratory resistance that increases the positive pressure within the airway. Thus, collateral ventilation is stimulated, making the airway patent during the entire expiratory phase [13, 14].

For the proper functioning of OOAF devices, it must be taken into account the amplitude of the oscillation (difference between the values of the highest and lowest pressure generated through Acapella®), frequency of oscillation (number of oscillations per second), and positive expiratory pressure (PEP $\geq$ 10 cmH$_2$O) generated [13, 15].

Flutter® is a portable instrument that combines stabilization of the airways and favoring bronchial hygiene, generates positive expiratory pressure, and causes endobronchial vibrations during expiration through the device, mobilizing mucus. Pressure fluctuations prevent bronchial collapse facilitating expectoration [8, 16]. It is recommended for the treatment of patients with bronchial hypersecretion [8]. The pressure, vibration, and PEP exerted through the Flutter® and Shaker® are dependent on the expiratory flow maintained by the patient and the balance between the angulation of the devices attached to the patient and the force of gravity incident on the device, which promotes interruptions in the passage of air through the movement of a sphere of steel inside these devices that reverberate with the thoracic vibration [8, 13, 17].

30.3 Conclusion

Bronchial hygiene maneuvers are resources widely used by physical therapists in the context of intensive care, with the aim of assisting in mucociliary clearance and preventing complications resulting from the accumulation of secretions in the airways.

The role of physiotherapy is extensive, and it is part of the multidisciplinary care offered to patients, being considered an efficient therapeutic resource in the treatment of patients undergoing mechanical ventilation, with the objective of promoting the removal of retained pulmonary secretions, reducing intrapulmonary shunt, and recruiting areas collapsed, in addition to improving the compliance of the respiratory system.

References

1. Fahy JV, Dickey BF. Função e disfunção do muco das vias aéreas. Nova Engl J Med. 2010;363:2233–47. https://doi.org/10.1056/NEJMra0910061.
2. Belli S, Prince I, Savio G, et al. Técnicas de desobstrução das vias aéreas: a escolha certa para o paciente certo. Front Med. 2021;8:544826. https://doi.org/10.3389/fmed.2021.544826.
3. Nici L, Donner C, Wouters E, Zuwallack R, Ambrosino N, Bourbeau J, et al. Declaração da American Thoracic Society/European Respiratory Society sobre reabilitação pulmonar. AMJ Respir Crit Care Med. 2006;173:1390–413. https://doi.org/10.1164/rccm.200508-1211ST.
4. Costa D. Fisioterapia respiratória básica. Atheneu: Editora; 1999. p. 127.
5. McCarren B, Alison JA, Herbert RD. Vibração e seu efeito no sistema respiratório. Aust J Physiother. 2006;52:39–43. https://doi.org/10.1016/S0004-9514(06)70060-5.

6. Main E, Prasad A, Schans C. Fisioterapia torácica convencional comparada a outras técnicas de desobstrução das vias aéreas para fibrose cística. Cochrane Database Syst Rev. 2005;1:CD002011. https://doi.org/10.1002/14651858.CD002011.pub2.
7. Gallon A. Avaliação da percussão torácica no tratamento de pacientes com produção copiosa de escarro. Respir Med. 1991;85:45–51. https://doi.org/10.1016/S0954-6111(06)80209-X.
8. Sarmento GJV. O ABC da fisioterpia respiratória. 2nd ed. Manole: Editora; 2015. p. 537.
9. Menkes HA, Traystman RJ. Ventilação colateral. Am Rev Respir Dis. 1977;116:287–309.
10. App EM, Kieselmann R, Reinhardt D, Lindemann H, Dasgupta B, King M, et al. Alterações na reologia do escarro na doença pulmonar da fibrose cística após dois tipos diferentes de fisioterapia: flutter vs drenagem autogênica. Peito. 1998;114:171–7. https://doi.org/10.1378/peito.114.1.171.
11. Rand S, Aurora P, Main E. PEP therapy in secretion management. Clin Nurs Patient Care. 2015. Available from https://hospitalhealthcare.com/hhe.
12. Mueller G, Bersch-Porada I, Koch-Border S, Raab AM, Jonker M, Baumberger RM, Michel F. Laboratory evaluation of four different devices for secretion mobilization: Acapella choice, green and blue versus water bottle. Respir Care. 2014;59(5):673–7.
13. Couto AS. Efeito Etgol e Acapella sobre aeração e ventilação pulmonar avaliada através da tomografia por impedância elétrica em indivíduos com fibrose cística. Dissertação. Universidade Federal Pernambuco. Recife, 2016, p. 171.
14. Morrison L, Agnew J. Oscillating devices for airway clearance in people with cystic fibrosis. Cochrane Database Syst Rev. 2014;7:CD006842.
15. Dos Santos AP, Guimaraes RC, De Carvalho EM, Gastaldi AC. Mechanical behaviors of Flutter VRP1, Shaker, and Acapella devices. Respir Care. 2013;58(2):298–304.
16. Antunes LCO, et al. Comparação da eficácia da fisioterapia respiratória convencional com o Flutter® VRP1 em pacientes com bronquiectasia. Salusvita. 2001;20(1):11–21.
17. Volsko TA, Difiore J, Chatburn RL. Performance comparison of two oscillating positive expiratory pressure devices: Acapella versus Flutter. Respir Care. 2003;48(2):124–30.

Airway Clearance: Cough-Assisted Devices

31

Hugo Miranda, Sofia Miranda, Inês Machado Vaz, and Nélson Barros

31.1 Introduction

Muscle weakness is a frequent problem in intensive care units (ICU) [1] and can be due to primary neuromuscular disorders, like *myasthenia gravis* or amyotrophic lateral sclerosis (<0.5% of all ICU admissions). However, much more frequently that weakness develops as physical sequelae while patients are being treated for other conditions. In fact, admissions to the ICU, due to the severity of the motive of admission, co-morbidities, and associated technical and pharmacological interventions, can result in significant physical, cognitive, and behavioral sequelae [1–3], collectively named post-intensive care syndrome (PICS).

One of the main physical sequelae is intensive care unit-acquired weakness (ICUAW) [4]. It is characterized by a flaccid tetraparesis with respiratory muscle involvement, as well as prolonged deconditioning and functional incapacity.

Data from health institutions worldwide [2] indicates incidences varying between 25 and 31%, which correspond roughly to 3.25–6.1 million new cases per year. Several risk factors have been already identified, such as multiple-organ failure, previous co-morbidities, and the usage of drugs like corticosteroids. Although its pathophysiology isn't already completely understood, it seems to be multifactorial and can be related to such mechanisms as muscle atrophy or autophagy deregulation.

H. Miranda (✉) · N. Barros
Serviço de Medicina Intensiva do Centro Hospitalar de Trás-os-Montes e Alto Douro, Vila Real, Portugal
e-mail: hmiranda@campus.ul.pt

S. Miranda
Serviço de Medicina Interna do Hospital do Divino Espírito Santo, Azores, Portugal

I. M. Vaz
Serviço de Medicina Física e Reabilitação do Centro Hospitalar de Trás-os-Montes e Alto Douro, Vila Real, Portugal

A. M. Esquinas (ed.), *Humidification in the Intensive Care Unit*,
https://doi.org/10.1007/978-3-031-23953-3_31

287"

Even though multiple clinical, imaging, electromyographic, and histological criteria are used to its diagnosis, there isn't a gold standard yet. The main manifestations include flaccid tetraparesis and neuromuscular respiratory failure, the latter often presenting as inability to wean off mechanical ventilation [4]. More recently, the existence of various presentation patterns that may coexist was suggested and includes polyneuropathy, myopathy, sarcopenia, and diaphragmatic dysfunction. These manifestations can develop quickly, even in few days after admission to the ICU.

Considering its high incidence and great morbimortality, several interventions have been suggested to prevent its development and its complications. The compromise of the cough reflex ranks amongst its most frequent complications.

31.2 The Importance of the Cough Reflex in the Critically Ill Patient

Cough represents a physiological defense mechanism responsible for aiding the mobilization and, most importantly, the expulsion of secretions to the proximal airways. This mechanism has two crucial purposes: keeping the airways free from foreign bodies and, in the case of pathological conditions such as respiratory infections, eliminating the excess secretions.

In order to have an effective cough reflex, a certain sequence of physiological events that allow an adequate secretion mobilization is necessary. Succinctly, the patient should inspire profoundly (until 85–90% of the total lung capacity) firstly, with a following brief closure of the glottis, that will contribute to increase transitorily the intra-thoracic pressure. After that, the glottis opening along with the abdominal contraction will generate a expulsive force, with flows typically greater than 360 L/min, that allows the mobilization of secretions to the proximal airways with its subsequent elimination [5].

However, multiple mechanisms condition cough efficacy in the ICU. Amongst the most frequently affected mechanisms, we can find:

1. Inspiratory phase compromise (e.g., restrictive syndromes resulting from inspiratory muscle weakness)
2. Glottic competence compromise and effective apnea (e.g., artificial airway)
3. Expiratory phase compromise (e.g., generalized muscle weakness with abdominal involvement)

In the absence of this protective mechanism, the patients are more vulnerable to secretion retention, alveolar ventilation changes, atelectasis, and recurrent respiratory infections, which contribute to a progressive increase of the respiratory morbidity [6, 7]. In fact, the inefficacy of the cough reflex can become so relevant that an inability to wean off mechanical ventilation can occur, leading to longer hospital stays and all their consequences [8].

Therefore, when a patient can't produce an effective cough, it becomes necessary to employ techniques that reinforce or substitute altogether that mechanism. In respiratory physiotherapy, the airway clearance techniques can be divided in two groups: *peripheral* (stimulates the secretion mobilization from the peripheral to the central airways) and *central techniques* [6] (increases the secretion elimination in the central airways through cough potentiation).

In this chapter, the authors will only explore the proximal techniques, focusing mainly on those that imply the use of mechanical devices.

31.3 Proximal Techniques

The proximal techniques have the cough potentiation through inspiration or expiration assistance or both as a primary objective. Such techniques, frequently designated as "cough augmentation," rely on cough support or simulation as a means to increase the flow at the peak and thus facilitate the elimination of the secretions from the larger airways. Figure 31.1 shows summarily the different forms of proximal techniques at our disposal at the moment.

31.3.1 Expiratory Assistance

The objective of the expiratory assistance is to help the expiratory muscles create sufficient intra-thoracic and intra-abdominal pressures in order to generate an expiratory flow, promoting the mobilization of the secretions as consequence. The

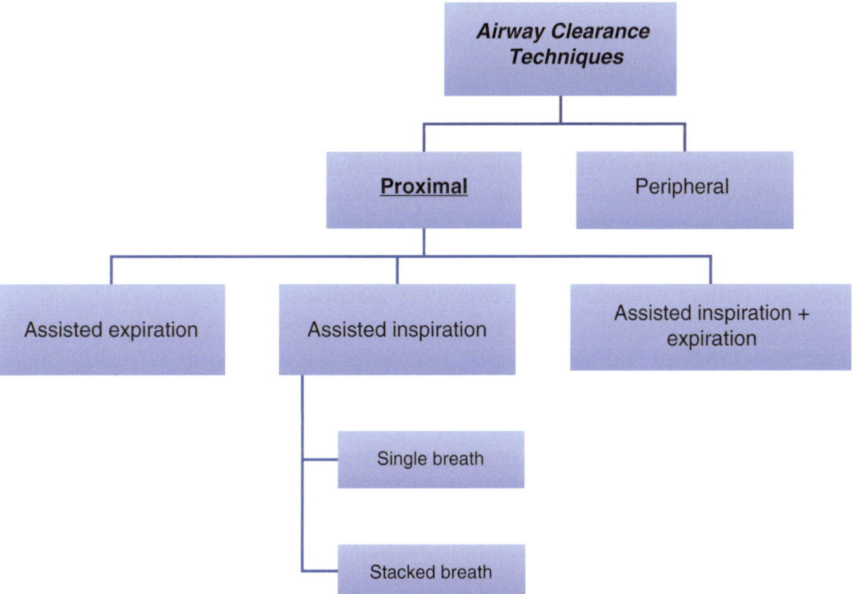

Fig. 31.1 Proximal airway clearance techniques

expiratory assistance can be divided in two types: *manual* (based on the use of external mechanical forces or compressions applied to the thoraco-abdominal region during the expiration) and through the *usage of a mechanical device* [6, 7, 9] (e.g., mechanical insufflator-exsufflator).

31.3.1.1 Mechanical Devices

The mechanical insufflator-exsufflator belongs to this group of devices and allows the generation of an isolated negative pressure (exsufflation) that is only applied during the expiration. Such pressure is applied through a full face mask or through a mouthpiece connected to an artificial airway.

Studies [5, 6, 9] indicate that this technique improves the flow during the cough peak, helping the patient eliminate the secretions. In spite of its usefulness, this technique has an inferior efficacy when compared to the combined assistance.

31.3.2 Inspiratory Assistance

The main goal of this technique is to increase the inspiratory lung volumes as a form of potentiate the cough effect. In fact, the recruiting of the inspiratory volumes generates an expiratory flow bias. This phenomenon can be explained by the optimization of the width-tension relation of the expiratory muscles [9], as the inhalation of a bigger air volume before the compressive and expiratory phases of the cough promote the development of a greater intra-thoracic pressure and subsequent flow during the cough peak (a higher expiratory than inspiratory flow is registered).

The inspiratory assistances can be divided in two groups: *single breath* (e.g., inspiration, expiration, inspiration, expiration) and *stacked breath* [6, 9] (e.g., inspiration, inspiration, inspiration, expiration).

31.3.2.1 Single Breath

Single breath consists of a technique where the vital inspiratory capacity is increased through the utilization of various devices (e.g., bag-valve-mask, volumetric ventilators, mechanical insufflator-exsufflator, or intermittent positive pressure devices). The patient is therefore forced to do a prolonged inspiration and then is instructed to cough (with or without manual expiratory assisted cough).

An increased inspiratory flow is thus generated that, along with the expiratory muscle recruitment and static recoil, potentiates the creation of a frankly higher expiratory volume than would be expected from a non-assisted cough.

31.3.2.2 Stacked Breath

Stacked breath consists of a technique where the patient is subjected to multiple inspirations, with no expiration between them, until achieving the maximal insufflation capacity. Only then is the patient instructed to cough (with or without manual expiratory assisted cough).

Such a technique is only possible through the utilization of several devices, like volumetric ventilators or a bag-valve-mask. However, the fact the glottis has a crucial role in this type of technique precludes its application on specific situations, where the single breath should be preferred [6].

31.3.3 Combined Assistance: Inspiratory + Expiratory

The combined cough assistance stimulates the cough mechanisms through the delivery of a positive pressure (insufflation) and through the creation of a negative pressure (exsufflation). The sequential application of these two types of pressure, only separated by very brief pauses, potentiates the mobilization and expulsion of the secretions on an extremely effective manner. Besides that, the fact that this technique can be used in patients with spontaneous ventilation, intubated or tracheostomized resorting to specific interfaces, has fostered its increasing utilization in the ICU.

This type of assistance can be divided in two groups: *inspiratory assistance combined with manual expiratory cough assistance* (more time and resource consuming and less efficacious) and *mechanical insufflation-exsufflation devices* (MIED).

The authors opted to focus on the MIED due to its generalized utilization, simpler user interface, and proven effectiveness in patients admitted to the ICU. Its main indications, contraindications, complications, and programming set-ups will be addressed on the following pages.

31.3.3.1 Mechanical Insufflation-Exsufflation Devices

Its utilization implies the creation of a rapid change of positive to negative pressures, as to simulate the airflow alterations that occur during the spontaneous cough reflex. From a conceptual point of view, this kind of devices compensates not only the inspiratory weakness but also the expiratory capacity of the patients, generating a transthoracic pressure gradient capable of facilitating the secretions mobilization.

Indications, Contraindications, and Complications

According to the literature [5–7], the main physiological indications for its utilization are:

- Inability to generate flow peaks greater than 160–200 L/min
- Vital capacity <50% than expected or <1500 mL

As such, it becomes evident that the main clinical indication is the absence of an effective cough reflex. That becomes even more noticeable in the presence of certain pathologies [9], such as:

- Neuromuscular disorders/polyneuropathy
- Chest wall disorders
- Diaphragmatic dysfunction
- Thoracic or abdominal trauma or peri-operatory
- Bronchopulmonary diseases

However, not all patients benefit from its utilization. Therefore, it's important to be able to recognize which patients have formal contraindications [6, 7, 9]:

- Recent barotrauma
- Non-drained pneumothorax
- Bullous emphysema
- Lung abscess
- Recent upper gastrointestinal surgery
- Increased intracranial pressure
- COPD or severe asthma
- Recent lobectomy
- Vomit
- Abundant hemoptysis

Even though it's not a formal contraindication, the need of oxygen supplementation or the presence of cardiovascular instability or bronchospasm implies an additional precaution when using this kind of devices.

At last, knowing the potential complications associated with these devices is also very important. They can be divided in the following manner [9]:

- *Respiratory system*: pneumothorax, pneumomediastinum, hemoptysis (mucosal lesion in the presence of adherent secretions), and/or small airway collapse
- *Cardiovascular system*: bradycardia and hypotension
- *Musculoskeletal system*: chest wall pain (more frequent when associated with manually assisted cough)
- *Gastrointestinal system*: nausea, vomit, and abdominal bloating

Of all those, the more frequently described in literature are hypotension and chest wall pain.

Necessary Material

The pressure gradient can be delivered through an artificial airway (orotracheal tube or tracheostomy cannula) or through a natural airway (using adequate interfaces). So the treatment is possible, and it's necessary to know what material is required to initiate it:

- An antibacterial filter
- A simple tube
- An adaptor to oxygen delivery, if necessary
- An adequate interface (oronasal mask or a mouthpiece)
- Mechanical insufflator-exsufflator

Technical Optimization

Before initiating the technique, the patient should ideally be positioned on Fowler's, so as to facilitate its execution. It should be executed 2 h after or 30 min before the meals. If aerosolized therapy is also needed, it should be given 30 min before the initiation of the cough-assisted maneuver [6].

Variables and Its Thresholds

The current MIED models can be used in one of two ways:

1. *Manual*: the operator is responsible for manually alternating between inspiration and expiration, which implies coordination with the patient's ventilation.
2. *Automatic*: the device is responsible for the automatic alternation between inspiration, expiration, and time pause.

On the other hand, it's also important to recognize which are the parameters to set up [5, 6, 9] on the device, as well as the values to define. On a succinct manner, these devices imply the adjustment of:

- *Pressure* (unit—cmH_2O)
  - Inhalatory: upper pressure threshold during insufflation
  - Exhalatory: upper pressure threshold during exsufflation
- *Time* (unit—seconds)
  - Inhalatory: necessary time interval to achieve the defined inhalatory pressure
  - Exhalatory: necessary time interval to achieve the defined exhalatory pressure
  - Time pause: transitional time interval since the achievement of the inhalatory positive pressure until the beginning of the application of the exhalatory negative pressure
- *Inspiratory flow* (unit—L/min), which can be set up in low, moderate, and high flow

Table 31.1 shows on a more schematic way the thresholds of the parameters to set up on the cough-assisted device.

Regarding the *inhalatory flow*, it can vary between *200* and *600* L/min, but higher flows are typically preferred in the presence of an artificial airway. The inspiratory flow should however be adjusted in agreement to the patient's individual needs/tolerance.

There are still two characteristics in these devices that are worthy to point out:

- *Cough-trak:* it consists of a trigger system where the sequence of the applied pressures is synchronized with the patient's inhalatory effort. This parameter's

Table 31.1 Defined limits for the variables of the insufflation-exsufflation mechanical devices

Variable	Possible thresholds	Increments
Inhalatory pressure	0–70 cmH_2O	From 1 on 1 cmH_2O
Exhalatory pressure	0–70 cmH_2O	From 1 on 1 cmH_2O
Inhalatory time	0–5 s	From 0.1 on 0.1 s
Exhalatory time	0–5 s	From 0.1 on 0.1 s
Pause time	0–5 s	From 0.1 on 0.1 s

goal is to increase the efficacy on the pressure delivery. However, in order for it to be used, the device has mandatorily to be on *automatic mode*.

- *Oscillation*: it can be applied during both the inspiratory and the expiratory phases. Its goal is to increase the secretion mobilization and its subsequent drainage. If this option is activated, the operator should set up the *frequency* (indicates the pulse distribution velocity) and the *amplitude* (indicates the pulse variation from the defined basal pressure). Typically, frequency should vary between 1 and 20 Hertz (Hz) and frequency between 1 and 10 cmH$_2$O. Contrarily to the cough-trak, this option *can be used with both the manual and the automatic modes.*

How to Program the Device and Apply the Treatment?
- This technique should be initiated at low inspiratory and expiratory pressures (±20 cmH$_2$O) with ±5 cmH$_2$O increments at each 2–3 cycles. *If a natural airway is being used, pressures of ±30–40 cmH$_2$O are generally enough. If an artificial airway is being used, high pressures (±50–70 cmH$_2$O) are generally necessary to* overcome the resistance created by the orotracheal tube/tracheostomy cannula.
- The automatic mode implies the definition of an *inspiratory time between 1 and 3 s*, an *expiratory time between 0.5 and 2 s*, and a *pause time between 0.5 and 2 s*. It is important to remember that time pause cannot be set up on the manual mode and in the presence of cough-trak, as it is programmed by the operator or the device, respectively.
- The operator should opt for a *low inspiratory flow* in the presence of *a natural airway*, but a *higher inspiratory flow* is preferred in the presence of an *artificial airway* [6].
- The oscillation should be started at *a high frequency (20 Hz) and low amplitude (1 cmH$_2$O)*, during the inspiratory phase. Tolerance should be constantly evaluated, and only after being ascertained should the operator consider the need to prolong it to the expiratory phase.
- In the adult patient, *four to six treatment sessions* should be ideally performed, with each session having *four to six cough cycles* (cough cycle = inspiratory time + time pause + expiratory time).
- A pause of 2–5 s can be taken between cough cycles, if the operator wishes to. Pauses of 30–60 s should be taken between sessions.
- *Each session should be concluded with an insufflation.* Such procedure will guarantee the maintenance of an appropriate residual functional capacity, especially in patients who exhibit more pronounced muscular weakness.

31.4 Outcomes

In spite of the current lack of robust scientific evidence, the literature supports the utilization of cough-assisted devices [7, 8, 10] as they seem to have a beneficial role in the ICU, reflected on shorter periods of mechanical ventilation, reduced number of reintubations, shorter ICU stays after extubation, and reduced infectious complications. All of this highlights the importance of this technique as an ICU routine and the need of trained personnel that enhances even further its benefits.

31.5 Main Obstacles

Two recent studies [11, 12], that focused on the realization of inquiries to healthcare professionals, tried to understand the problems faced concerning the adherence to these techniques. Both revealed that unfamiliarity with the equipment and the lack of robust scientific evidence and trained personnel were the main obstacles to their implementation.

A deeper analysis of these studies showed that reduced population samples, the lack of double-blind clinical trials, and the utilization of non-standardized interventions are some of the many factors that contribute to the current low level of evidence.

31.6 Conclusion

Cough-assisted techniques are safe and effective procedures, whose implementation is fairly simple on any ICU. Even though lacking at the moment, the existent scientific evidence demonstrates that its utilization can improve the ventilatory weaning protocols, as well as reduce the morbimortality in patients with a deficient cough reflex. This underlines the enormous importance of promoting more robust studies that allow the consolidation of the current evidence, helping foster its generalized use in the ICU in return.

Key Points
- Cough augmentation techniques are very useful in ICU, especially in patients with ICUAW and protracted ventilatory weaning.
- Healthcare professional training is crucial to its correct implementation in the ICU.
- The importance of the recognition of its indications and contraindications cannot be overstated.
- Inspiratory and expiratory pressures and times should be individualized for each patient.
- These techniques can also be utilized in patients with tracheostomies or with orotracheal tubes, even though it requires higher pressures as the smaller diameter of the cannula generates higher resistance.

References

1. Jolley SE, Bunnell AE, Hough CL. ICU-acquired weakness. Chest. 2016;150(5):1129–40. https://doi.org/10.1016/j.chest.2016.03.045.
2. Schefold JC, Wollersheim T, Grunow JJ, Luedi MM, Z'Graggen WJ, Weber-Carstens S. Muscular weakness and muscle wasting in the critically ill. J Cachexia Sarcopenia Muscle. 2020;11(6):1399–412. https://doi.org/10.1002/jcsm.12620.

 3. Vanhorebeek I, Latronico N, Van den Berghe G. ICU-acquired weakness. Intensive Care Med. 2020;46(4):637–53. https://doi.org/10.1007/s00134-020-05944-4.
 4. Wang W, Xu C, Ma X, Zhang X, Xie P. Intensive care unit-acquired weakness: a review of recent progress with a look toward the future. Front Med. 2020;7:1–9. https://doi.org/10.3389/fmed.2020.559789.
 5. Spinou A. A review on cough augmentation techniques: assisted inspiration, assisted expiration and their combination. Physiol Res. 2020;69:S93–S103. https://doi.org/10.33549/physiolres.934407.
 6. Chatwin M, Toussaint M, Gonçalves MR, et al. Airway clearance techniques in neuromuscular disorders: a state of the art review. Respir Med. 2018;136:98–110. https://doi.org/10.1016/j.rmed.2018.01.012.
 7. Morrow B, Argent A, Zampoli M, Human A, Corten L, Toussaint M. Cough augmentation techniques for people with chronic neuromuscular disorders. Cochrane Database Syst Rev. 2021;4(4):CD013170. https://doi.org/10.1002/14651858.CD013170.pub2.
 8. de Cássia Nunes L, Rizzetti DA, Neves D, et al. Mechanical insufflation/exsufflation improves respiratory mechanics in critical care: randomized crossover trial. Respir Physiol Neurobiol. 2019;266:115–20. https://doi.org/10.1016/j.resp.2019.05.008.
 9. Fernández-Carmona A, Olivencia-Peña L, Yuste-Ossorio ME, Peñas-Maldonado L. Ineffective cough and mechanical mucociliary clearance techniques. Med Intensiva. 2018;42(1):50–9. https://doi.org/10.1016/j.medin.2017.05.003.
 10. Swingwood E, Stilma W, Tume L, et al. The use of mechanical insufflation-exsufflation in invasively ventilated critically ill adults: a scoping review protocol. Syst Rev. 2020;9(1):1–5. https://doi.org/10.1186/s13643-020-01547-8.
 11. Swingwood E, Tume L, Cramp F. A survey examining the use of mechanical insufflation-exsufflation on adult intensive care units across the UK. J Intensive Care Soc. 2020;21(4):283–9. https://doi.org/10.1177/1751143719870121.
 12. Rose L, Adhikari NK, Poon J, Leasa D, McKim DA. Cough augmentation techniques in the critically ill: a Canadian national survey. Respir Care. 2016;61(10):1360–8. https://doi.org/10.4187/respcare.04775.

Salvatore Musella and Elena Sciarrillo

The management of bronchial secretions is one of the main problems encountered in a wide spectrum of medical conditions ranging from respiratory disorders (for example, COPD, cystic fibrosis, bronchiectasis), neuromuscular disorders, and patients undergoing either thoracic or abdominal surgery.

Mucus production and cough are important for airway defense and protection of the lower respiratory tract against inhaled irritations, but excessive mucus obstructs airways, and excessive cough has been associated with several complications.

A wide range of treatments, techniques, and devices are present in scientific literature for managing bronchial encumbrance in respiratory physiotherapy; there is insufficient evidence to affirm the superiority of one technique over another [1]; the choice must rather be made on the level of cooperation of the patient, on his physical condition, on the peak cough expiratory flow, on the degree of obstruction, and on the localization of mucus (proximal or peripheral).

For these reasons, over the past few years, in addition to manual airway clearance techniques, we have witnessed the development of assist mechanical devices.

The purpose of this chapter is to describe the devices that use high-frequency oscillations and how they favor the clearance of the airways in subjects with respiratory problems. High-frequency chest wall oscillation (HFCWO) and compression (HFCWC) is part of the high-frequency airway clearance-assisted techniques acting on lungs as indicated by an increased transrespiratory pressure associated with an increase of inspiratory flow or by a decreased transrespiratory pressure associated with an increase in expiratory flow. Differently, unassisted methods rely on passive exhalation energy to generate chest wall oscillations (for example, Flutter, Acapella) [2].

S. Musella (✉) · E. Sciarrillo
UOC Fisiopatologia E Riabilitazione Respiratoria – Monaldi Hospital, Naples, Italy

UO 1° Utsir Covid – Cotugno Hospital, Naples, Italy

Those allowing chest wall oscillation and compression are essentially rigid chest cuirasses, inflatable vests, and mechanical units connected to them that are external to the chest wall; these systems are used for lung disease treatment and prevention, in particular for those characterized by impaired mucus clearance and/or cough, where patients are at risk of acquiring acute bronchitis or pneumonia.

The chest cuirass system introduced in 1983 and described by Hayek for the very first time (Hayek external high-frequency oscillation—concept and practice, 1993) is achieved through a rigid chest cuirass connected to a compressor that can deliver either a positive or a negative pressure to produce high-frequency, small-volume oscillation in the airways. HFCWO uses a chest cuirass to generate biphasic changes in transrespiratory pressure. In any case (positive or negative pressure pulses or both), the general idea is to get air behind secretions and move them toward the larger airways, where they can be coughed up and expectorated.

The Hayek oscillator operates at a frequency ranging from 1 to 17 Hz. This device offers a control over inspiratory-expiratory ratio (1:6 to 6:1) and inspiratory pressure (from - 70 cmH_2O + 70 cmH_2O) [3].

HFCWC involves an inflatable vest wrapped around the chest. A high-output compressor rapidly inflates and deflates the vest through some hoses. During the inflation phase, a pressure is exerted on the body surface (in the range of about 5–20 cmH_2O), which forces the chest wall to compress and generates a short burst of expiratory flow. Pressure pulses are overlapped to a small positive pressure baseline (about 12 cmH_2O). On deflation, the chest wall recoils to its resting position, which causes an inspiratory flow. The HFCWC operates at 2–25 Hz and generates an esophageal pressure and airflow oscillations. HFCWC can generate volume changes from 17 to 57 mL and flows up to 1.6 L/s, which lead to "mini-coughs" to mobilize secretions. Sessions may last about 20–30 min and consist of short time intervals at different compression frequencies, separated by huff coughs [2, 4, 5].

Other airway clearance techniques require active patient participation. For example, autogenic drainage and active cycle of breathing technique both involve a combination of breathing exercises performed by the patient. Positive expiratory pressure therapy requires patients to exhale through a resistor to produce positive expiratory pressures during a prolonged period of exhalation. Instead, HFCWO and HFCWC are passive oscillatory devices designed to provide airway clearance without the active participation of the patient.

HFCWC causes flow oscillation, which is an effective way to clear mucus from the airways through different mechanisms [6]:

- It modifies the mucus viscoelasticity, reducing its adhesiveness and viscosity.
- It encourages the gas-liquid interactions in the airways.
- It produces bigger expiratory flow peaks than inspiratory flow peaks, causing secretions to move from peripheral to proximal airways.
- It increases the ciliary activity.

The most appropriate frequency value to address a better airway clearance ranges between 11 and 15 Hz [7], and it gets close to the physiological ciliary beat frequency (13 Hz).

Tomkiewicz et al. on the other hand observed that viscosity decreased after 30 min of oscillating at a 22 Hz frequency.

Basing on these premises, HFCWC needs to be tuned to increase the treatment efficacy [8].

As a matter of fact, Warwick and Hansen [9] tuned HFCWC in patients with CF by evaluating the ratio between frequency, volume, and flow and arbitrarily selected the frequency values that provided the three highest flows and the three largest volumes. Patients were then prescribed a 30-min treatment, consisting of those 6 frequency values set up for 5 min each. The treatment resulted in positive effects on FVC and FEV1.

Oscillation frequencies and applied pressures were selected basing on volume and expiratory flow values; in fact, the peak expiratory flow/peak inspiratory flow ratio has to be >1.1 for the mechanical devices to operate an effective airway clearance.

The frequency and the pressure values providing the highest flow and volume are to be chosen according to the patient comfort.

King et al. [7] while using HFCWC measured high peak oscillatory flow rates compared to a cough. The observed expiratory airflow rates were on average higher than inspiratory flows and were sufficiently strong to produce a mucus-airflow interaction.

Cystic fibrosis [10] is caused by abnormal chloride ion transport on the apical surface of epithelial cells in exocrine gland tissues. The abnormal composition of secretions from affected epithelial surfaces results in increased viscosity. It has been theorized that HFCWC devices are particularly effective in clearing the abnormal secretions of cystic fibrosis because vibratory shear forces facilitate expectoration by reducing the viscosity of these secretions, much in the same way that shaking jello causes it to become fluid.

A 2017 Cochrane review [11] evaluates the effectiveness of oscillatory devices as used in cystic fibrosis for airway clearance.

Outcomes included pulmonary function, sputum weight and volume, individual preference, quality-of-life measures, and number of hospitalizations per study period.

The authors concluded that oscillatory devices can be effective in clearing secretions; however, despite a noticeable improvement in sputum volume, there was no statistically significant evidence that suggested the use of these devices opposite to other physiotherapy techniques, considering respiratory function as the primary outcome in the short term.

In addition to this, Darbee et al. [12] assessed that HFCWO is efficacious in improving pulmonary function, ventilation distribution, and gas mixing for subjects who had CF and who were experiencing an acute exacerbation of their pulmonary disease.

In patients with non-cystic fibrosis bronchiectasis, HFCWO) therapy is used, whereas any other airway clearance techniques or devices have proved ineffective.

Barto et al. [13] showed that from a registry of 2596 adult bronchiectasis patients, those with NCFB using HFCWO therapy were associated with reductions in patient-reported exacerbation rates, hospitalizations, antibiotic use, and improvements in respiratory symptoms and quality of life. Importantly, these benefits were also observed in the frequent exacerbator subgroup. Moreover, the improvements in hospitalization rates, consistent with self-reported quality-of-life measures, suggest that the patient health improvement is supported for at least a year after the therapy initiation.

Patients with neuromuscular diseases frequently develop weakness of the respiratory muscles that leads to difficulty in coughing and respiratory secretions clearance, leading to mucus plugging and pulmonary infections [14]. Techniques aiming to secretion clearance are widely recommended and can include both mucus-mobilizing techniques and assisted cough techniques. Many mucus-mobilizing approaches are impractical and ineffective in patients with neuromuscular disease due to their immobility and/or to their lack of ability to generate sufficient expiratory flow or lip-sealing around a mouthpiece. HFCWO devices move secretions from peripheral airways toward central airways. The evidence in favor of HFCWO in neuromuscular patients comes largely from case studies, case series, and a few small clinical trials: Yuan et al. [15] in a controlled randomized trial in the cerebral palsy or neuromuscular disease pediatric population showed excellent safety and tolerability for high-frequency chest wall oscillation and may positively affect health-related outcomes and prevent respiratory infections.

In an exploratory randomized, controlled trial, Lange et al. [16] evaluate changes in respiratory function in patients with amyotrophic lateral sclerosis (ALS) after using high-frequency chest wall oscillation. The group study has ALS Functional Rating Scale respiratory subscale score ≤ 11 and ≥ 5 and forced vital capacity (FVC) $\geq 40\%$ predicted. This study showed that using HFCWO for only 3 months produced a significant improvement in the feeling of breathlessness, increased secretion mobilization, and a trend toward slowing the decline of forced vital capacity. Although there were significant decreased of peak expiratory flow in nonusers, Longhini et al. [17] led a study on 60 patients (30 normosecretive patients and 30 hypersecretive patients requiring regular aspirations) in invasive mechanical ventilation through an endotracheal tube and found that using HFCWO 10 minute/day at a frequency of 10 Hz may improve the hypersecretive patient ventilation especially in the back area, without compromising the gas exchanges.

In conclusion, high-frequency chest wall oscillation and compression systems are efficacious and well-tolerated alternatives to the classic airway clearance techniques and are useful with non-compliant patients and in peripheral airway secretion accumulation (Fig. 32.1).

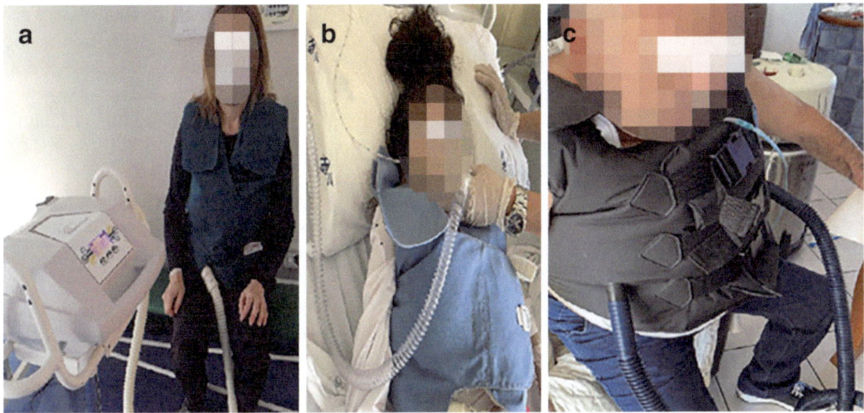

Fig. 32.1 Example of treatment with HFCWC. From left to right: (**a**) Adult cystic fibrosis, (**b**) neuromuscular disorder in association with NIV, and (**c**) non-cystic fibrosis bronchiectasis *Pseudomonas aeruginosa* colonization

References

1. Belli S, Prince I, Savio G, Paracchini E, Cattaneo D, Bianchi M, et al. Airway clearance techniques: the right choice for the right patient. Front Med (Lausanne). 2021;8:544826. https://doi.org/10.3389/fmed.2021.544826.
2. Chatburn RL. High-frequency assisted airway clearance. Respir Care. 2007;52(9):1224–35.
3. Fink JB, Mahlmeister MJ. High-frequency oscillation of the airway and chest wall. Respir Care. 2002;47(7):797–807.
4. Chang HK, Weber ME, King ME. Mucus transport by high-frequency nonsymmetrical oscillatory airflow. J Appl Physiol. 1988;65(3):1203–9. https://doi.org/10.1152/jappl.1988.65.3.1203.
5. King M, Zidulka A, Phillips D, Wright D, Gross D, Chang HK. Tracheal mucus clearance in high-frequency oscillation: effect of peak flow rate bias. Eur Respir J. 1990;3(1):6–13.
6. Dosman CF, Jones RL. High-frequency chest compression: a summary of the literature. Can Respir J. 2005;12(1):37–41. https://doi.org/10.1155/2005/525813.
7. King M, Phillips DM, Gross D, Vartian V, Chang HK, Zidulka A. Enhanced tracheal mucus clearance with high frequency chest wall compression. Am Rev Respir Dis. 1983;128:511–15. https://doi.org/10.1164/arrd.1983.128.3.511.
8. Tomkiewicz RP, Biviji A, King M. Effects of oscillating air flow on the rheological properties and clearability of mucous gel simulants. Biorheology. 1994;31(5):511–20. https://doi.org/10.3233/bir-1994-31501.
9. Warwick WJ, Hansen LG. The long-term effect of high-frequency chest compression therapy on pulmonary complications of cystic fibrosis. Pediatr Pulmonol. 1991;11(3):265–71. https://doi.org/10.1002/ppul.1950110314.
10. Hanssens LS, Duchateau J, Casimir GJ. CFTR protein: not just a chloride channel? Cells. 2021;10(11):2844. https://doi.org/10.3390/cells10112844.
11. Morrison L, Innes S. Oscillating devices for airway clearance in people with cystic fibrosis. Cochrane Database Syst Rev. 2017;5(5):CD006842. https://doi.org/10.1002/14651858.CD006842.pub4.
12. Darbee JC, Kanga JF, Ohtake PJ. Physiologic evidence for high-frequency chest wall oscillation and positive expiratory pressure breathing in hospitalized subjects with cystic fibrosis. Phys Ther. 2005;85(12):1278–89. https://doi.org/10.1093/ptj/85.12.1278.

13. Barto TL, Maselli DJ, Daignault S, Stiglich J, Porter J, Kraemer C, et al. Real-life experience with high-frequency chest wall oscillation vest therapy in adults with non-cystic fibrosis bronchiectasis. Ther Adv Respir Dis. 2020;14:1753466620932508. https://doi.org/10.1177/1753466620932508.

14. Lechtzin N, Wolfe LF, Frick KD. The impact of high-frequency chest wall oscillation on healthcare use in patients with neuromuscular diseases. Ann Am Thorac Soc. 2016;13(6):904–9. https://doi.org/10.1513/AnnalsATS.201509-597OC.MID:26999271.

15. Yuan N, Kane P, Shelton K, Matel J, Becker BC, Moss RB. Safety, tolerability, and efficacy of high-frequency chest wall oscillation in pediatric patients with cerebral palsy and neuromuscular diseases: an exploratory randomized controlled trial. J Child Neurol. 2010;25(7):815–21. https://doi.org/10.1177/0883073809350223.

16. Lange DJ, Lechtzin N, Davey C, David W, Heiman-Patterson T, Gelinas D, et al. High-frequency chest wall oscillation in ALS: an exploratory randomized, controlled trial. Neurology. 2006;67(6):991–7. https://doi.org/10.1212/01.wnl.0000237439.78935.46.

17. Longhini F, Bruni A, Garofalo E, Ronco C, Gusmano A, Cammarota G, et al. Chest physiotherapy improves lung aeration in hypersecretive critically ill patients: a pilot randomized physiological study. Crit Care. 2020;24(1):479. https://doi.org/10.1186/s13054-020-03198-6.

Humidification Recommendations in High-Frequency Percussive Ventilation

Andreína Vasconcelos

33.1 Introduction

Humidification of inhaled gases has been standard of care in mechanical ventilation for a long period of time. In the past, a variety of reports described important airway damage by applying dry gases during artificial ventilation. Consequently, it has been utilizing external humidifiers to compensate for the lack of natural humidification mechanisms when the upper airway is bypassed. Humidifiers add molecules of water to gas in order to avoid the consequences associated with lack of humidification in mechanically ventilated patients. They are classified as active or passive based on the presence of external sources of heat and water (active humidifiers) or the utilization of patients' own temperature and hydration to achieve humidification in successive breaths (passive humidifiers).

High-frequency percussive ventilation (HFPV) is a specific mode of high-frequency ventilation (HFV) that was developed in the early 1980s by FM Bird. Initially applied in the treatment of patients with acute respiratory failures after smoke inhalation and in burns patients. Further studies showed an improvement in gas exchange in cases refractive to conventional mechanical ventilation (CMV) like patients with acute respiratory distress syndrome (ARDS), pediatric, and neonate patients.

In this chapter we aim to describe the basic principles of airway humidification during invasive mechanical ventilation of patients, and also it describes the most frequently humidifiers used. Finally, we abording these aspects in the HFPV mode.

A. Vasconcelos (✉)
Centro Hospitalar do Baixo Vouga, Aveiro, Portugal

A. M. Esquinas (ed.), *Humidification in the Intensive Care Unit*,
https://doi.org/10.1007/978-3-031-23953-3_33

33.2   Physiological Airway Control of Heat and Humidity

Humidity is usually characterized in terms of absolute or relative humidity. Absolute humidity (AH) is the mass of water in a given volume of air expressed in milligrams per liter (mg/L). Relative humidity (RH) is the ratio of AH to the maximum amount of water vapor capacity at a specific temperature. Whenever the amount of gas contained in a sample is equal to its water vapor capacity, the RH is 100% and the gas is completely saturated which is defined as maximum absolute humidity, and at 37 °C it is approximately 44 mg/L. It is important to understand that water vapor capacity of a sample will increase exponentially to the temperature, so if the AH remains constant, RH will decrease whenever the temperature increases, and it will increase when the temperature decreases.

Heat and moisture exchange is one of the most important functions of the respiratory system. The connective tissue of the nose is characterized by a rich vascular system of numerous and thin-walled veins. This system is responsible for warming the inspired air to increase its humidity carrying capacity. As the inspired air goes down the respiratory tract, it reaches a point at which its temperature is 37 °C and its relative humidity is 100%. This point is known as the isothermic saturation boundary (ISB), and it is usually located 5 cm below the carina. The respiratory mucosa is lined by pseudostratified ciliated columnar epithelium and with numerous goblet cells. These cells, as well as submucosal glands underneath the epithelium, are responsible for maintaining the mucous layer that serves as a trap for pathogens and as an interface for humidity exchange. At the level of the terminal bronchioles, the epithelium turns into a simple cuboidal type with minimal goblet cells and scarce submucosal glands. Hence, the capacity of these airways to carry on the same level of humidification maintained by upper airways is limited.

After endotracheal intubation, as the upper airway loses its capacity to heat and moisture inhaled gas, the ISB is shifted down the respiratory tract. This imposes a burden on the lower respiratory tract that it is not well prepared for the humidification process so, during mechanical ventilation, humidification is imperative when an upper airway is being replaced. Adequate humidification through an artificial airway should provide enough heat and water delivery to the respiratory tract, so that heat and water loss is kept at a minimum. Consequently, delivery of partially cold and dry medical gases brings about potential damage to the respiratory epithelium, manifested by increased work of breathing, atelectasis, thick and dehydrated secretions, airway obstruction, and alveolar derecruitment.

Current American Association for Respiratory Care (AARC) guidelines recommend that heated humidifiers used with mechanical ventilators produce a minimum temperature of 30 °C and 30 mg/L of AH. The American Society for Testing and Materials (ASTM) and the International Organization for Standardization (ISO) standards are more stringent requiring manufactures of heated humidifiers to produce a minimum of 33 mg/L of AH. The ASTM and ISO do not have a minimum temperature requirement for heated humidifiers; however, their minimum AH of 33 mg/L at full saturation requires at least a temperature of 31 °C.

33.3   Types of Humidifiers

In order to avoid the consequences associated with lack of humidification in mechanically ventilated patients, a variety of devices (humidifiers) have been introduced in clinical practice. They add molecules of water to gas, and they are classified as active or passive based on the presence of external sources of heat and water (active humidifiers) or the utilization of patients' own temperature and hydration to achieve humidification in successive breaths (passive humidifiers).

33.3.1 Active Humidifiers: Heated Humidifiers

Active humidifiers are devices composed of an electric heater on which a plastic casing with a metallic base is placed in which sterile water is stored. When the base is warmed, the water temperature increases by convection. Some active humidifiers are self-regulated by a mechanism consisting of a heating wire (heated-wire breathing circuit) that keeps the gas temperature constant during its passage through the circuit and a wire with two temperature sensors connected to the exit of the heater (distal) and to a part of the circuit (close to the patient) to control the system temperature. It should be taken into account that while heated-wire breathing circuit keeps the temperature stable throughout its route and decrease the condensation, the lack of control exposes the patient to risks such as a higher incidence of occlusion of the artificial airway.

33.3.1.1   Bubble Humidifiers

The flow of entering air is forced to pass through a tube that leads to the lower part of the casing. The gas exiting from the distal end of the tube (under the water surface) forms bubbles that gain humidity and temperature as they rise to the water surface. The amount of water in the container and the flow rate are factors affecting the humidity content of the gas. Simply expressed, if the water column in the container is taller, the gas-water interface will increase. Inversely, as the circulating flow increases, the device performance drops. They exhibit high resistance to airflow imposing higher work of breathing than pass-over ones. Furthermore, they may generate microaerosol. These types of devices are no longer used.

33.3.1.2   Pass-over Humidifiers

The airflow passes over the water surface, which is hot, and the circulating gas gains heat and humidity from the gas-water interface formed. In comparison with the previously described device, pass-over humidifiers have lower resistance. It is important to consider that the water temperature in the enclosure will be a determining factor for humidity. A variant of the pass-over humidifier is the "wick" humidifier, in which a porous membrane that absorbs humidity (such as blotting paper) is dipped into water surrounded by the heating element, keeping the membrane constantly saturated with water vapor. The dry gas enters the chamber, makes contact with the wick, and is loaded with more water vapor than in the basic system because the gas-liquid interface is larger. Another variant is the hydrophobic membrane humidifier, where dry gas passes through the membrane, and due to the membrane properties, only water vapor passes through. The dry gas is loaded with water vapor and exits the chamber.

33.3.1.3 Counter-Flow Humidifier

The water is heated outside the vaporizer. During its passage through the chamber of the humidifier, the air is moisturized and warmed to body temperature. After being heated, water is pumped to the top of the humidifier, enters the inside of the humidifier through small diameter pores, and then runs down a large surface area while the gas flows in counter direction.

33.3.1.4 Inline Vaporizer

These humidifiers use a small plastic capsule where water vapor is injected into the gas in the inspiratory limb of the ventilator circuit immediately proximal to the patient wye. In addition to the water vapor, gas heating is supplemented by a small disk heater in the capsule. Water is delivered to the capsule by a peristaltic pump housed in a controller. The amount of water sent to the capsule is set by the clinician based on minute volume through the circuit. Both temperature and humidity are adjustable and displayed constantly. The proximity to the wye connection obviates the requirement for heated wires and external temperature probes.

33.3.2 Passive Humidifiers

Heat and moisture exchangers (HMEs) are also called artificial noses because they mimic the action of nasal cavity in gas humidification. The working principle for these devices is based on their capacity to retain heat and humidity during expiration and to deliver at least 70% of them to the inhaled gas during subsequent inspiration. This "passive" function can be achieved by different mechanisms, and the classification of these devices is based on their mechanisms. Due to the working principle of a passive humidifier, it should always be placed before the "Y" part of the circuit, allowing the device to contact the inspired and expired air during each ventilation cycle which makes the passive humidifier part of the instrumental dead space (VD).

33.3.2.1 Heat and Moisture Exchangers (HMEs)

Heat and moisture exchangers are simple condensers constructed with elements made of disposable foam, synthetic fiber, or paper, with a significant surface area that can generate an effective temperature gradient through the device delivering heat on each inspiration. From the field of filtration, hydrophobic HMEs were made to repel the humidity and to retain the heat of the expired gas, delivering it in the next inspiration.

33.3.2.2 Hygroscopic Condenser Humidifiers (HCHs) or Hygroscopic Heat and Moisture Exchangers (HHMEs)

In contrast with HMEs, HCHs or HHMEs are devices made with synthetic fiber coated by a hygroscopic chemical product (calcium chloride or lithium chloride), which absorbs expired water vapor and delivers it to the inspired gas, optimizing the delivery of humidity. The synthetic fiber also helps decrease the accumulation of condensation in a device-dependent position.

33.3.2.3 Heat and Moisture Exchangers with Filter

These devices are made with materials needed for moisturizing and heating based on their working principle (hydrophobic or hygroscopic); in addition, they contain an electrostatic filter. Filters are flat layers of fiber material (modacrylic or propylene) that act as a barrier to the gas flow; at the same time, the filtration performance is optimized by applying material with electrostatic charge. The available types of filters are heat and moisture exchanger filters (HMEFs), hygroscopic condenser humidifier filters (HCHFs), or hygroscopic heat and moisture exchanger filters (HHMEFs).

33.3.2.4 Combined Heat and Moisture Exchangers

Hygroscopic and hydrophobic elements are used to create a combined HME. The performance in terms of absolute humidity is better in HCHs than in HMEs. However, the performances are similar between HCHs and combined HMEs.

33.3.3 Special Humidifiers

33.3.3.1 Humidifiers for Aerosol Therapy

The HME for aerosol therapy (Gibeck Humid-Flo®) is an HME that has the property of remaining inline during the application of aerosols in mechanical ventilation, avoiding the opening of the circuit and potentially reducing the contamination of tubing and the exposure of healthcare staff to contaminated gases. This type of humidifier has two modes, "HME and AEROSOL," which can be selected by rotating the central axis of the device. By choosing HME, the device acts as a conventional passive humidifier. In aerosol mode, the humidifier part is skipped; therefore, the aerosol goes directly to the patient without coming into contact with the humidifier material. However, the AH delivered with this device is at least questionable since it delivers 30.4 mg/L but with a VT of 1000 mL.

33.3.3.2 Heat and Moisture Exchanger Booster

The HME Booster® is a type of hybrid active humidifier consisting of a passive humidification system and a "T" connector containing a self-regulated heater and a small-volume chamber for continuous infusion of distilled water (consuming approximately 250 mL every 3 days). The upper part of the device has a hydrophobic membrane that only allows the passage of water when it has evaporated toward the tubing. Therefore, the humidity from the water evaporated on the membrane is aggregated during inspiration, improving the gas conditions by approximately 3–4 mg/L (depending on the VT, *I/E* ratio, and the type of HME used). During the expiratory phase, heat and humidity are retained by the passive properties of the humidification system. The VD of the device is approximately 9 mL. It stands out as advantages: easy to use, eliminates excessive condensation in the tubing, could be useful for hypothermic patients, and has a bacterial filter (active humidifiers do not have a bacterial filter). As disadvantages, it does not include temperature monitoring, increases resistance, and requires a source of electrical energy (potential risk of burns and/or electric shocks).

33.3.3.3 Active Hygroscopic Heat and Moisture Exchangers

This device consists of an HHME in a heated casing in the shape of a cone with a radiator and an electronic controller. There is a line between the device and the water source, another line between the radiator and the controller, and a third heating line between the device and the controller. The casing contains a paper element that provides a surface for humidity transfer to the gas. A water source drips continuously on the paper element, and the casing heat makes the liquid evaporate, increasing the humidity of the inhaled gas. The device is electronically controlled through a water and temperature control unit used to program the volume per minute of the patient. Some of the proposed advantages are eliminating condensation from the inspiration branch and avoiding the use of water traps. In addition, if the water source is depleted, this device continues working like an HHME (providing approximately 28–31 mg/L AH). The active HHME provides temperatures of 36–38 °C and 90–95% relative humidity. The AH provided by the device is similar to the HME or active humidifiers but with lower water use and less condensation. The VD of the device is 73 mL, and the resistance is 1.7 cmH$_2$O/L/s. The disadvantages of this product are the possibility of skin burns and greater VD compared with a heated humidifier or only an HHME.

33.4 Principles of HFPV

During normal spontaneous breathing and CMV, gas movement occurs due to convection and molecular diffusion. Convection is the bulk flow of gas through the anatomical VD as the result of a pressure gradient caused by diaphragm contraction during normal breathing or from positive pressure ventilation. Diffusion is the movement of gas molecules down a concentration gradient in the distal parts of the airway and alveoli. Based on these mechanisms, alveolar ventilation theoretically can only occur if the VT exceeds VD. High-frequency ventilation is characterized by breathing frequencies higher than 1 Hz where VT of 1–3 mL/kg is less than the VD.

HFPV may be defined as flow-regulated time-cycled ventilation that creates controlled pressure and delivers a series of high-frequency subtidal volumes in combination with low-frequency breathing cycles. HFPV was delivered via volumetric diffusive respirator (VDR-4; Percussionaire Corporation, Sandpoint, Idaho, USA). The system is classified as a pneumatically driven, time-cycled, high-frequency flow interrupter, intermittent mandatory ventilation. It is equipped with a high-frequency flow generator connected to the device (the phasitron) that provides the interface between the patient and the machine.

The ventilator is connected to a high-pressure air generator, fed by two normal sources of oxygen and air. Two inspiratory circuits, a high-pressure and a low-pressure circuit, branch off the ventilator. The low-pressure circuit is connected to two systems located downstream from one another, the humidifier and the nebulizer. The two circuits are connected to the phasitron from which the expiratory circuit branches. The phasitron also has a system for real-time recording and visualization of pressure delivered to the patient. Measurement is made distal to the high-pressure pulsatile flow source, which is located near the connection to the endotracheal tube.

The phasitron constitutes the heart of this mode of ventilation. It is composed of a hollow cylinder in which the airflow from the high-pressure circuit causes a spring-controlled piston to move back and forth. The low-pressure inspiratory circuit supports a flow volume delivery that is inversely proportional to the pressure reached at the level of the airways; in other words, when the system approaches the desired pressure level, the fraction of delivered air comes almost exclusively from the high-pressure circuit. The phasitron has two safety valves, an inspiratory and an expiratory valve, which ensure that the set pressure is maintained at the level of the airways; the third expiratory safety valve is connected to the volume reservoir. In this way, the circuit remains constantly open to room air and allows the patient to enter at any phase of the breathing cycle, without further increasing the working pressure. Here it is important to underline that the circuit can be used in both pediatric and adult patients.

Ventilator parameter settings include pulsatile flow rate, oscillatory continuous positive airway pressure (CPAP), PEEP, inspiratory time, expiratory time, pulse frequency, and pulse inspiratory and expiratory (I/E) ratio. The sliding Venturi precisely stacks the injected subtidal volumes at the high-frequency rate set, for the inspiratory time selected. The inspiratory time is time cycled off, allowing a drop to oscillatory CPAP/PEEP for the selected expiratory time. High-frequency rates may be varied from 80 to 1000 cycles per minute with the VDR-4.

HFPV has been used to improve gas exchange in patients with adult respiratory distress syndrome (ARDS) failing conventional ventilation while increasing mean airway pressure and decreasing peak airway pressure without affecting hemodynamics. Previous studies have shown HFPV to be effective in reducing intracranial pressure in traumatic brain injury, treating lung injury associated with burns and inhalational injury, reducing time on extra-corporeal membrane oxygenation, recruiting lung volume and improving hypoxemia in pulmonary resection, and improving oxygenation and providing lung protective ventilation in pediatric acute respiratory failure. HFPV was also used as salvage therapy in patients after cardiac surgery and in morbidly obese patients.

33.5 Humidification During HFPV

Adequate humidification delivery during HFV modes has been a challenge because of the gas flow delivery characteristics of high-frequency ventilators when compared with the gas flow delivery characteristics of conventional ventilators. HFPV delivers higher gas flow rates at higher respiratory rates, posing a difficult task because major portions of gas flow bypass-heated pass-over humidifier systems intended to provide minimal AH to the patient. Inadequate humidification during HFPV causes mucus plugging, loss of airway patency, and/or endotracheal tube (ETT) occlusion.

Patients on HFPV can be vulnerable to inadequate humidification for two reasons. First, unlike most mechanical ventilators, which direct the gas through a heated humidifier for delivery at the circuit Y-piece, in HFPV the gas goes directly to the circuit Y-piece, permitting most of the gas to bypass a humidifier before reaching the patient. Second, an HFPV-independent continuous (bias) gas flow must be used in which the gas passes via tubing to the humidifier and then to the circuit Y-piece. The resulting gas mixture may or may not have acceptable heat and humidity.

Allan et al. [1] was concerned about the risk of inadequate humidification during HFPV. So, they studied five humidifiers [two heated pass-over (MR730 and MR850), one heated wick (ConchaTherm Hi-Flow), one heated countercurrent membrane (2000i), and an unheated continuous jet nebulization (tracheobronchial jet nebulizer)] during HFPV with a lung model, at bias gas flows of 10, 30, and 50 L/min, and compared the results to those from a comparator ventilator/humidifier setup and to the minimum temperature (30 °C) and humidity (30 g/L) recommended by the AARC, at both regular room temperature and a high ambient temperature. Temperature was measured at the humidifier outflow point and at the artificial carina. Of the 7 HFPV/humidifier combinations, 2 (the MR850 at a bias flow of 50 L/min and the ConchaTherm Hi-Flow with VDR nebulizer) provided a carinal temperature equivalent to the comparator setup at room temperature, whereas 1 HFPV/humidifier combination (the ConchaTherm Hi-Flow with modified programming, at bias flows of 30 and 50 L/min) provided a higher carinal temperature. At high ambient temperature, all of the setups delivered lower carinal temperature than the comparator setup. Only two setups (the ConchaTherm with modified programming at a bias flow of 50 L/min and the ConchaTherm Hi-Flow with VDR nebulizer) provided carinal humidification equivalent to the comparator setup, without regard to ambient temperature; the other humidifiers were less effective. The ConchaTherm with modified programming and the ConchaTherm with the VDR nebulizer provided the most consistent humidification.

Intensive care units that use the VDR-4 ventilator have tried adding a pass-over or wick-style humidifiers to the Injectron nebulizer (Percussionaire Corp., Sandpoint, ID) on the VDR-4, combining two wick-style humidifiers, and adding acetylcysteine or heparin to try and manage thick secretions with patients on HFPV. This represents all the known humidification schemes that are used with HFPV.

Tiffin et al. [2] tested a novel inline vaporizing humidifier and two gas-water interface humidifiers during HFPV using the new VDR-4 Fail-safe Breathing Circuit Hub to determine whether delivered humidification could be improved. This new humidification system, the Hydrate Omni™, delivers water vapor into the gas flow of the ventilator circuit rather than water droplets as delivered by the gas-water interface humidifiers. Measurements of AH and gas temperature were made on the three different humidification systems using a test lung model under standard ambient conditions. The authors found that when using the novel inline vaporizer, it provided better humidification when compared with the standard gas-water interface humidifier during HFPV using the new VDR-4 breathing circuit.

HFPV's distinctive gas flow mechanism may impair gas heating and humidification, so all humidification systems should be tested with HFPV prior to clinical use.

End Practical: Key Messages
- Airway humidification represents a key intervention in mechanically ventilated patients.
- Inappropriate humidifier settings or selection of devices may negatively impact clinical outcomes by damaging airway mucosa, prolonging mechanical ventilation, or increasing work of breathing.
- Humidifier devices may function passively or actively, depending on the source of heat and humidity. Depending on the clinical scenario, humidifier selection may change over time. Therefore, knowledge of the advantages and disadvantages of each of these devices is essential for respiratory care practitioners.
- HFPV may be defined as flow-regulated time-cycled ventilation that creates controlled pressure and delivers a series of high-frequency subtidal volumes in combination with low-frequency breathing cycles. It is equipped with a high-frequency flow generator connected to the device (the phasitron) that provides the interface between the patient and the machine.
- HFPV has been used to improve gas exchange in patients with ARDS failing conventional ventilation while increasing mean airway pressure and decreasing peak airway pressure without affecting hemodynamics. HFPV has also shown to be effective in reducing intracranial pressure in traumatic brain injury, treating lung injury associated with burns, and inhalational injury.

References

1. Allan PF, Hollingsworth MJ, Maniere GC, Rakofsky AK, Chung KK, Naworol GA, Ward JA, Perello M, Morris MJ. Airway humidification during high-frequency percussive ventilation. Respir Care. 2009;54(3):350–8. Erratum in: Respir Care. 2009 Jul;54(7):978. PMID: 19245729.

2. Tiffin NH, Short KA, Jones SW, Cairns BA. Comparison of three humidifiers during high-frequency percussive ventilation using the VDR-4® Fail-safe Breathing Circuit Hub. J Burn Care Res. 2011;32(3):e45–50. https://doi.org/10.1097/BCR.0b013e318217f864. PMID: 21422945.

Biphasic Cuirass Ventilation for Airway Secretions

34

Gary W. Mefford

The physical interventions and tools of application for chest physical therapy including volume expansion and pulmonary secretion clearance are utilized to enhance many patients' compromised ability to maintain clear airways. These interventions are directed toward some portion of a spectrum of effects considered as key to effective secretion clearance therapy. Consider this spectrum to represent the treatments employed within our secretion clearance toolkit. On one end of the spectrum is secretion modification, in the middle of the spectrum is mobilization, and at the other end is expectoration. In order to understand the utility of any tool or technique used to enhance secretion clearance completeness, one must recognize where that technique falls within this spectrum. This discussion will cover this spectrum, the tools that fall within the ranges of the spectrum with an ultimate focus on the secretion clearance support functions, and other clinical advantages of treatment with the Hayek RTX Biphasic Cuirass Ventilator. It will also show how the unique combination of HFCWO and cough support via cuirass provides airway clearance that uniquely supports the full range of the secretion clearance intervention spectrum.

In the absence of illness, the body manages normal flow of pulmonary secretions without difficulty and adequately supports elevated requirements of most short-term respiratory illnesses without secretion retention. Therefore, retained secretions in the lungs can be the result of pathology, pulmonary muscle weakness, or poor overall health.

Poor lung health can be particularly compromising. Weak patients' lungs may worsen over time as they are unable to clear even normal volumes of secretions. Patients with muco-proliferative illnesses may have normal personal airway clearance capability, but high volumes of sputum combined with other symptoms of their

G. W. Mefford (✉)
Clinical Operations and Sales, Hayek Medical Devices, London, UK
e-mail: Gary.mefford@hayekmedical.com; http://www.hayekmedical.com

A. M. Esquinas (ed.), *Humidification in the Intensive Care Unit*,
https://doi.org/10.1007/978-3-031-23953-3_34

313

illness can overwhelm their reserves. The worst periods can fatigue even the well-conditioned. Lung infections result from the body's inability to manage secretion production that exceeds its ability to mobilize and expectorate. This inability can also cause secretions to accumulate even when the lungs are not producing excess amounts. Most patients with unaddressed retained secretions will have pulmonary deterioration due to reoccurrences of pneumonias that result in lung injury over time.

Physical conditioning and rehabilitation interventions designed to maximize the effectiveness of the lungs and upper airways for getting rid of excessive pulmonary secretions of the body can benefit capable patients.

These types of interventions are geared toward increasing cough effectiveness by improving inspiratory and expiratory strengths and capacities as well as chest wall mobility. Therapies designed to improve a patient's cough and lung clearance techniques can be highly beneficial for the overall airway clearance program. The healthier and more skilled the patient is with self-administered physical airway clearance techniques, the more of the secretion clearance spectrum they are able to provide for themselves.

34.1　The Secretion Clearance Spectrum: Modification > Mobilization > Expectoration

Secretion Modification At this end of the spectrum, medications and techniques are directed generally at thinning thick, tenacious, and sticky retained secretions so that they may be restored to normal viscosity and motility. Mucolytic medications, optimal humidification of inspired gas, and oscillatory airflow techniques are therapies with the goal of creating a thinner viscosity mucous gel layer. This allows secretions to mobilize upward more readily with less patient effort. Mucolytics and hypertonic NaCl solutions may vary in effectiveness depending on the drug and the specific effect on the characteristics of the sputum's unique qualities related to the underlying cause of the secretions present. These are prescribed with a goal of creating a more mobile mucous blanket. High humidity and high-flow nasal cannulas allow delivery of gas that meets or nearly meets the patient's inspiratory demand. The gas delivered is humidified at or near 100% BTPS. This high level of humidity can have a thinning effect on thick secretions as they become hydrated by the saturated inspired gas. Positive pressure ventilation (PPV), whether non-invasive or invasive, should generally be applied with humidification to prevent thickening of secretions. Oscillatory airflow techniques can be extrathoracic, such as high-frequency chest wall compressors (HFCWC) via air bladder vests or high-frequency chest wall oscillators via the biphasic cuirass. They can also be applied with mask or mouthpiece, as with oscillating PEP and positive percussive medication delivery devices. These various oscillating therapies modify secretions by creating an oscillatory flow wave throughout the airways, causing turbulence in the gel layer that alters the mucoid bonds resulting in a thinning effect [1]. Secretion modification is at one end of the spectrum of the secretion clearance toolkit.

Secretion Mobilization Pulmonary secretion retention resolution is not as simple as catching up mucus clearance with mucus production. In order for secretions to be made available at the main bronchi and trachea for clearance from the lungs, they need to be mobilized from the distal regions where they pool and create airway obstruction. Therapeutic tools and techniques such as active cycle breathing (ACB), autogenic drainage (AD), forced expiratory techniques (FET), positioning, clapping, oscillatory techniques, and intermittent positive pressure breathing (IPPB) or positive pressure techniques that mimic IPPB are utilized to create a secretion mobilization effect. These tools and techniques move secretions from the alveoli, terminal bronchioles, and distal airways up to larger airways. The final goal is expectoration or clearance from the lungs. ACB and AD, once mastered, can be self-administered by patients that have adequate strength and airway conductance to generate enough flow to create secretion upward movement without excessive use of reserves. Positioning and percussive clapping is the classic chest physical therapy. This technique requires a trained caregiver for the clapping. Specific drainage positions are known to facilitate drainage of specific regions of the lungs. Caregivers can administer clapping and FET for all lung fields or for specific trouble regions. This can be combined with ACB in capable patients to enhance mobilization. The position changes required for the patients and the physical consistency needed for the caregivers can be exhausting. Some drainage positions may destabilize the patient, depending on position used, severity, location of retained secretions, and degree of VQ mismatch.

Oscillatory techniques, previously discussed in secretion modification, can also be considered to have a potential beneficial effect on mobilization. As the patient utilizes the therapy, the puffs of gas created generate an upward wafting effect on the gel layer. Oscillatory PEP devices include the advantage of positive pressure opening airways beyond secretions allowing the oscillating expiratory flow to create a pressure wave. This opens airways distal to secretions allowing gas to flow from below bringing secretions upward with it. Oscillatory treatments with vest- or air bladder-type devices quickly squeeze and release the chest repeatedly to create the effect of high-frequency chest wall compression (HFCWC). With the Hayek biphasic cuirass, negative and positive pressure alternates within the shell to create true high-frequency chest wall oscillation (HFCWO) [2]. Intra-cuirass pressures balance between negative and positive to deliver true oscillation. Due to the similarity of the way the cuirass supports ventilation to natural breathing, the airways are generally more open. This facilitates secretion flow rather than inhibits as may occur with positive airway pressure (PAP) support tools.

Secretion mobilization is a key component of effective airway clearance efforts. In order to clear the lungs of any significant amount of retained secretions, effective mobilization from distal to large airways must occur. The ACB techniques cover a range on the secretion clearance spectrum that includes expectoration and mobilization in more mobile patients with less advanced needs. The standard therapy for mobilization of mucus to the large airways has been postural drainage and percussion (PD&P). This therapy supports secretion clearance mainly from the mobilization portion of the spectrum. The clapping may have, at most, a marginal effect on sputum viscosity. The oscillating therapies facilitate upward mobilization by creating puffs of gas flow that move secretions. Normal or supported cough must follow for complete clearance.

Expectoration Once retained pulmonary secretions are modified to normally flowing viscosity, and mobilized to the larger airways, in order to have the most complete airway clearance possible, the mobilized sputum must be cleared from the airways or expectorated. The natural cough is the primary and most desirable means of creating expectoration. When ineffective or inadequate, the natural cough can be supported in many ways. If the cough is failing, then the secretion clearance program is failing. Support of cough can be achieved via several techniques depending on the nature of the cough failure. The natural cough consists of several phases, each playing an important role in expectoration. When selecting ways that can support efforts to normalize or enhance cough effectiveness, these cough phases and related failures should be considered. For this discussion, we will consider a normal cough to occur in the following phases: (1) deep inspiration, (2) glottic closure, (3) pressure build, (4) glottic release/modulation, (5) expiratory flow generation, and (6) secretion expulsion. Below are the phases and how they can be supported for increased completeness of expectoration.

Deep Inspiration In order to generate an effective expiratory cough flow, adequate inspiratory volume must be achieved. Cough supporting interventions will nearly always emphasize a deep inspiration. For patients with poor natural inspiratory volume, mechanical support of this must be provided. For others, maximum effect possible is desired, and they find mechanical support brings greater efficiency to the airway clearance process. Increased treatment effectiveness can shorten treatment session duration and frequency of need. Mechanical support of a deeper inspiration for cough is achieved either by a positive pressure breath (IPPB techniques, in-exsufflator device, manual resuscitator bag, or ventilator) or by a negative pressure breath (Hayek cuirass).

Glottic Closure In a natural cough sequence, once the lungs are full, the glottis closes in part or in full, modulating expiratory flow and creating flow bursts. Patients with an open tracheostomy will not be able to utilize glottic flow burst. Peak expiratory cough flows in the absence of glottic closure, and modulation may be decreased.

Pressure Build With an effective natural cough, muscles of expiration are brought into use and intrathoracic pressure spikes. With weak, fatigued, or compromised patients, cough pressure generation is poor. The muscles needed cannot generate adequate contraction to create enough flow to move secretions. This can be supported by manual cough assist techniques, in-exsufflation techniques, or the expiratory portion of the cough phase of the airway clearance module on the Hayek

Biphasic Cuirass Ventilator. All expiratory support techniques provide a maximum effect following provision of a deep breath.

Glottic Release/Modulation The glottis is then released partially or completely. Glottic release can occur in single, near-complete exhalations or intermittently causing multiple bursts of flow with each cough breath. Glottic flow modulation, other capabilities, and reflexes can be diminished when a tracheostomy tube has been in place for prolonged periods and may need time to recover. In order to restore the patients' ability, speech therapy airway, swallow interventions, tracheal decannulation trials, and tracheostomy removal may be of benefit.

Expiratory Flow Generation In a healthy cough, the activated muscles of exhalation contract to create a burst or series of bursts of gas flow in synchrony with glottic modulation. For individuals unable to effectively contract these muscles, expiratory flow support can be provided by manual or mechanical cough assist techniques. The manual techniques may include abdominal thrusts, rib springing, or expiratory chest shivers applied during release of a deep inspiration. Mechanical means of expiratory cough flow support can be provided with an in-exsufflator during exsufflation or with the expiratory phase of the cough portion of the secretion clearance module on the Hayek RTX.

Secretion Expulsion The flow of secretions up the upside-down tree of the lungs ultimately arrives at the trachea. As secretions accumulate near the carina, the need to cough is sensed. A cough occurs with the purpose of carrying secretions from the airways. A purposeful goal-directed cough will generally create greater expectoration with less drain on reserves than uncontrolled spontaneous coughing.

Some of the interventions that help with the individual areas of modification, mobilization, or expectoration of secretions do little outside a single zone of the secretion clearance intervention spectrum. Some others perform at multiple places in the spectrum and may spread across a wider range of benefits.

Therapeutic intervention with the Hayek Biphasic Cuirass Secretion Clearance-timed treatment module covers all three. It utilizes true HFCWO for modification and mobilization of respiratory secretions, establishing better flow and then cycles to assist with cough.

Hayek biphasic cuirass for complete secretion clearance compared to other forms of secretion clearance assistance tools.

Oscillatory Wave Form The majority of the "vest"-type devices on the market utilize *high-frequency chest wall compression* (HFCWC) and may refer to it as *high-frequency chest wall oscillation* (HFCWO). However, oscillation requires both a negative and a positive pressure applied to the chest wall. "Vest"-type devices are not able to provide anything other than a positive pressure deflection. "High-frequency chest wall oscillation uses a chest cuirass to generate biphasic changes in trans-respiratory pressure" [2]. The RTX, by virtue of the rigid cuirass, flexible seal, and the high-frequency oscillation of the gas flow wave form generated by the power unit and applied to the chest wall through the cuirass, provides true HFCWO. This oscillatory wave applied to the lungs through the cuirass and chest wall provides a secretion thinning effect, as well as an increase in the transport of the patient's retained secretions up to the large bronchi and trachea for expectoration. The disadvantage of chest wall compression versus true oscillation is that over the duration of a therapy session, the high-frequency compressions have the potential to cause patient discomfort and dyspnea. This is presumably due to compression of lung volumes during the therapy. It has been shown in animal studies that this may cause reduction in FRC "…HFCWC resulted in a marked decrease (up to 50%) in end-expiratory lung volume with significantly lower PaO_2, lower compliance, and higher alveolar-arterial oxygen gradient…" [3].

This compressive effect may not be favorable with patients that have or are prone to alveolar collapse, which is a characteristic of the majority of the patients requiring secretion clearance treatment. The oscillatory wave provided by the RTX is frequently found much more tolerable by patients. Discomfort and dyspnea are rare, presumably due to the maintenance and protection of full lung volumes, while a higher intrathoracic intensity is delivered.

Assisted Cough At the completion of each phase of *high-frequency chest wall oscillation*, the Hayek biphasic cuirass provides cough assistance by the same non-invasive cuirass interface. This is accomplished by the power unit advancing to the next phase where negative pressure is applied to the chest wall creating a full lung inflation, followed by a positive pressure against the chest wall facilitating a strong expiratory gas flow. The elements of a good cough are a deep breath and a strong forced expiratory cough effort which are enhanced by this phase. The patient can perform huff cough and forced cough maneuvers in synchrony with the positive pressure deflections, thereby producing increased expiratory cough flows. This allows expectoration of secretions that were loosened and mobilize up the bronchial tree by the previous phase of oscillation. Even patients with no ability to generate a cough flow can have effective flows with this type of expiratory support. The majority of patients who retain secretions and fail to expectorate, refractory to all other secretion clearance therapies, will be productive using this combined oscillation and cough assist method. No "vest"-type device can provide this type of assistance. Other device-related forms of cough support typically require a facial or direct to artificial airway interface and utilize positive pressure to create lung inflation. This is not as natural or as well-distributed throughout the lungs as the negative pressure lung inflation provided by the cuirass.

Pulmonary Support The RTX can be adjusted via the same cuirass interface to provide various levels of well-tolerated non-invasive support of ventilation (NIV). The NIV support of the biphasic cuirass ventilation (BCV) modes can provide patients' muscles of respiration with periods of rest. The continuous negative or continuous negative extrathoracic pressure (CNEP) mode can be used for lung recruitment sessions either routinely or episodically for as long as indicated, allowing reversal of atelectatic changes, and effecting small airway caliber increases resulting in improved airflows such as forced expiratory volume/1 s (FEV1). NIV support with BCV can help improve measures of strength and endurance of the pulmonary muscle groups, allowing greater availability of system reserves when needed for activities of daily living. The utility of CNEP for volume expansion and airway clearance therapy create additional possible strategies for restoring lung function. No "vest"-type device or other mechanical secretion clearance assistance tool can provide this. Another benefit of the cuirass interface is that it allows application concomitantly with other ventilatory support techniques such as aerosol therapy, high-humidity high-flow oxygen, NIPPV, and PPV providing secretion clearance support during the use of other ventilation support methods.

Conclusion Secretion clearance can be enhanced via many highly varied techniques and medications. Each targets goals within the secretion clearance spectrum, whether focused on a single portion or range. The Hayek RTX, as a secretion management tool, provides unparalleled potential as far as comfort, effectiveness, and efficiency. The cuirass applied high-frequency oscillatory wave thins and advances secretions to the large airways and combines with its assisted cough function to facilitate expectoration.

The Hayek RTX is the lung tool that covers the full secretion clearance spectrum. Secretion clearance is considered a hallmark of good pulmonary care for patients with symptoms of, or who are prone to, pulmonary secretion retention. Additionally, the ability of the RTX to provide non-invasive ventilatory support, via its biphasic modes, and lung recruitment via a sustained inflation increase, is a unique benefit. When indicated, it can be used without requiring a mask or a tracheostomy but will work with either present, if needed.

When lungs are at risk for secretions building up in the distal airways, and the goal is to clear them as thoroughly as possible, they must be modified and mobilized so they can be moved on their way upward and out of the system. The Hayek BCV Secretion Clearance Module offers significant advantages for weak patients or those seeking a highly effective therapy for maximizing lung health with effective secretion management applications. The Hayek biphasic cuirass provides a unique mechanical secretion clearance support tool. It provides an alternative therapy that covers more of the spectrum of interventions that can help pulmonary secretions on their way up the upside-down pulmonary tree (Figs. 34.1 and 34.2).

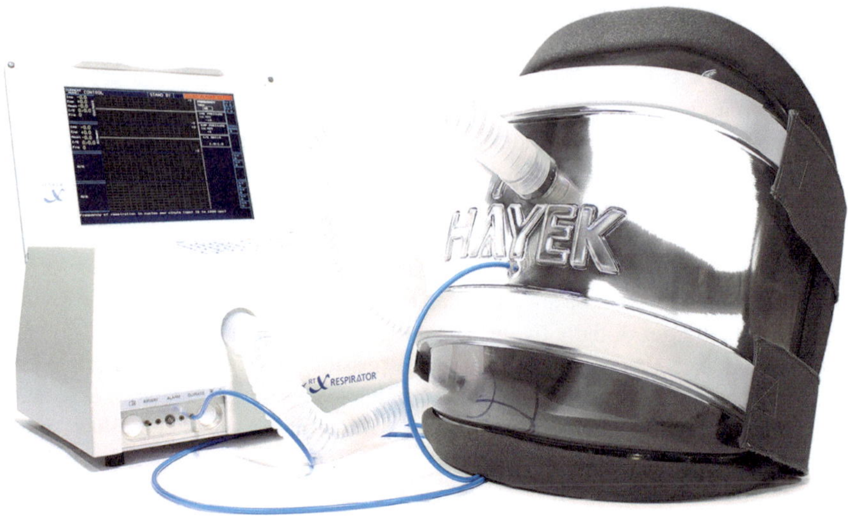

Fig. 34.1 The Hayek Biphasic Cuirass provides a unique mechanical secretion clearance support tool and an alternative therapy that covers more of the spectrum of interventions that can help with pulmonary secretions

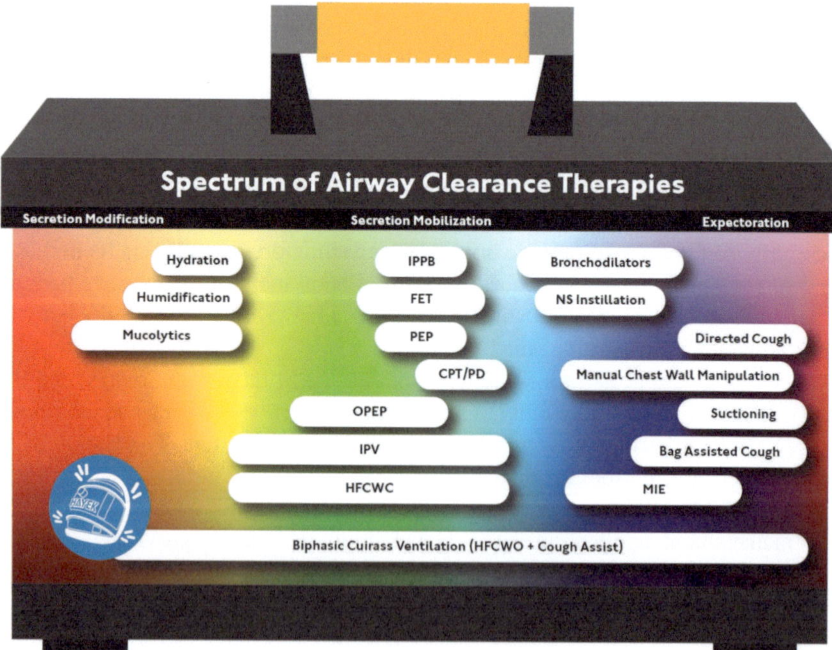

Fig. 34.2 The Hayek RTX Biphasic Cuirass Ventilator with HFCWO and Cough support via cuirass provides airway clearance that supports the full range of the secretion clearance intervention spectrum

References

1. Hamid Q, Shannon J, Martin J. Physiologic basis of respiratory disease. Hamilton: BC Decker Inc; 2005. p. 410.
2. Chatburn RL. High-frequency assisted airway clearance. Respir Care. 2007;52(9):1224–35; discussion 1235–7. PMID: 17716388. http://rc.rcjournal.com/content/respcare/52/9/1224.full.pdf.
3. Eyal F, Hayek Z, Armengol J, Jones R. High frequency chest wall compression in cats with normal lungs. Pediatr Res. 1987;21:183–7. http://www.ncbi.nlm.nih.gov/pubmed/3547282.

Aerosol Therapy and Humidification 35

Elena Fernández Fernández and Ronan MacLoughlin

35.1 Humidification in the Intensive Care Unit

As discussed in greater detail throughout this book, humidification of the patient airway is a critical component of many respiratory support interventions, especially in those patients in receipt of therapy over extended periods. Broadly, humidification is classified as (a) active or (b) passive. Active humidification typically employs the use of a heating plate which is used to vaporize sterile water, hence the common term of heated humidification (HH). This heated vapor is then introduced to the patient airways on appliance of the positive pressure or gas flow during the inhalation phase of the breath. The heater element is typically placed away from the patient, for reasons of practicality and safety. Given its placement, it is also less likely that the patient's own secretions will contaminate the heated water column. Passive humidification makes use of heat and moisture exchangers (HMEs) which are essentially compiled of a hydrophobic porous material that allows for patient-appropriate gas flows to pass through, but not the patient's own exhaled moisture. They capture heat and moisture from the patient's exhaled gas and return up to 70%

The original version of this chapter was previously published non-open access. A Correction to this chapter is available at https://doi.org/10.1007/978-3-031-23953-3_38

E. F. Fernández
Medical Affairs, Aerogen Limited, Galway, Ireland

R. MacLoughlin (✉)
Research and Development, Science and Emerging Technologies, Aerogen Limited, Galway, Ireland

School of Pharmacy and Biomolecular Sciences, Royal College of Surgeons in Ireland, Dublin, Ireland

School of Pharmacy and Pharmaceutical Sciences, Trinity College, Dublin, Ireland
e-mail: rmacloughlin@aerogen.com

A. M. Esquinas (ed.), *Humidification in the Intensive Care Unit*,
https://doi.org/10.1007/978-3-031-23953-3_35

of both to the next inhalation [1–4]. Often, these HMEs are primed with sterile water prior to use as part of the manufacturing process. HMEs are placed between the patient wye and patient interface, for example, the endotracheal tube or tracheostomy tube. HME may also be combined with a filter layer in order to prevent microbiological contamination of the patient ventilatory circuit. This potential for contamination stems from the increased likelihood of patient secretions impacting on the HME itself and thereafter migrating through the porous materials to the oxygen source side. Such HMEs are referred to as HMEF.

The comparative clinical efficacy with respect to active (HH) versus passive (HME) humidification systems has been reported to be similar. In one meta-analysis and meta-regression of randomized controlled trials, no superiority of HMEs or HHs, in terms of artificial airway occlusion, pneumonia, and mortality, was found. It was noted that a trend favoring HMEs was observed in studies including a high percentage of patients with pneumonia diagnosis at admission and those with prolonged mechanical ventilation [5]. A randomized multicenter trial investigating the impact of HH or HME on ventilator-associated pneumonia rates in adults found no difference between the two [6]. A more recent study in 20 subjects positive for SARS-Cov-2 reported a greater incidence of endotracheal tube occlusions (ETOs) with HH. Following an investigation, a strong correlation between heater plate temperatures of the HH and humidity delivered was seen. Subsequently, measures to avoid under-humidification were implemented (including heater plate temperature monitoring), and no more ETOs occurred [7]. Similar variability in humidification levels has been noted also for various combinations of gas flow rate, humidifier type, and circuit type [8]. Intuitively, it would be expected that variations in humidification levels would have varying effects on hygroscopic growth of aerosol droplets. Finally, unconditioned gases, that is to say, no heating and no humidity added above ambient or dry, are not generally used in neonates for reasons that include the increased body temperature recorded in infants with HH and the resulting reduction in cases of hypothermia on admission to the neonate ICU [9]. HH versus HME was assessed in one recent study in rabbits and found that HH increased the highest absolute humidity levels, followed by HME, with unconditioned gases recording the lowest. The study concluded that the use of a T-piece resuscitator with HME could be a good alternative to HH given that positive-pressure ventilation is used ideally for short periods of time in the delivery room [10].

HH and HME may be used together inadvertently, and this dual humidification in ventilation circuits is considered an under-recognized error in the ICU, in operating room, or during patient transfer, and correspondingly there have been reports of critical airway occlusions within 24 h [11, 12]. In this scenario, unless the aerosol device is placed between the HME and endotracheal tube, no aerosol would likely be delivered to the patient given the HME would prevent aerosol transit to the patient.

One other consideration in the selection of either HH or HME that does not relate to humidification is the potential effect on ventilatory function and gas exchange. In 24 patients with acute respiratory failure (ARF), Jaber et al. report a negative effect of HME usage. They found that the increased dead space of the HME decreased the efficiency of non-invasive ventilation (NIV) in those patients [13]. As these effects would likely happen over time, the implication for aerosol therapy is that the delivered dose would change over time also.

In a prospective, randomized, controlled physiologic study in difficult-to-wean chronic respiratory failure (CRF) patients, HME usage was associated with significantly increased inspiratory effort variables as well as dynamic intrinsic positive end-expiratory pressure and severe respiratory acidosis. The authors, therefore, concluded that the type of airway humidification device used may negatively influence the mechanical efficacy of ventilation and, unless the pressure support ventilation level is considerably increased, the use of a heat and moisture exchanger should not be recommended in difficult or potentially difficult-to-wean patients with CRF [14]. Additional dead space and variation in ventilation function, as identified in those studies, have been shown to affect the amount of aerosol delivered to the patient lung [15, 16].

35.2   Aerosol Therapy Combined with Humidification

Aerosol therapy during respiratory support in the intensive care unit (ICU) is a commonly prescribed intervention in the treatment of both respiratory (local targeting) and non-respiratory (systemic targeting) conditions. International surveys on aerosol therapy in the ICU suggest that between 90% and 99% of healthcare professionals (HCPs) administer aerosol therapy during both invasive and non-invasive mechanical ventilations and approximately 24% administer aerosol therapy during high-flow nasal oxygen (HFNO) therapy [17–19]. The direct access to the lung offers the potential for targeted high-dose delivery direct to the site of action, for example, topical administration of bronchodilators, ionic solutions, steroids, mucociliary modulators and anti-infectives, or targeting the site of absorption for systemically acting drugs, such as prostanoids, anticoagulants, and diuretics.

From these surveys, the primary aerosol delivery devices used in the ICU include pressurized metered dose inhalers (pMDI), Venturi jet nebulizers (JN), and vibrating mesh nebulizers (VMN). Each may be included in the patient circuit during mechanical ventilation, both invasive and non-invasive. However, following from COVID-19 renewed focus on HCP safety during aerosol therapy, the VMN has become the favored device as it has been shown to maintain a closed ventilator circuit during drug refill, unlike the JN which must be disassembled for drug refill, nor does the VMN need to be removed from the circuit between doses, as is the case with pMDI [20, 21]. This is reflected in several guidance and recommendation documents issued around the world [22–28]. Whilst no additional steps are mandated during HH, between 22% (international) and 62.7% (China) of HCPs reported that they turned off the humidifier during concurrent use of aerosol therapy [17, 18]. Concurrent use of each of pMDI, JN, and VMN has been described in the literature, and apart from selected HME, there are no contraindications against their use. All three of these aerosol device types are also suited for use with HH circuits and with no specific contraindications against their use. Figures 35.1, 35.2, and 35.3 detail the potential placement location options for aerosol delivery devices (indicated by

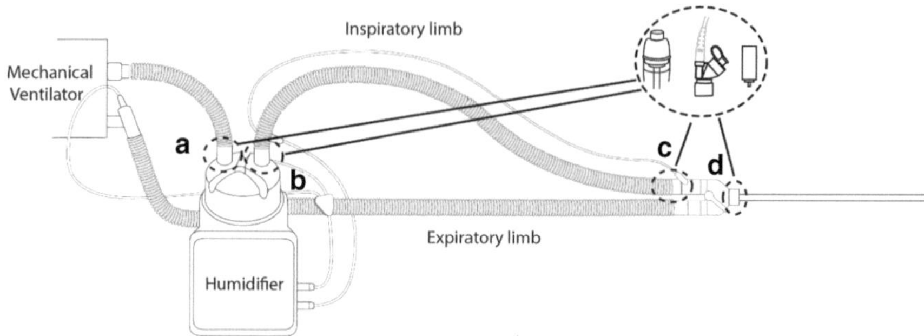

Fig. 35.1 Locations where aerosol devices may be included in the active, heated humidified (HH) mechanical ventilation setup. (**a**) Ventilator or dry side of humidifier, (**b**) patient or wet side of humidifier, (**c**) inspiratory limb at the patient wye, and (**d**) between the patient wye and patient interface, e.g., endotracheal tube (shown here), tracheostomy

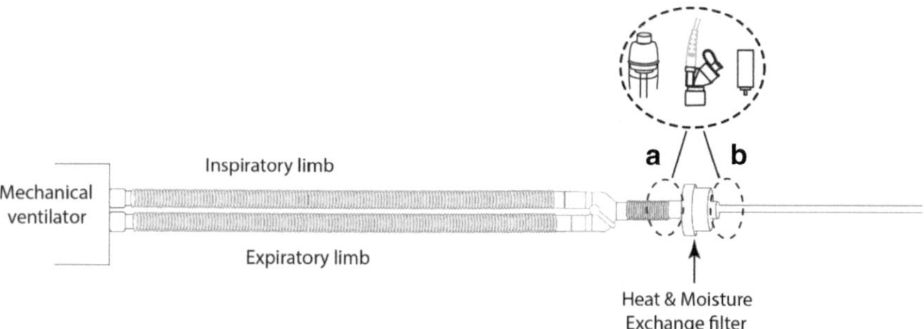

Fig. 35.2 Locations where aerosol devices may be included in the passive, heat and moisture exchange (HME) mechanical ventilation setup. (**a**) Ventilator side of the HME. *Note*: This is only suitable when aerosol therapy is being administered in combination with a bypass HME or HME that allows aerosol to pass through the porous materials. (**b**) Patient side of the HME, between HME and patient interface, e.g., endotracheal tube (shown here), tracheostomy

the device in the dotted circle) in the HH mechanical ventilation, HME mechanical ventilation, and HFNO configurations, respectively.

HME may require additional interventions on behalf of the HCP. For example, increased frequency of HME replacement given the potential for increased resistance to flow across the HME as the exhaled fraction of medical aerosol makes the HME wetter over time. It must be noted however that this exposure to exhaled medical aerosol is not necessarily catastrophic, and the outcome will vary by drug, dosing regimen, and HME type (large surface area pleated paper versus small surface area sponge) [29, 30]. Indeed, some HME manufacturers, such as Intersurgical (UK) and PALL (USA), indicate that a selection of their HME is suitable for repeated use in combination with aerosol therapy and maintain the same (typically 24 h) life as those HME not approved for use with aerosol therapy.

HME designs exist that facilitate concurrent aerosol therapy, without the need for removal of the HME or the potential increased frequency of replacement. One such

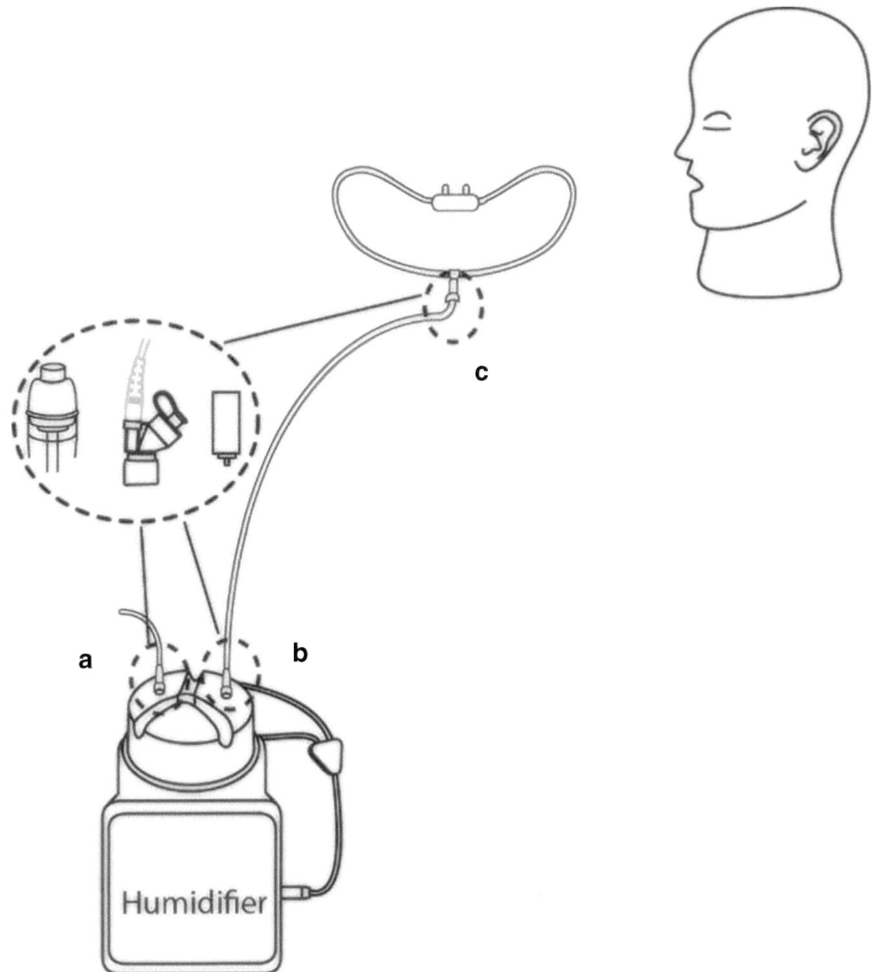

Fig. 35.3 Locations where aerosol devices may be included in the high-flow nasal oxygen (HFNO) setup. (**a**) Gas source/dry side of the humidifier, (**b**) patient/wet side of the humidifier, and (**c**) between the patient circuit and patient interface, e.g., nasal cannula (shown here), tracheostomy, mask

design is known as the bypass HME where a manually actuated mechanical valve can direct air through the HME membrane or, during aerosol therapy, bypass the membrane so that it does not come into contact with the exhaled medical aerosol. Examples of bypass HMEs include, but are not limited to, CircuVent® HME/HCH (ICU Medical, USA), AirLife® Filtered Bypass HME (Vyaire Medical, USA), and Gibeck® Humid-Flo® HME (Teleflex, USA).

There is also an alternate HME design that claims compatibility with aerosol therapy but relies on the porous materials, with no filter as opposed to a bypass mechanism. In this design, aerosol droplets pass through the porous materials. The

ThermoFlo® HN (Arc Medical, Ireland) claims only a "moderate" reduction in aerosol delivery through the HME with no significant increase in resistance measures.

VMN is the predominant delivery device used during HFNO as it does not influence gas flow or applied pressures, facilitates constant applied pressure during the drug refill process, and is increasingly recommended for use and integrated into self-contained blower-based HFNO systems [19, 31, 32]. Those systems include the Fisher & Paykel Airvo™ system, the Vapotherm Precision Flow Hi-VNI™, and Inspired Medical O2FLO™ system as examples. JN are contraindicated against for connection to HFNO systems by some manufacturers given that the additional air required for the nebulizer's operation alters gas flow and the titered oxygen mixes, especially at lower applied gas flow rates. HFNO systems are exclusively HH systems that incorporate the humidifier in the patient circuit and with gas flowing in one direction only. Thus, HME usage during HFNO is nil.

35.3 Effect of Humidification on Aerosol Drug Delivery

Across all respiratory interventions whether invasive or non-invasive, there are several contributors to aerosol drug delivery performance, such as aerosol device, patient interface, aerosol generator position in the circuit, gas flow rates, and breathing and ventilation parameters that have been shown to affect aerosol drug delivery to the patient lung in the critical care setting [31, 33–39]. However, what remains less clear is whether the hygroscopic growth of aerosol droplets that happens when aerosol is exposed to a humidified patient circuit has an appreciable effect on the dose delivered to the lung. A review of the published literature suggests that there is little consensus between (a) the various published human studies, (b) the chosen respiratory support intervention (e.g., HFNO or MV), and (c) the in vitro bench studies. Selected studies are summarized below in order to inform the readers understanding of the current state of the art.

35.4 Effect on Aerosol Droplet Diameters

Hygroscopic growth of aerosols itself is well described in the literature where, briefly, the greater the temperature and relative humidity, the greater the increase in droplet diameter, and thus the greater the droplet mass (mass median aerodynamic diameter (MMAD)) [40–44]. In relation to aerosol-mediated drug delivery, an increase in droplet and mass increases the ballistic aerosol fraction within the patient circuit that is then more likely to impact and rain out, thus becoming unavailable to the patient for inhalation as an aerosol, or in the case of a spontaneous breathing patient inhaling via mouthpiece, the larger droplets may deposit high up in the respiratory tract [34, 45]. This basic understanding is likely the rationale for HCPs being noted to turn off humification during aerosol therapy.

The timescale for water condensation on a growing droplet can depend not only on the starting droplet size and the rate of gas-phase moisture transport but also on the surface and bulk composition of the droplet [46]. Thus, growth can be controlled to some degree by formulation design, for example, the addition of fatty acids or amphiphilic surfactants [47]. Empirical characterization of the timescale for droplet growth was performed in one study for saline, tobramycin plus saline, and tobramycin alone. Droplets were seen to grow from approximately 1 μm to between 3 and 4 μm (depending on the formulation) within 5–6 s when relative humidity was raised from 50% to 99.5% [48]. This is a significant increase in droplet diameter and such growth, or at least a portion of it is entirely feasible as a droplet is transported down a HH HFNO circuit or the inspiratory limb of a HH mechanical ventilator circuit.

Interestingly, exploitation of hygroscopic growth of therapeutic aerosols for increased aerosol delivery has been proposed. In these systems, small droplets capable of distal distribution within the lung are generated and, as they are exposed to the humid environment of the lung, undergo hygroscopic growth. As a consequence, these now bigger heavier droplets deposit on the lung surface on exhalation [49, 50].

35.5 Spontaneous Breathing: Mouthpiece

A small number of human studies have been published looking at the effect of hygroscopic growth itself and do provide some insight into the combination of humidification and aerosol therapy. One dynamic SPECT study in six spontaneously breathing healthy subjects (no respiratory intervention) assessed the effect of hygroscopic growth on aerosol deposition in the lung. Changes in regional deposition with increasing hygroscopic growth were recorded [51]. In line with the published literature looking at differences in regional deposition with differing droplet sizes, the results in this study revealed significant differences in aerosol deposition resulting from the controlled hygroscopic growth of droplets, thus demonstrating the potential effect of humidification on aerosol therapy [52].

35.6 Spontaneous Breathing: HFNO

To these authors' knowledge, there is no study that has looked directly at the comparative effect of both HH and HME on aerosol droplet size under fully controlled study conditions; however, it has been investigated under HFNO conditions where the gas was both heated and unheated. In that study, the MMAD of the aerosol droplets was significantly higher in the HH condition. With respect to aerosol delivery to the lung, unheated gas was associated with aerosol delivery performance similar to that recorded for heated humidified gas but only at 10 L/min. At higher gas flow rates (30 and 50 L/min), aerosol delivery performance was significantly higher when the gas was unheated [53]. A small preliminary bench study of the effect of humidifier temperature was conducted during HFNO, and no difference was noted in aerosol delivery for two temperatures (34 and 37 °C) when assessed across three gas flow rates (10, 30, and 60 L/min) [54].

35.7 Mechanical Ventilation

There are several published in vitro reports on the impact of humidification on aerosol delivery performance during mechanical ventilation; however, the findings are not all in agreement.

Lin et al. demonstrated on the bench that turning off the humidifier for up to 40 min prior to pMDI administration on ventilator did not increase aerosol delivery [55]. This finding was contrary to that of Lange and Finlay where on ventilator an increase in pMDI MMAD was seen with increasing temperature and relative humidity, resulting in a significant reduction in inhaled mass [43].

Studies directly comparing several different aerosol generator devices in humidified and non-humidified ventilator circuits have also been conducted. These also suggest that in a non-humidified circuit the inhaled dose was greater than that with a humidified circuit, and this was consistent across each of pMDI, ultrasonic nebulizer (USN), JN, and VMN [56].

The effect of HME design has also been assessed. Ari et al. studied the aerosol delivery performance of a VMN when used concurrently with three different types of bypass HME. Results indicate that there was no difference between the CircuVent, Humid-Flo, and AirLife [57]. This in vitro study also looked at the effect of simulated exhaled humidity from the patient in an effort to understand what effects that may have on reported aerosol delivery. It was noted that when simulated exhaled humidity was added to the ventilator circuit, aerosol drug delivery was significantly reduced but more consistent. The authors posit that the simulated exhaled humidity may make the bench setup more consistent with the circuit environment of the real ventilated patient. In another, preliminary bench study, the choice of HME design with varying materials (pleated paper, sponge, filter) was not seen to have a significant effect on the amount of aerosol delivered to the end of the endotracheal tube [58]. Separately, a single study reported the aerosol loss whilst passing through the ThermoFlo was in the order of <40%, with no significant increase in airflow resistance [25]. Considering this finding, it is clear that when assessing the potential effect of the type of humidification (HH or HME), one must also consider the intricacies of the components involved. Here the HME design, not passive humidification, was the cause of the reduced aerosol delivery.

In a randomized crossover design involving 36 asthmatic patients in receipt of mechanical ventilation, urinary salbutamol was used as a measure of the amount of aerosol delivered to the lung under "dry" and "humidified" (HH) conditions. In this study, no significant difference was noted between the two. The authors suggest that in vitro reports overestimate the impact of dry non-humidified versus heated humidified conditions on the delivery of aerosol during invasive mechanical ventilation, thus further undermining the practice of turning the humidifier off [59].

A further study conducted by the same group in 72 asthmatic subjects receiving invasive mechanical ventilation compared VMN to pMDI, under 2 humidity conditions, that is to say, with and without humidification. Results indicated that VMN resulted in a trend to shorter ICU days compared to pMDI and that this trend held for both humidification conditions [60].

Moraine et al. investigated the placement of an USN (a) before the humidifier (which was turned on) and (b) at the end of the inspiratory limb, at the patient wye, with the humidifier turned off during aerosol delivery. In this 38-subject study, the pulmonary bioavailability of ipratropium, assessed by urine concentrations of the drug, was similar for both conditions, suggesting again that in the clinical setting, there may be little beneficial effect in turning off the humidifier [61].

Similar findings were again noted during a study of 48 COPD patients in receipt of single-limb non-invasive ventilation (NIV). Assessing the effect of turning off the humidifier, no difference was seen in the urine levels of salbutamol compared to having the humidifier on [62]. This group also reports no difference in a bench model of single-limb NIV, under three heat and humidification conditions, that is to say, (a) no heat and no humidification, (b) humidification with no-heat, and (c) heat with humidification [63]. Importantly, those findings were replicated in an ex vivo setup wherein subjects inhaled ipratropium via an aerosol capture filter and the potential dose of inhaled ipratropium quantified [62].

A final NIV study in 36 COPD patients in receipt of automatic continuous positive airway pressure (auto-CPAP) looked at the effect of humidification on salbutamol levels in the urine following delivery using VMN, JN, and pMDI. The findings in this study once again recorded no difference in the urinary excreted salbutamol levels post inhalation between the humidified and dry conditions [64].

A summary of the relevant studies relating to the effect of humidification on aerosol therapy is illustrated in Table 35.1.

In summary, studies in invasively and non-invasively mechanically ventilated patients observed no significant difference in the amount of drug delivered to the lung, which is counter to the findings of the study conducted in spontaneously breathing patients and several of the published in vitro and in silico studies. This may suggest that other factors contribute to the experimental findings, such as lack of paired controls for variables such as position of nebulizer in the circuit, the combination of humidification on or off and where the nebulizer is positioned, and the use of simulated exhaled humidity. In addition, variables not discussed here but mentioned in the literature include the pre-conditioning of the circuit for sufficient amounts of time to allow for the HH or HME or un-humidified conditions to reach a point at which they are truly representative of the intended state and experimental setup for each intervention that are consistent with those seen in a clinical practice. Finally, given that the majority of the in vivo and a portion of the in vitro studies suggest that there is no difference in clinical endpoint or reported dose delivered, the practice of turning the humidifier off during aerosol therapy in order to maximize the delivered dose should be reconsidered. Indeed, any potential increase in the efficiency of aerosol delivery must be weighed against the potential deleterious effects of ventilation with under humidified dry gases [65, 66].

Table 35.1 Graphical summary of the findings on the effect of humidification on aerosol therapy reported by studies cited in this chapter. Effect is defined as a statistically significant value in the respective studies

Reference	Study type	Measure	No effect	Effect Humidity	Effect No humidity	p value
Hadrell et al. [40]	In vitro	Droplet size analysis		▬		NS
Peng et al. [42]	In vitro	Droplet size analysis		▬		NS
Lang et al. [43]	In vitro—MV	Predicted delivered dose -pMDI		▬		<0.01
Lin et al. [55]	In vitro—MV	Predicted delivered dose -pMDI	▬			NS
Ari et al. [56]	In vitro—MV	Predicted delivered dose			▬	<0.01
Ari et al. [57]	In vitro—MV	Predicted delivered dose - VMN			▬	<0.01
Ari et al. [57]	In vitro—MV	Predicted delivered dose - exh humidity	▬			>0.5
Batemen et al. (2016)	In vitro—MV	Predicted delivered dose - VMN	▬			0.488
Murphy et al. [38]	In vitro—HFNO	Predicted delivered dose -VMN	▬			>0.5
Saeed et al. [63]	In vitro—NIV	Predicted delivered dose		▬		NS
Chan et al. (2004)	In vivo imaging—tidal	Deposition pattern		▬		NS
Alcoforado [53]	In vivo imaging— HFNO	Lung dose - 30 + 50 LPM			▬	0.015/<0.001
Alcoforado [53]	In vivo imaging— HFNO	Lung dose -10 LPM	▬			0.531
Moustafa et al. [59, 60]	In vivo— human MV	Urinary salbutamol	▬			NS
Moustafa et al. [59, 60]	In vivo— human MV	Urinary salbutamol	▬			<0.5
Moraine et al. [61]	In vivo— human MV	Urinary ipratropium	▬			<0.5
Saeed et al. [62]	In vivo— human NIV	Urinary salbutamol	▬			NS
Abdelrahim et al. [64]	In vivo— human CPAP	Urinary salbutamol	▬			NS

pMDI pressurized metered dose inhaler, *VMN* vibrating mesh nebulizer, *MV* mechanical ventilation, *HFNO* high-flow nasal oxygen, *NIV* non-invasive ventilation, *CPAP* continuous positive airway pressure

References

1. Kacmarek RM, Stoller JK, Heuer AJ, Chatburn RL, Kallet RH. Egan's fundamentals of respiratory care. Amsterdam: Elsevier; 2017.
2. Wilkes AR. Heat and moisture exchangers and breathing system filters: their use in anaesthesia and intensive care. Part 1—history, principles and efficiency. Anaesthesia. 2011;66:31–9.
3. Wilkes AR. Heat and moisture exchangers and breathing system filters: their use in anaesthesia and intensive care. Part 2—practical use, including problems, and their use with paediatric patients. Anaesthesia. 2011;66:40–51.
4. Wilkes AR. The moisture-conserving performance of breathing system filters in use with simulated circle anaesthesia breathing systems. In: Anaesthetic Research Society meeting, Bristol; 1997. https://doi.org/10.1111/j.1365-2044.2004.03613.x.
5. Vargas M, Chiumello D, Sutherasan Y, Ball L, Esquinas AM, Pelosi P, Servillo G. Heat and moisture exchangers (HMEs) and heated humidifiers (HHs) in adult critically ill patients: a systematic review, meta-analysis and meta-regression of randomized controlled trials. Crit Care. 2017;21:1–14.
6. Lacherade JC, Auburtin M, Cerf C, et al. Impact of humidification systems on ventilator-associated pneumonia: a randomized multicenter trial. Am J Respir Crit Care Med. 2012;172:1276–82. https://doi.org/10.1164/rccm200408-1028OC.
7. Lavoie-Bérard CA, Lefebvre JC, Bouchard PA, Simon M, Lellouche F. Impact of airway humidification strategy in mechanically ventilated COVID-19 patients. Respir Care. 2022;67:157–66.
8. Plotnikow GA, Villalba DS, Calvo EP, Quiroga C, Navarro E. Performance of invasive mode in different heated humidification systems with high-flow nasal cannula. Respir Care. 2022.
9. McGrory L, Owen LS, Thio M, Dawson JA, Rafferty AR, Malhotra A, Davis PG, Kamlin COF. A randomized trial of conditioned or unconditioned gases for stabilizing preterm infants at birth. J Pediatr. 2018;193:47–53.
10. Bernatzky A, Galletti MF, Fuensalida SE, Mariani GL. Heated humidifier versus heat-and-moisture exchanger during positive pressure ventilation with a T-piece resuscitator in rabbits. Respir Care. 2020;65:1295–300.
11. Doyle A, Mariyaselvam M, Wijewardena G, English N, Gent E, Young P. The simultaneous use of a heat and moisture exchanger and a heated humidifier causes critical airway occlusion in less than 24 hours. J Crit Care. 2015;30:863.e1–3.
12. Patel V, Mariyaselvam MZA, Peutherer C, Young PJ. Accidental dual humidification in intensive care units: repeated alerts and system changes are not enough. J Crit Care. 2018;47:159–63.
13. Jaber S, Chanques G, Matecki S, Ramonatxo M, Souche B, Perrigault P-F, Eledjam J-J. Non-invasive ventilation. Intensive Care Med. 2002;28:1590–4.
14. Girault C, Breton L, Richard JC, Tamion F, Vandelet P, Aboab J, Leroy J, Bonmarchand G. Mechanical effects of airway humidification devices in difficult to wean patients. Crit Care Med. 2003;31:1306–11.
15. Dugernier J, Wittebole X, Roeseler J, Michotte JB, Sottiaux T, Dugernier T, Laterre PF, Reychler G. Influence of inspiratory flow pattern and nebulizer position on aerosol delivery with a vibrating-mesh nebulizer during invasive mechanical ventilation: an in vitro analysis. J Aerosol Med Pulm Drug Deliv. 2015;28:229–36.
16. Bennett WD, Scheuch G, Zeman KL, Brown JS, Kim C, Heyder J, Stahlhofen W, Ze-Man KL. Bronchial airway deposition and retention of particles in inhaled boluses: effect of anatomic dead space. J Appl Physiol (1985). 1998;85(2):685–94.
17. Ehrmann S, Roche-Campo F, Sferrazza Papa GF, Isabey D, Brochard L, Apiou-Sbirlea G. Aerosol therapy during mechanical ventilation: an international survey. Intensive Care Med. 2013;39:1048–56.
18. Sun Q, Chang W, Liu X, Xie J, Qiu H, Yang Y, Liu L Aerosol therapy during mechanical ventilation in intensive care units: a questionnaire-based survey of 2203 ICU medical staff in China. J Intensive Med. 2022. https://doi.org/10.1016/J.JOINTM.2022.04.003.

19. Li J, Tu M, Yang L, Jing G, Fink JB, Burtin C, de Andrade AD, Gong L, Xie L, Ehrmann S. Worldwide clinical practice of high-flow nasal cannula and concomitant aerosol therapy in the adult ICU setting. Respir Care. 2021;66:1416–24.

20. Joyce M, McGrath JA, Eain MMG, O'Sullivan A, Byrne M, Macloughlin R. Nebuliser type influences both patient-derived bioaerosol emissions and ventilation parameters during mechanical ventilation. Pharmaceutics. 2021;13(2):199. https://doi.org/10.3390/pharmaceutics13020199.

21. Mac Giolla Eain M, Joyce M, MacLoughlin R. An in vitro visual study of fugitive aerosols released during aerosol therapy to an invasively ventilated simulated patient. Drug Deliv. 2021;28:1496–500. https://doi.org/10.1080/10717544.2021.1951893.

22. Fink JB, Ehrmann S, Li J, et al. Reducing aerosol-related risk of transmission in the era of COVID-19: an interim guidance endorsed by the International Society of Aerosols in Medicine. J Aerosol Med Pulm Drug Deliv. 2020;33:300–4.

23. Cinesi Gómez C, Peñuelas Rodríguez Ó, Luján Torné M, et al. Recomendaciones de consenso respecto al soporte respiratorio no invasivo en el paciente adulto con insuficiencia respiratoria aguda secundaria a infección por SARS-CoV-2. Archivos de Bronconeumología. 2020;56:11–8.

24. Respiratory Care Committee of Chinese Thoracic Society. Expert consensus on preventing nosocomial transmission during respiratory care for critically ill patients infected by 2019 novel coronavirus pneumonia. Zhonghua Jie He He Hu Xi Za Zhi. 2020;43:288–96.

25. British Thoracic Society COVID-19: information for the respiratory community | British Thoracic Society | Better lung health for all. https://www.brit-thoracic.org.uk/covid-19/covid-19-information-for-the-respiratory-community/. Accessed 2 Aug 2022.

26. Halpin DMG, Criner GJ, Papi A, Singh D, Anzueto A, Martinez FJ, Agusti AA, Vogelmeier CF. Global initiative for the diagnosis, management, and prevention of chronic obstructive lung disease. The 2020 GOLD Science Committee report on COVID-19 and chronic obstructive pulmonary disease. Am J Respir Crit Care Med. 2021;203:24–36.

27. Kumar P, Kulkarni AP, Govil D, Dixit SB, Chaudhry D, Samavedam S, Zirpe KG, Bn Gopal P, Kar A. Airway management and related procedures in critically ill COVID-19 patients: position statement of the Indian Society of Critical Care Medicine. Indian J Crit Care Med. 2020;24(8):630–42. https://doi.org/10.5005/jp-journals-10071-23471.

28. Federazione delle Associazioni dei Dirigenti Ospedalieri Internisti. COVID-19 | GUIDA CLINICO-PRATICA FADOI FADOI è orgogliosa di presentare la Guida Clinico-Pratica sull'infezione da SARS-CoV-2 in italiano, completa di bibliografia, a cura del Gruppo Giovani FADOI.

29. Jiang Z, Liang H, Peng G, Wang S, Zhang B, Sun Q, Xu Y, Zeng H, Huang J. Effect of IFN-α and other commonly used nebulization drugs in different nebulization methods on the resistance of breathing circuit filters under invasive mechanical ventilation. Ann Transl Med. 2022;10:189.

30. Kelly P, O'Sullivan A, Sweeney L, MacLoughlin R. Assessment of passive humidifier performance following on-ventilator aerosol therapy. In: 5.1 airway pharmacology and treatment. European Respiratory Society; 2016. p. PA956.

31. Li J, Fink JB, MacLoughlin R, Dhand R. A narrative review on trans-nasal pulmonary aerosol delivery. Crit Care. 2020;24:506.

32. Miller AG, Gentile MA, Tyler LM, Napolitano N. High-flow nasal cannula in pediatric patients: a survey of clinical practice. Respir Care. 2018;63:894–9.

33. Bennett G, Joyce M, Sweeney L, MacLoughlin R. In vitro study of the effect of breathing pattern on aerosol delivery during high-flow nasal therapy. Pulm Ther. 2019;5(1):43–54. https://doi.org/10.1007/s41030-019-0086-x.

34. Bennett G, Joyce M, Sweeney L, MacLoughlin R. In vitro determination of the main effects in the design of high-flow nasal therapy systems with respect to aerosol performance. Pulm Ther. 2018;4(1):73–86. https://doi.org/10.1007/s41030-018-0054-x.

35. Naughton PJ, Joyce M, Mac Giolla Eain M, O'Sullivan A, MacLoughlin R. Evaluation of aerosol drug delivery options during adult mechanical ventilation in the COVID-19 era. Pharmaceutics. 2021;13:1574.

36. Berlinski A, Randy Willis J. Albuterol delivery by 4 different nebulizers placed in 4 different positions in a pediatric ventilator in vitro model. Respir Care. 2013;58:1124–33.
37. Bennett G, Joyce M, Fernández EF, MacLoughlin R. Comparison of aerosol delivery across combinations of drug delivery interfaces with and without concurrent high-flow nasal therapy. Intensive Care Med Exp. 2019;7:20.
38. Murphy B, Eain MMG, Joyce M, Fink JB, MacLoughlin R. Evaluation of aerosol drug delivery with concurrent low and high flow nasal oxygen. ERJ Open Res. 2022;8(4):00220-02022.
39. Fernández Fernández E, Joyce M, O'Sullivan A, MacLoughlin R. Evaluation of aerosol therapy during the escalation of care in a model of adult cystic fibrosis. Antibiotics. 2021;10:472.
40. Hadrell AE, Davies JF, Miles REH, Reid JP, Dailey LA, Murnane D. Dynamics of aerosol size during inhalation: hygroscopic growth of commercial nebulizer formulations. Int J Pharm. 2014;463:50–61.
41. Li L, Sun S, Parumasivam T, Denman JA, Gengenbach T, Tang P, Mao S, Chan HK. L-Leucine as an excipient against moisture on in vitro aerosolization performances of highly hygroscopic spray-dried powders. Eur J Pharm Biopharm. 2016;102:132–41.
42. Peng C, Chow AHL, Chan CK. Study of the hygroscopic properties of selected pharmaceutical aerosols using single particle levitation. Pharm Res. 2000;17(9):1104–9.
43. Lange CF, Finlay WH. Overcoming the adverse effect of humidity in aerosol delivery via pressurized metered-dose inhalers during mechanical ventilation. Am J Respir Crit Care Med. 2000;161(5):1614–8.
44. Haddrell AE, Lewis D, Church T, Vehring R, Murnane D, Reid JP. Pulmonary aerosol delivery and the importance of growth dynamics. Ther Deliv. 2017;8:1051–61.
45. Legh-Land V, Haddrell AE, Lewis D, Murnane D, Reid JP. Water uptake by evaporating pMDI aerosol prior to inhalation affects both regional and total deposition in the respiratory system. Pharmaceutics. 2021;13:941.
46. Davies JF, Haddrell AE, Miles REH, Bull CR, Reid JP. Bulk, surface, and gas-phase limited water transport in aerosol. J Phys Chem A. 2012;116:10987–98.
47. Hickey AJ, Martonen TB. Behavior of hygroscopic pharmaceutical aerosols and the influence of hydrophobic additives. Pharm Res. 1993;10:1–7.
48. Rovelli G, Miles REH, Reid JP, Clegg SL. Accurate measurements of aerosol hygroscopic growth over a wide range in relative humidity. J Phys Chem A. 2016;120:4376–88.
49. Son Y-J, Longest PW, Tian G, Hindle M. Evaluation and modification of commercial dry powder inhalers for the aerosolization of a submicrometer excipient enhanced growth (EEG) formulation. Eur J Pharm Sci. 2013;49:390–9.
50. Worth Longest P, Tian G. Development of a new technique for the efficient delivery of aerosolized medications to infants on mechanical ventilation. Pharm Res. 2015;32:321–36.
51. Chan H-K, Eberl S, Daviskas E, Constable C, Young I. Changes in lung deposition of aerosols due to hygroscopic growth: a fast SPECT study. J Aerosol Med. 2002;15:307–11.
52. Usmani OS, Biddiscombe MF, Barnes PJ. Regional lung deposition and bronchodilator response as a function of β_2-agonist particle size. Am J Respir Crit Care Med. 2005;172:1497–504.
53. Alcoforado L, Ari A, Barcelar J, Brandão S, Fink J, de Andrade A. Impact of gas flow and humidity on trans-nasal aerosol deposition via nasal cannula in adults: a randomized cross-over study. Pharmaceutics. 2019;11:320.
54. Murphy B, O'Sullivan O, Bennett G, Fernández Fernández E, MacLoughlin R. P16 effect of humidifier temperature during high flow nasal therapy on concurrent aerosol drug delivery with a vibrating mesh nebuliser. In: Clinical developments in non-invasive ventilation and sleep. London: BMJ Publishing Group Ltd and British Thoracic Society; 2021. p. A75.1.
55. Lin H-L, Fink JB, Faarc R, Zhou Y, Cheng Y-S. Influence of moisture accumulation in inline spacer on delivery of aerosol using metered-dose inhaler during mechanical ventilation. Respir Care. 2009;54(10):1336–41.
56. Ari A, Areabi H, Fink JB. Evaluation of aerosol generator devices at 3 locations in humidified and non-humidified circuits during adult mechanical ventilation. Respir Care. 2010;55:837–44.

57. Ari A, Alwadeai KS, Fink JB. Effects of heat and moisture exchangers and exhaled humidity on aerosol deposition in a simulated ventilator-dependent adult lung model. Respir Care. 2017;62:538–43.
58. Bateman RM, Sharpe MD, Jagger JE, et al. 35th international symposium on intensive care and emergency medicine. Crit Care. 2015;19(Suppl 1):P1–P578.
59. Moustafa IOF, Ali MRAA, Al Hallag M, Rabea H, Fink JB, Dailey P, Abdelrahim MEA. Lung deposition and systemic bioavailability of different aerosol devices with and without humidification in mechanically ventilated patients. Heart Lung. 2017;46:464–7.
60. Moustafa IOF, ElHansy MHE, Al Hallag M, Fink JB, Dailey P, Rabea H, Abdelrahim MEA. Clinical outcome associated with the use of different inhalation method with and without humidification in asthmatic mechanically ventilated patients. Pulm Pharmacol Ther. 2017;45:40–6.
61. Moraine J-J, Truflandier K, Vandenbergen N, Berré J, Mélot C, Vincent J-L. Placement of the nebulizer before the humidifier during mechanical ventilation: effect on aerosol delivery. Heart Lung. 2009;38:435–9.
62. Saeed H, Mohsen M, Salah Eldin A, Elberry AA, Hussein RR, Rabea H, Abdelrahim ME. Effects of fill volume and humidification on aerosol delivery during single-limb noninvasive ventilation. Respir Care. 2018;63:1370–8.
63. Saeed H, Mohsen M, Fink JB, Dailey P, Salah Eldin A, Abdelrahman MM, Elberry AA, Rabea H, Hussein RRS, Abdelrahim MEA. Fill volume, humidification and heat effects on aerosol delivery and fugitive emissions during noninvasive ventilation. J Drug Deliv Sci Technol. 2017;39:372–8.
64. Abdelrahim M. Effects of heat and humidification on aerosol delivery during auto-CPAP noninvasive ventilation. Arch Pulmonol Respir Care. 2017;3:011–5.
65. Sottiaux TM. Consequences of under- and over-humidification. Respir Care Clin N Am. 2006;12:233–52.
66. Branson RD, Faarc R, Gentile MA. Is humidification always necessary during noninvasive ventilation in the hospital? Respir Care. 2010;55:209.

Airway Clearance in Critically Ill Patients

36

Joana Almeida Borges

Abbreviations

COPD	Chronic obstructive pulmonary disease
DNA	Deoxyribonucleic acid
FiO_2	Fraction of inspired oxygen
HFCWO	High-frequency chest wall oscillation
I/E	Inspiratory/expiratory
ICU	Intensive care unit
IPV	Intrapulmonary percussive ventilation
LVR	Lung volume recruitment
MI-E	Mechanical insufflation-exsufflation
NAC	*N*-acetylcysteine
PEEP	Positive end-expiratory pressure
PEF	Peak expiratory flow
PEP	Positive expiratory pressure
PIF	Peak inspiratory flow

36.1 Introduction

Airway clearance techniques for critically ill patients improve mucociliary clearance, and their role is not well defined.

Mucociliary dysfunction in patients requiring mechanical ventilation occurs for multiple direct and indirect mechanisms, including anesthetic medications,

J. A. Borges (✉)
Pulmonology Department, Centro Hospitalar e Universitário de Coimbra, Coimbra, Portugal

© The Author(s), under exclusive license to Springer Nature Switzerland AG 2023

A. M. Esquinas (ed.), *Humidification in the Intensive Care Unit*,
https://doi.org/10.1007/978-3-031-23953-3_36

epithelial damage from endotracheal tube cuffs, lack of humidification, high FiO_2, inflammation, immobility, and/or atelectasis. Cough is also impaired by expiratory muscle weakness and the mechanically prevented glottic closure by the endotracheal tube [1, 2].

Flow bias becomes a major mechanism responsible for airway clearance in the absence of cough. In mechanically ventilated patients, peak inspiratory flow (PIF) is usually greater than peak expiratory flow (PEF) which creates an inspiratory flow bias and leads mucus into the lungs [3].

Data supporting the use of these therapies in the mechanically ventilated patients is limited and mainly based on expert opinions.

Mucus clearance therapies in this population aim to break the cycle of chronic inflammation and prevent extubation failures. They include both pharmacological and non-pharmacological therapies and are divided into mucoactive and cough augmentation strategies [1].

36.2 Mucoactive Therapies

These therapies are grouped into expectorants and mucolytics, which are used to hydrate and decrease the viscosity of mucus and to increase cough.

There are also mucoregulators (like carbocisteine) that decrease the production of mucus and mucokinetics (like ambroxol) that work by increasing mucus transport by acting on the cilia [4].

They can be used in patients requiring mechanical ventilation, particularly those with excessive secretions and whose extubation is approaching, and in combination to improve results. Their routine use in ICU patients is not supported by the literature [1, 5], and they cause no significant adverse events [6].

Mucoactive agents showed no effect on the duration of mechanical ventilation, hospital stay, days without ventilation, and mortality, but they reduced the ICU length of stay [4].

36.2.1 *N*-acetylcysteine (NAC)

Nebulized NAC works like a mucolytic by cutting the disulfide bonds that link the mucin oligomers. It can increase the risk of bronchospasm because of its acidic pH, so lower concentrations of NAC should be used or used after bronchodilatation [1, 5, 6].

36.2.2 Dornase Alfa

Dornase alfa has been used as a mucolytic and is an enzyme that cleaves DNA polymers. This therapy demonstrated a decrease in the duration of mechanical ventilation, ICU length of stay, and atelectasis. It showed no difference in reintubation rate [1, 5].

36.2.3 Hypertonic Saline

Nebulized hypertonic saline functions as a mucolytic and an expectorant. This therapy works by increasing water content [4] and has shown to reduce mechanical ventilation time [1].

36.3 Cough Augmentation Strategies

In mechanically ventilated patients, impaired cough and secretion clearance are of prognostic importance as they are associated with a higher risk of extubation failure.

Cough augmentation techniques are mostly indicated to secretion clearance. Pneumothorax and rib fracture were the most frequent absolute contraindications for mechanical insufflation-exsufflation and manually assisted cough, respectively. Mucus plugging requiring tracheostomy inner cannula change was the most common complication of these methods [7] (Table 36.1).

The types of interfaces depend on the method used and can either be applied noninvasively through a mask or mouthpiece or invasively through a tracheostomy or endotracheal tube [7].

In patients undergoing invasive mechanical ventilation, the combination of techniques (like manual hyperinflation, postural drainage, and endotracheal suction) has demonstrated beneficial effects [8].

Table 36.1 Indications, contraindications, and complications for cough augmentation strategies

Indications	Absolute and relative contraindications	Complications
– Secretion clearance	– Pneumothorax	– Mucus plugging requiring tracheostomy inner cannula change
– Weaning from invasive mechanical ventilation	– Rib fracture	– Chest pain
– Weaning from noninvasive ventilation	– Increased intracranial pressure	– Hypotension
– Prevent reintubation	– Recent thoracic or abdominal surgery	– Arrhythmias
– Prevent intubation	– Hemoptysis	– Mucus plugging requiring endotracheal tube change
	– Nausea and vomiting	– Pneumothorax or pneumomediastinum
	– Impaired consciousness	– Hemoptysis
	– Bullous emphysema	
	– Severe asthma and COPD	

36.3.1 Mechanical Insufflation-Exsufflation (MI-E)

MI-E is a method of airway clearance that simulates the airflow characteristics of a natural cough: a deep inspiration with positive pressure, followed by a rapid and forced negative pressure exsufflation that moves secretions for suctioning.

There are a number of devices commercially available, and they are designed for intermittent use. Maximal inspiratory and expiratory pressures as well as inhalation, pause, and exhalation times (Ti, Tp, and Te) are previously selected to obtain an effective expiratory flow [9].

It has been recommended for use in patients mechanically ventilated with signs of secretion retention and with a weak cough (peak cough flow <160 L/min) to facilitate weaning or to reduce the risk of reintubation. The use of these devices improved lung compliance [2, 3].

Mucus plugging requiring tracheostomy inner cannula change is the most frequent complication.

A cough sequence is the continuous application of several cough cycles (Ti + Tp + Te), usually between 8 and 12 cycles. Between each cough sequence, an interval of 2 min is recommended. MI-E should be applied at least three times per day and whenever the patient needs it [9].

36.3.2 Manually Assisted Cough

This method provides increased air compression in the lungs by applying a timed abdominal or costal thrust to the glottic opening. Chest pain is a frequent complication, and manually assisted cough implies specific knowledge [7].

36.3.3 Lung Volume Recruitment (LVR)

LVR (also termed air-stacking) consists of an insufflation of the lungs without exhalation until maximum insufflation capacity, either via the ventilator or an adapted resuscitation bag with a one-way valve [10].

The increased end-inspiratory volume aims at assisting with secretion removal by promoting cough effectiveness [2, 3]. It has a low rate of hemodynamic and respiratory adverse events, hypotension being the most frequent.

Ventilator hyperinflation is preferable to manual hyperinflation because it avoids positive end-expiratory pressure (PEEP) loss, and hypoxemia [8].

36.3.4 High-Frequency Chest Wall Oscillation (HFCWO)

HFCWO vest involves an external oscillatory compression of the chest wall leading to expiratory flows that exceed inspiratory flows.

In mechanically ventilated patients, it improved mucus clearance and oxygenation and decreased atelectasis and peak airway pressures after its use [1].

36.3.5 Oscillatory Positive Expiratory Pressure

Positive expiratory pressure (PEP) therapies include intrapulmonary percussive ventilation (IPV) and unassisted modalities like flutter valves and acapella devices.

IPV is a non-continuous form of high-frequency ventilation (60–600 cycles/min) delivered by a pneumatic device that provides quick bursts of sub-physiological tidal breaths. High-frequency breaths and larger expiratory flow create shear forces that cause dislodgement of the airway secretions [11].

The total recommended treatment time is up to 20 min to reduce the risk of hyperventilation. Parameters that determine IPV include working pressure, percussion frequency, I/E ratio, and proximal pressure [9].

IPV was associated with improvement of oxygenation and lung compliance and lower ICU length of stay and incidence of respiratory infections in critically ill patients [2, 8].

Expiratory resistance devices with a one-way valve provide a constant pressure during expiration. Exhaled air causes vibrations within the device that are transmitted to the lung and promote bronchial drainage of secretions [1].

36.3.6 Manual Percussion

Manual percussion of the chest wall during expiration in mechanically ventilated patients is used to move secretions from distal to more proximal areas (central airways). It can be associated with postural drainage to improve oxygenation and lung compliance [2, 8].

A summary of pros and cons of the previously described techniques is shown in Table 36.2.

Table 36.2 Pros and cons of some cough augmentation strategies

Technique	Pros	Cons
Mechanical insufflation-exsufflation	– Prevention of reintubation	– Expensive
	– Better and faster airway clearance	– May be deleterious for patients at risk of lung collapse (i.e., high PEEP levels) or severe hypoxemia
	– Preferred by patients to suction	
Manually assisted cough	– Reduced the need of suction	– Implies trained nurses
	– Easy technique to teach	
Lung volume recruitment	– Low cost	– Implies trained personnel
	– Simple technique	
	– Improved oxygenation and static lung compliance	
	– Low rate of hemodynamic repercussions	
Unassisted positive expiratory pressure therapies (PEP)	– Low cost	
	– Preferred by patients with postural drainage and percussion	
Intrapulmonary percussive ventilation	– Improved oxygenation and expiratory muscle performance	– Expensive
Manual percussion	– Improved ventilation	– Implies some pain and anxiety
	– Reduced airway obstruction and atelectasis	– Increase of oxygen consumption
	– Preferred by patients with PEP	– Atelectasis and bronchoconstriction as adverse effects

36.4 Postural Drainage

This technique consists in facilitating the movement of secretions within the bronchial tree due to the force of gravity, placing the patient in different positions.

Its use optimizes oxygenation and ventilation/perfusion, increases lung volume, reduces respiratory work, and minimizes cardiac work [8].

Patient positioning (e.g., semi-recumbent position) can be a strategy to reduce the risk of secondary respiratory bacterial infections [12].

36.5   Endotracheal Suction

Endotracheal suction is a standard-of-care method for clearing airway secretions and stimulates coughing in ventilated patients. Instillation of 0.9% saline by the endotracheal tube before suction is helpful by loosening secretions and decreasing its viscosity [5].

It has limited efficacy since it is only able to aspirate secretions up to mainstem bronchi [2]. It is therefore reasonable to first perform other techniques to mobilize secretions from peripheral to central airways [10].

Closed suction systems may be preferable due to their efficiency and the reduced number of suction-induced complications.

This technique is considered a measure to prevent ventilator-associated pneumonia [8] and has also shortened the duration of mechanical ventilation [12]. However, it can cause scarring and bleeding of the tracheal mucosa and precipitate oxygen desaturation, hemodynamic instability, and increased intracranial pressure.

36.6   Other Therapies

Adequate heating and humidifying inspiratory gas are also important for mucociliary clearance [2].

Macrolide and inhaled antibiotics are therapies used to directly target inflammation and infection that are poorly studied to help mucus clearance in this population [1].

36.7   Conclusion

The impaired mechanisms of airway clearance in critically ill patients are mucociliary transport and cough. Therapies include mucoactive and cough augmentation strategies.

More evidence regarding the efficacy and safety of airway clearance techniques in critically ill patients is needed. Combination therapy offers the best results in this group of patients.

These techniques could improve extubation protocols and prevent reintubation in critically ill patients with ineffective cough.

References

1. Goetz RL, Vijaykumar K, Solomon GM. Mucus clearance strategies in mechanically ventilated patients. Front Physiol. 2022;13:834716.
2. Makhabah DN, Ambrosino N. Airway clearance in the intensive care unit. EMJ Respir. 2013;1:135–9.

3. Volpe MS, Guimarães FS, Morais CCA. Airway clearance techniques for mechanically ventilated patients: insights for optimization. Respir Care. 2020;65(8):1174–88.
4. Anand R, McAuley DF, Blackwood B, et al. Mucoactive agents for acute respiratory failure in the critically ill: a systematic review and meta-analysis. Thorax. 2020;75:623–63.
5. Papacostas MF, Luckett P, Hupp S. The use of pulmonary clearance medications in the acutely ill patient. Expert Rev Respir Med. 2017;11(10):815–26.
6. Tarrant BJ, Maitre C, Romero L, et al. Mucoactive agents for adults with acute lung conditions: a systematic review. Heart Lung. 2018;48(2):141–7.
7. Rose L, Adhikari NK, Poon J, et al. Cough augmentation techniques in the critically ill: a Canadian National Survey. Respir Care. 2016;61(10):1360–8.
8. Goñi-Viguria R, Yoldi-Arzoz E, Casajús-Sola L, et al. Fisioterapia respiratoria en la unidad de cuidados intensivos: Revisión bibliográfica. Enferm Intensiva. 2018;29(4):168–81.
9. Fernández-Carmona A, Olivencia-Peña L, Yuste-Ossorio ME, et al. Tos ineficaz y técnicas mecánicas de aclaramiento mucociliar. Med Intensiva. 2018;42(1):50–9.
10. Pathmanathan N, Beaumont N, Gratrix A. Respiratory physiotherapy in the critical care unit. Contin Educ Anaesth Crit Care Pain. 2015;15(1):20–5.
11. Hassan A, Lai W, Alison J, et al. Effect of intrapulmonary percussive ventilation on intensive care unit length of stay, the incidence of pneumonia and gas exchange in critically ill patients: a systematic review. PLoS One. 2021;16(7):e0255005.
12. Battaglinia D, Robbaa C, Caiffa S, et al. Chest physiotherapy: an important adjuvant in critically ill mechanically ventilated patients with COVID-19. Respir Physiol Neurobiol. 2020;282:103529.

Airway Clearance in Tracheostomized Patients

37

Maria Barbagallo and Eleonora Schiappa

Abbreviations

cmH_2O	Centimeters of water
CPT	Chest physical therapy
d	Day
EFA	Expiratory flow accelerator
ETS	Endotracheal suctioning
FET	Force expiratory technique
FiO_2	Fraction of inspired oxygen
h	Hours
ICP	Intracranial pressure
ICU	Intensive care unit
IPV	Intrapulmonary percussive ventilation
LCI	Lung collapse index
MH	Manual hyperinflation
MI-E	Mechanical insufflation-exsufflation
min	Minutes
PaO_2	Arterial oxygen partial
PaO_2/FiO_2 ratio	Ratio of arterial oxygen partial pressure (PaO_2 in mmHg) to fractional inspired oxygen (FiO_2 expressed as a fraction, not a percentage)
PEEP	Positive end-expiratory pressure
PEP	Positive expiratory pressure
RCT	Randomized controlled trial

M. Barbagallo (✉) · E. Schiappa
Department of Anesthesiology and Critical Care, University Hospital of Parma, Parma, Italy
e-mail: mbarbagallo@ao.pr.it; eschiappa@ao.pr.it

© The Author(s), under exclusive license to Springer Nature Switzerland AG 2023

A. M. Esquinas (ed.), *Humidification in the Intensive Care Unit*,
https://doi.org/10.1007/978-3-031-23953-3_37

37.1 Introduction

Tracheotomy has become a routine procedure in intensive care units (ICUs) [1]. Tracheostomy is associated with loss of moistening and warming of inhaled air from the upper airways, and this often correlates with reduced patient mobility, impaired chest movements, reduced ventilation, and impaired/ineffective cough. As a result of these changes, there is an increased mucus production in the airways with an inability to remove the secretions by the patient [1].

Mechanically ventilated patients present increased mucus production and impairment of mucociliary clearance owing to the mechanical effect of artificial airways, high fractions of inspired oxygen, lesions caused by tracheal suctioning, inadequate humidification, and drugs (including paralyzing agents) [2–4]. Relative immobility of the mechanically ventilated patient confined to bed can lead to atelectasis, impaired cough, and retained secretions [1]. Finally, muscle weakness associated with prolonged ICU stay may also contribute to secretion retention [1].

The care of these patients involves the need for frequent daily aspirations through the tracheostomy cannula [1]. Endotracheal suctioning (ETS) is one of the most common procedures performed in patients with artificial airways [3]. It involves the mechanical aspiration of pulmonary secretions from an artificial airway to prevent its obstruction [3, 5]. There are several modes of aspiration including open-circuit suction, closed-circuit suction, and minimally invasive (shallow) or deep suctioning [1]. However, this procedure is invasive and unpleasant, with risk of side effects (e.g., injury to the airway mucosa), and it requires the intervention of trained nursing staff and/or a dedicated caregiver [1].

Airflow obstruction secondary to retained secretions increases the work of breathing, produces ventilation-perfusion mismatch, and can result in gas exchange abnormalities. Retained secretions can serve as a source of infection and inflammation [6]. Thus, respiratory care and physiotherapy are important components in the treatment of critically ill patients [6]. In particular, early intervention may prove effective in avoiding complications and improving the prognosis for patients admitted to ICUs [7].

Secretion management in the mechanically ventilated patient consists primarily of adequate humidification, airway suctioning, and mobilization [3, 6]. When these routine methods fail, a variety of interventions are used to enhance airway clearance with the goal of improving lung mechanics and gas exchange and preventing atelectasis and infection [8].

Conventional chest physical therapy (CPT) is frequently used, and it can be applied to the intubated patient. It includes postural drainage, percussion, vibration, continuous rotational therapy, and manual hyperinflation (MH) [6]. More recently, several alternatives to these conventional techniques have been developed. These include positive expiratory pressure (PEP), flutter valve, intrapulmonary percussive ventilation, and high-frequency chest wall oscillation [7]. Assisted mucus-clearing techniques are also usually performed daily and include Free Aspire and mechanical insufflation-exsufflation [7].

37.2   Discussion and Analysis Main Topic

37.2.1 Conventional Chest Physiotherapy

Chest physiotherapy is one of the most frequently performed interventions in the intensive care unit and is considered important to achieve successful weaning from the ventilator [9]. Several physiotherapy techniques are used to facilitate an adequate bronchial drainage in these patients, mainly depending on the patient's compliance and staff expertise [9]. One of the primary objectives of chest physiotherapy is to improve airway clearance [1].

37.2.1.1   Postural Drainage

Postural drainage comprises the promotion of bronchial drainage by making use of gravity [10]. The potential positions are determined by the individual clinical problem because the movement and mobilization of an intubated patient in the ICU are restricted by the presence of various drains and lines connected to the patient. For this reason it is sometimes difficult to place such a patient in the correct postural drainage position for the specific area of the lung that requires drainage [10].

37.2.1.2   Continuous Rotational Therapy

Continuous rotational therapy refers to the use of specialized beds that continuously and slowly turn a patient along the longitudinal axis, up to an angle of 60° onto each side, with the degree and speed of rotation pre-programmed [5]. The therapy is achieved by the entire platform of the bed rotating (also known as kinetic therapy) or by the inflation and deflation of compartments in the mattress (also known as oscillating beds). The rationale for the use of continuous rotational therapy is that it will prevent dependent airway closure, atelectasis, and stagnation of pulmonary secretions, including subsequent infection that are believed to result from prolonged immobility [5].

There is abundant literature on the use of rotating beds designed to prevent ventilator-associated pneumonia and treat atelectasis [3]. However, the study of these beds' effect on secretion clearance has been limited. Davis et al. compared secretion clearance, lung mechanics, and gas exchange in paralyzed patients with acute respiratory distress syndrome randomized to receive manual turning, manual turning with percussion and postural drainage, continuous lateral rotation or continuous lateral rotation with percussion, and postural drainage performed by the pneumatic cushions of the bed. Each of 20 patients received each treatment, in a randomized order, for 6 h. The combination of continuous lateral rotation and percussion and postural drainage produced more secretions in this small group of paralyzed patients, but no other benefit was identified [11].

37.2.1.3   Percussion and Vibration

The literature on percussion and vibration in mechanically ventilated patients is poor [3]. Percussions may be performed manually (using cupped hands) by clapping the chest wall over the affected area of the lung [3, 5, 9]. Vibrations may be applied manually or via mechanical devices by vibrating, shaking, or compressing the chest wall during the expiratory phase [3]. These techniques are believed to increase clearance of airway secretions by the transmission of an energy wave through the chest wall [9]. In the mechanically ventilated patient with retained secretions, chest clapping is supposed to mechanically loose secretions [3]. There is no known mechanism by which percussion can improve atelectasis, unless it is by removal of mucus plugs. In an RCT that included mechanically ventilated ICU subjects, Chen and colleagues compared mechanical chest vibration (via vibration pad used in supine position, 60 min/session, 6 times/day over 72 h) plus routine positioning in 50 subjects, to routine positioning alone in 45 subjects. The differences in sputum weight were significant between groups, with greater sputum in the intervention group. The lung collapse index of the vibration group was significantly improved, compared with the positioning group at 72 h [4].

37.2.1.4 Manual and Ventilator Hyperinflation

Manual hyperinflation (MH) involves delivering tidal volumes to airway pressures of 40 cmH_2O or a tidal volume (TV) that is 50% greater than that delivered by the ventilator. This is followed by a quick release of pressure on expiration, leading to a rapid flow of air, simulating the effect of a cough [5, 9]. Ventilator hyperinflation is achieved by altering the ventilatory settings to gradually increase tidal volume. It may produce the same effects as manual hyperinflation whilst maintaining the PEEP level and controlling airway pressure limits [12]. Hyperinflation is used with the aim of preventing pulmonary collapse, re-expanding collapsed alveoli, improving oxygenation and lung compliance, and increasing movement of pulmonary secretions toward the central airways [9]. It is not without risk, so it is recommended that during MH, airway pressure and/or TV be monitored, in addition to hemodynamic status, because high airway pressure and large lung volumes produce adverse hemodynamic effects and can injure the lung via barotrauma and/or volutrauma [3]. Contraindications include severe bronchospasm, pneumothorax, and increased intracranial pressure [5]. Physiotherapists have used manual hyperinflation for many years for mobilizing excess pulmonary secretions, reinflating areas of atelectasis, and improving oxygenation. Several studies have shown improved compliance and oxygenation after manual hyperinflation, but the findings about changes in secretion volume have been inconsistent [3].

Although manual hyperinflation has been shown to be an effective technique in the management of intubated patients, it has several limitations [12]. These include disconnection of the patient from the ventilator resulting in loss of PEEP, poor control of airway pressure and flow, and the fraction of inspired oxygen being 1.0. These limitations are eliminated with ventilator hyperinflation. Berney et al. found that hyperinflation using the ventilator is as effective as manual hyperinflation in clearing excess pulmonary secretions and improving static pulmonary compliance [12].

Ventilator hyperinflation was found to be as good as manual hyperinflation in sputum clearance and improving static pulmonary compliance. This suggests that both should be equally effective in treating atelectasis [12].

37.2.2 Alternative Techniques

Over the last few years, new medical devices have become available on the market to facilitate the ascent of the secretions from the lower airways [1]. Proposed mechanisms of action of these devices include a decrease in the viscoelastic properties of mucus and the creation of short bursts of increased expiratory flow acceleration that assist mucus clearance [6].

37.2.2.1 PEP

PEP was first developed as an airway clearance technique in Denmark in the 1970s. PEP devices can be categorized as low-pressure devices (5–20 cmH$_2$O at mid-exhalation) and high-pressure devices (26–102 cmH$_2$O via forced expiratory maneuvers after maximal inspiration) [6]. Oscillatory PEP was first developed in Switzerland as the flutter device, but there are now similar devices from other manufacturers, such as Acapella and Quake.

37.2.2.2 Flutter Valve

The flutter valve (Varioraw SARL, Scandipharm Inc, Birmingham, AL) is shaped like a pipe with a hardened plastic mouthpiece at one end, a plastic protective, perforated cover at the other end, and a high-density stainless steel ball resting on a plastic circular cone under the perforated cover. When the patient exhales through the flutter, the steel sphere moves up and down inside the pipe, generating oscillations in expiratory pressure and airflow that vibrate the airway walls, probably diminishing the mucus adhesiveness and decreasing the collapsibility of the airways and accelerating airflow [2]. Exhaling through the device creates oscillations in the airway, the frequency of which can be modulated by changing the inclination of the pipe [8].

This device was initially designed to assist the removal of bronchial secretions in patients with cystic fibrosis. Because of the low cost and ease of implementation of the flutter valve, it has been largely used in respiratory therapy outpatient services and mechanically ventilated patients to treat a range of pulmonary hyper-secretive conditions [2].

In a crossover RCT that included 20 mechanically ventilated subjects with pulmonary infection and hypersecretion in an adult ICU, Chicayban et al. compared flutter to normal-pressure controlled ventilation [2]. The subjects received normal ventilation or two 15-min sessions of flutter, separated by a 6-h wash-out period. At follow-up immediately after the intervention, secretion production and static compliance were greater in the flutter group. The most accepted explanation for the higher compliance observed after the application of flutter valve is the displacement of secretions from the peripheral airway to more central areas, promoting the expansion/recruitment of collapsed units [2]. According to Volsko et al., positive pressure oscillations produce abrupt variations in the airway caliber, reducing the adherence of secretions to the bronchial wall and favoring their detachment and displacement. Furthermore, the increase in lung distention pressure promotes the expansion of poor ventilated or collapsed areas. This expansive effect increases collateral ventilation, surfactant renewal, and expiratory flow, yielding a better gas-liquid interaction [2].

Contrary to manual hyperinflation, this method does not require the patient's disconnection from the ventilator, thus avoiding the exposure of airways, interruption of ventilation and ventilatory monitoring, and collapse of airspaces. The coupling of the flutter valve to the expiratory port of the ventilator is a more practical procedure than some ventilator-induced hyperinflation protocols. However, its adjustment to the expiratory circuit of some ventilators may be difficult, and care should be taken to avoid auto-triggering because of abrupt expiratory flow variations [2].

37.2.2.3 Intrapulmonary Percussive Ventilation and High-Frequency Chest Wall Oscillation

Intrapulmonary and high-frequency chest wall oscillation techniques were presented by Rob Chatburn [6]. The available technologies in this category include intrapulmonary percussive ventilation, high-frequency chest wall compression, and high-frequency chest wall oscillation [6]. The potential mechanisms of action for intrapulmonary and high-frequency chest wall oscillation techniques include air-liquid shear forces (multiple "mini coughs"), radial displacement of the airway, mechanical rheological effects, and possibly increase in ciliary beating [6]. These devices apply a high-frequency percussion on the outside of the chest which, acting on the rheological properties of mucus and on the expiratory flows and liquid-gas interaction, promotes the mobilization of bronchial secretions [1, 8].

Intrapulmonary percussive ventilation (IPV) is a new technique designed to create a global effect of internal percussion of the lungs which aims at clearing the peripheral bronchial tree [7]. IPV uses a device that mobilizes secretions by rapidly oscillating a column of air via mouthpiece. Aerosolized medications can be delivered simultaneously [7].

The study of intrapulmonary percussive ventilation in mechanically ventilated patients has been limited to a few case reports [3]. Clini and colleagues evaluated the effectiveness of IPV in ICU subjects with tracheostomy recently weaned from mechanical ventilation [7]. The investigators allocated the subjects to either 15 days of IPV (2 sessions/day) plus CPT or CPT alone. In the IPV group, PaO_2 increased significantly from baseline, as did PaO_2/FIO_2 and maximal expiratory pressure. At day 15, 2 subjects in the CPT arm and 1 in the IPV arm had some pulmonary complications. At the 1-month follow-up, no IPV subjects had any complication, whereas two in the CPT group had pneumonia. The major effect induced by percussive ventilation was the significant improvement in the patients' oxygenation (PaO_2/FIO_2 ratio) which is highly correlated with a lesser degree of early and late complications [7].

This improvement was enhanced and speeded up compared with the usual physiotherapy, and it is likely that this effect depends on the mechanically induced high-flow rate, which provides a more rapid and profound removal of secretions. Percussive ventilation has also proved to be safe. None of the patients in the intervention, as in the control group, experienced dangerous effects such as acute airway hemorrhage during treatment or thereafter [7].

Another study tested the effectiveness of a mechanical chest vibration pad linked with repositioning every 2 h when used on mechanically ventilated critically ill patients [4]. Patients in the control group received routine positioning care, which included a change of position every 2 h by the ICU nurses. The position turning sequence was left lateral, supine, right lateral, and supine. Patients in the experimental group received routine positioning care plus mechanical chest vibration over 72 h. The chest vibration nursing intervention included placing a mechanical chest wall vibration pad on the patient's back for 60 min when the patient was turned into the supine position. The chest vibration intervention was performed 6 times a day, every 4 h over the 72 h. The vibration pad was placed from the shoulder to the sacrum. The vibration wave was generated from the pad (40 × 60 cm) in spiral, vertical, and horizontal directions. The patients lay on the pad with a blanket covering them. The results showed that for ventilated ICU patients, routine positioning care combined with 60 min of chest wall deep vibration when patients were in supine position was able to achieve a significant difference in 24-h dry sputum weight compared with a control group that received routine care only. The LCI (lung collapse index) in the experimental group also improved significantly at 48 and 72 h compared to that in the control group.

37.2.3 Assisted Mucus-Clearing Techniques

Cough-assisted devices are an alternative tool for those patients who have an impaired cough mechanism [1]. The main disadvantages of all these techniques are their complexity, high costs, the need of trained operators, possible side effects, and the discomfort perceived by the patient during the treatment. In addition, there is a need to determine which device to use based on the main mechanism underlying the excessive production versus the impaired removal of tracheobronchial secretions [1].

37.2.3.1 Insufflation-Exsufflation

Mechanical insufflation-exsufflation (MI-E) is gaining acceptance in ICUs for patients using ventilators [3, 6]. The device's objective is to maximize peak cough flow to attain sufficient airflow velocity for airway mucus shear and to promote cephalad flow of secretions; in other words, to simulate cough [6]. An earlier version of the device, the Cof-Flator, was available in 1952, but this technique did not really catch on until the Emerson CoughAssist In-Exsufflator was introduced in 1993.

The advantage of MI-E is that it applies negative pressure across the entire airway (both central and peripheral), in contrast to direct tracheal suction, which applies negative pressure to a small, localized area [6]. MI-E is perhaps the most physiologic recreation of a natural cough. It has been used to aid in the weaning from mechanical ventilation of patients with neuromuscular diseases. It appears to be more effective than direct tracheal suction for airway clearance in tracheostomized patients with amyotrophic lateral sclerosis [6].

37.2.3.2 Free Aspire

Free Aspire is a new device that uses expiratory flow accelerator (EFA®) technology [1]. The device generates an acceleration of the expiratory flow at tidal volume that, in turn, facilitates the non-invasive removal of excessive tracheobronchial secretions without the need for active collaboration from the patient [1]. Free Aspire uses vacuum technology to accelerate the expiratory flow. During the expiratory phase, the air expelled by the patient is accelerated due to the Venturi effect from the special connector. The acceleration is only activated during the expiratory phase, and the extent of acceleration is proportional to the flow of the expired air, according to the natural rhythm of the patient's breathing function. No negative pressure is generated inside the lungs, and so there is no risk of airways collapse as the technology is suction-free. Free Aspire does not require an efficient cough and, therefore, can be proposed also to patients with a weak cough reflex. The accelerated expiratory flow helps secretions to easily slide along the aqueous layer on the airway walls and so reach the cannula [1].

A pilot study from Belli et al. shows that the application of EFA technology in patients with tracheostomy tube is feasible and safe. Moreover, this study suggests that Free Aspire can reduce the need for deep aspirations through the tracheostomy cannula and, in general, the total number of invasive procedures [1].

This premise, combined with the absence of significant side effects, the improvement in symptoms, and a good tolerability by the patients, suggests that the treatment may help improve airway clearance.

A clear recommendation for evidence-based practice that can be made from a review of the literature is that hemodynamic status should always be carefully monitored to ensure there are no detrimental effects as a result of any physiotherapy intervention. Similarly, when appropriate, intracranial pressure (ICP) should be monitored during physiotherapy intervention. Although monitoring of metabolic status is not routinely used, physiotherapists should carefully consider each patient's reserve before any intervention in view of the evidence that physiotherapy may increase metabolic demand significantly [5].

37.3 Conclusions

Increased mucus production in the airways and the inability to remove the secretions are frequent problems in patients with tracheostomy. Mechanically ventilated patients present increased mucus production and impairment of mucociliary clearance owing to the mechanical effect of artificial airways. Respiratory care and physiotherapy are important components in the treatment of critically ill patients. Secretion management in the mechanically ventilated patient consists primarily of adequate humidification, airway suctioning, and mobilization, but when these routine methods fail, several types of alternative interventions exist to enhance airway clearance.

Chest physiotherapy is one of the most frequently performed interventions in the intensive care unit and includes postural drainage, percussion, vibration, continuous rotational therapy, and manual hyperinflation. Alternatives to these conventional techniques are positive expiratory pressure (PEP), flutter valve, intrapulmonary percussive ventilation, high-frequency chest wall oscillation, and assisted mucus-clearing techniques like mechanical insufflation-exsufflation.

Limited recommendations for evidence-based practice can be made about which treatment techniques should be used. There are insufficient data to enable physiotherapists to select treatment techniques using evidence-based practice for patients with specific pulmonary conditions. As far as the routine management of intubated ICU patients receiving mechanical ventilation is concerned, it is likely, despite the lack of evidence concerning suction, that majority of intubated patients will require regular suction to maintain a patent tracheostomy tube and to clear the central airways of secretions, regardless of the patient's underlying disease. However, the necessity for any other routine treatment beyond this (e.g., positioning, MH, vibrations, percussion) cannot currently be supported or refuted based on the available evidence. Whichever technique is used, it is important to assess the patient's reserve and always monitor hemodynamics, intracranial pressure, and airway pressure in order to avoid any complication.

> **Key Major Recommendations**
> - Mechanically ventilated patients present increased mucus production and impairment of mucociliary clearance, so respiratory care and physiotherapy are important components in the treatment of these patients.
> - Secretion management in the mechanically ventilated patient consists primarily of adequate humidification, airway suctioning, and mobilization.
> - Conventional chest physical therapy (CPT) is frequently used but, more recently, several alternatives have been developed.
> - There are insufficient data to enable physiotherapists to select treatment techniques using evidence-based practice for patients with specific pulmonary conditions.
> - Whichever technique is used. it is important to assess the patient's reserve and always monitor hemodynamics, intracranial pressure, and airway pressure in order to avoid any complication.

References

1. Belli S, Cattaneo D, D'Abrosca F, Prince I, Savio G, Balbi B. A pilot study on the non-invasive management of tracheobronchial secretions in tracheostomised patients. Clin Respir J. 2019;13(10):637–42.
2. Chicayban LM, Zin WA, Guimaraes FS. Can the flutter valve improve respiratory mechanics and sputum production in mechanically ventilated patients? A randomized crossover trial. Heart Lung. 2011;40(6):545–53.
3. Branson RD. Secretion management in the mechanically ventilated patient. Respir Care. 2007;52(10):1328–42; discussion 1327–1342.

4. Chen YC, Wu LF, Mu PF, Lin LH, Chou SS, Shie HG. Using chest vibration nursing intervention to improve expectoration of airway secretions and prevent lung collapse in ventilated ICU patients: a randomized controlled trial. J Chin Med Assoc. 2009;72(6):316–22.
5. Stiller K. Physiotherapy in intensive care: towards an evidence-based practice. Chest. 2000;118(6):1801–13.
6. Hess DR. Airway clearance: physiology, pharmacology, techniques, and practice. Respir Care. 2007;52(10):1392–6.
7. Clini EM, Antoni FD, Vitacca M, et al. Intrapulmonary percussive ventilation in tracheostomized patients: a randomized controlled trial. Intensive Care Med. 2006;32(12):1994–2001.
8. McCool FD, Rosen MJ. Nonpharmacologic airway clearance therapies: ACCP evidence-based clinical practice guidelines. Chest. 2006;129(1 Suppl):250S–9S.
9. Clini E, Ambrosino N. Early physiotherapy in the respiratory intensive care unit. Respir Med. 2005;99(9):1096–104.
10. Krause MW, Aswegen HV, De Wet EH, Joubert G. Postural drainage in intubated patients with acute lobar atelectasis: a pilot study. S Afr J Physiother. 2000;56(3):29–32.
11. Davis K Jr, Johannigman JA, Campbell RS, et al. The acute effects of body position strategies and respiratory therapy in paralyzed patients with acute lung injury. Crit Care. 2001;5(2):81–7.
12. Berney S, Denehy L. A comparison of the effects of manual and ventilator hyperinflation on static lung compliance and sputum production in intubated and ventilated intensive care patients. Physiother Res Int. 2002;7(2):100–8.

Correction to: Aerosol Therapy and Humidification

Elena Fernández Fernández and Ronan MacLoughlin

Correction to:
Chapter 35 in: A. M. Esquinas (ed.), *Humidification in the Intensive Care Unit*, https://doi.org/10.1007/978-3-031-23953-3_35

Chapter "Aerosol Therapy and Humidification" was previously published non-open access. It has now been changed to open access under a CC BY 4.0 license and the copyright holder updated to 'The Author(s)'. The book has also been updated with this change.

The updated original version of this chapter can be found at
https://doi.org/10.1007/978-3-031-23953-3_35

Index

© The Editor(s) (if applicable) and The Author(s), under exclusive license to
Springer Nature Switzerland AG 2023
A. M. Esquinas (ed.), *Humidification in the Intensive Care Unit*,
https://doi.org/10.1007/978-3-031-23953-3